20,001
Names
for Baby

20,001 NAMES for BABY

Carol McD. Wallace

AVON BOOKS NEW YORK

20,001 NAMES FOR BABY is an original publication of Avon Books.

AVON BOOKS
A division of
The Hearst Corporation
1350 Avenue of the Americas
New York, New York 10019

First Avon Books Trade Printing: May 1995
First Avon Books Mass Market Printing: March 1992

AVON TRADEMARK REG. U.S. PAT. OFF. AND IN OTHER COUNTRIES, MARCA REGISTRADA, HECHO EN U.S.A.

Printed in the U.S.A.

OPM   10   9   8   7   6   5   4   3

My thanks to my agent, Lynn Seligman, for cheerleading, to Rick for patience, and to my editor, Gwen Montgomery, for efficiency.

I am also grateful to the researchers who went before me, notably Leslie Dunkling and William Gosling, authors of *The Facts on File Dictionary of First Names*, and Connie Lockhart Ellefson, author of *The Melting Pot Book of Baby Names*.

Contents

Abbreviations

ix

Introduction

xi

PART 1
If It's A Girl . . .

1

PART 2
If It's A Boy . . .

205

Abbreviations

Af	African	*Jap*	Japanese
Arab	Arabic	*Lat*	Latin
Celt	Celtic	*masc*	masculine
com form	combining form	*Nig*	Nigerian
Czech	Czechoslovakian	*NAm Ind*	North American Indian
Dan	Danish	*Nor*	Norwegian
dim	diminutive	*OE*	Old English
Egypt	Egyptian	*OF*	Old French
Eng	English	*OG*	Old German
fem	feminine	*ONorse*	Old Norse
Fr	French	*Per*	Persian
Gael	Gaelic	*Pol*	Polish
Ger	German	*Port*	Portuguese
Gk	Greek	*Rus*	Russian
Haw	Hawaiian	*Scan*	Scandinavian
Heb	Hebrew	*Scot*	Scottish
Hung	Hungarian	*Sp*	Spanish
Ir	Irish	*Teut*	Teutonic
It	Italian	*var*	variant
		Viet	Vietnamese

Introduction

One of the first questions anybody asks about a newborn is, "What is the baby's name?" Faced with this tiny scrap of humanity, we want to put a name to it as if, by doing so, we welcome it to the realm of individuals. We always name the things we love. A small child will give names to even his tiniest toys or his well-chewed blanket, and the difference between "Blankie" and "the blanket" is an entire personality.

So when it comes to naming your baby, you want to get it right. You want to strike a fine balance between uniqueness and familiarity, honor a family member, reflect your ethnic heritage, avoid horrible nicknames, ensure that your child's name will never be misspelled. You'd like to name it for Granddad, but Granddad's name was Elmer. You thought Sally sounded nice until your best friend asked you if you're naming her for Gidget. The baby's due in six weeks and your spouse has vetoed every single suggestion. So you do what you always swore you wouldn't, and buy a baby name book.

There are many baby name books on the market. They give varying numbers of names, and varying amounts of information about the names. I believe that when it comes to picking a name, more is more. More choices can help you make *your* choice. I also think a simple alphabetical listing is easiest to use. I suspect most people simply browse through these books in the hope that the perfect selection will jump off the page at them. And who knows? Maybe sometimes it does.

More often, though, parents arrive at their final selection by a process of elimination. They rule out the bizarre names, the unfashionable names, the names that remind them of a second-grade bully. The process is highly emotional, because every name is wreathed with a cluster of associations that we may not even be aware of. Some of these associations are with public figures, which is why books like this one include examples of famous people under most listings. If you connect the name Hayley with a certain fresh-faced British girliness, that is probably because you saw Hayley Mills in *The Trouble With Angels* or *The Moonspinners*, even if you don't remember this momentous event.

We are also swayed, whether or not we'd like to think so, by fashion and class. Certain kinds of names are the ones used by any group at a certain time. In the 1980s, for instance, WASPy unisex names were enormously popular. The parents who named their babies Ashley or Whitney may not have been aware they were following a trend, but these names would not even have occurred to most parents twenty years earlier.

America takes its basic naming traditions, along with its language, from the British Isles. Before the Norman invasion in the eleventh century, England was inhabited by a mix of Celts and Germanic tribes. Many Old English names (like Albert or Randolph) are rooted in German languages. They tend to be attribute names, often characterizing prowess in battle. (The girls' names surviving from this era are usually later feminizations of the old forms, like Alberta.)

The Norman Conquest brought French names to England, and the gradual conversion of Britain to Christianity ushered in the use of saints' and Latin names, like Agnes or Vincent. But the great change in the Middle Ages was the formation of last names. The population increased, and a first name was no longer sufficient identification. John could mean one of three or four people in a community: but John Baker was the John who made the bread. Many of our last names and a good percentage of masculine first names come from this period. By and large, they are place names (John Woods) or occupational names (John Weaver), descriptive names (John White) or son-of names (John Johnson). The place names especially give a vivid glimpse of what life must have been like for the average Englishman at the time. The points of reference are humble, a stump or a willow tree or a stream that would nevertheless have been major landmarks in rural life.

The next great upheaval in naming practices came with the Reformation. Puritans felt it was popish to use saints' names, so they ransacked the Old Testament, bringing names like Ezra and Rebecca into fashion. Of course, there are many fewer female than male names in the Bible, so the Puritans also named their daughters for admired qualities or virtues like Constance or Hope. Since New England was settled by ardent Protestants, these names also took root in the northeastern colonies, and many of them survived well into the nineteenth century.

Through much of the eighteenth century America was still identified with Britain and followed its naming practices, which included the addition of a few Germanic names like Adelaide that were brought in the wake of the Hanoverian kings. But by the middle of the nineteenth century the habits of the two countries diverged. In England the middle class turned to the past and revived many of the Old English names that had been unused for centuries. At the same time many last names were adopted for use as first names, resulting in a generation of little boys named Carpenter or Wakefield. Meanwhile girls were often given flower names like Rose or Violet or Daisy, perfectly appropriate for the Victorian concept of girlhood.

In the United States, however, immigration began to make a mark. Irish, German, and Italian-born parents gave their children names that were redolent of the homeland, though the well-assimilated second generation often chose anglicized names. This tendency was particularly marked among Jewish immigrants several decades later who picked out Anglo-Saxon names like Sheldon and Alvin for their sons.

The elaborate three-syllable names of the turn of the century gave way to increasingly streamlined models as the twentieth century progressed. Made-up names like Darlene flourished, and children's names were increasingly drawn from popular culture. For instance, some parents consciously named a son Rick for the hero of *Casablanca*, while others, having seen the movie three nights before the baby's birth, no doubt decided to name Baby for Uncle Richard, and thought Rick would make a handy nickname. The popularity of certain names (like Samantha) closely followed the careers of a movie star or TV show. If nothing else, a star's fame guarantees that her name has been widely heard, so it doesn't sound completely outlandish when it's suggested for a baby.

Outlandish names, however, did become popular in the 1960s and 1970s. Cher Bono named her daughter Chastity. Frank Zappa's children are Moon Unit and Dweezil. The late actor River Phoenix has a brother named Leaf. Individuality was critical to counterculture parents, and traditional names began to drift out of favor.

This urge for uniqueness is still with us. Gone are the days of Tommy and Margaret and Susan and Peter. The names on kindergarten cubbies today are a dizzying cocktail of obscure Old Testament prophets, proud ethnic selections, creatively spelled favorites, and sheer inventions. Parents of the nineties want to be sure their children's names stand out.

There is already a countertrend afoot, though. Hospital nurseries are still full of babies named Chiarra and Zane, but the occasional truly old-fashioned choice is sneaking in. Molly is back. So is Theodore. I know little girls named Violet and Maisie. They're still unusual, but they come with a distinguished provenance. I think these are the names we'll be seeing more of in the next few years, though a parent who really wanted his baby to have an unusual name would choose, believe it or not, John or Mary.

Pick a Name, Any Name

There are any number of ways to choose a name for a baby. One of the most common is to use an old family name. If the family tie is strong enough, parents are often willing to overlook an unfashionable aura or an unpleasant meaning. If all the menfolk for five generations have been named Brendan, who are you to complain that the name means "stinking hair"?

But inspiration need not be limited to the family tree. Pick an attribute (brilliant mind: Hubert). Pick a birthstone (Ruby) or an astrological connection (Pisces, the water sign: Undine). Pick an ethnic favorite or the name of the Italian city where the baby was conceived. Name the baby for your favorite poet or an interesting saint.

Or simply leaf through this book and make a list, then pare the list down. Cut out the choices that won't work well with the baby's last name, or that have unacceptable nicknames. For instance, you might insist on calling your son Hugh, but sooner or later someone is going to call him Huey, and it may stick. If you're using a middle name, make sure the three initials together don't spell something odious. And when you're down to a handful of finalists, try the playground test. Can you imagine yourself bellowing the name across a crowded playground? If you feel self-conscious, it will never do.

As the pregnancy moves into its later months, you'll hear two questions over and over: "Do you know what you're having?" and "Have you thought about names?" You'll answer these questions as you like, of course. But bear in mind that people will feel perfectly free to tell you what they think about your choice of names—*before* you have the baby. If you wait until after the infant's already been named Osbert, nobody will be rude enough to criticize. If you're set on an unusual name, this might be the best strategy.

There's no use starting on the process too early. Maybe you can settle on the perfect name by the thirty-fourth gestational week, but there are plenty of parents who start doing their Lamaze breathing without a final selection. There's nothing wrong with making your choice after you've met the little one. And even if you think you've decided, it wouldn't hurt to tuck this book into your hospital bag just in case you have second thoughts.

Finding the perfect name for your baby can be difficult,

but the beauty of the process is this: By the time the baby is a few months old, his personality erases all other associations the name may hold. The second grade bully or the much-loved poet fade away, and the name becomes, quite simply, the name of your child. And you will have made the right choice.

20,001 Names for Baby

If It's
A Girl . . .

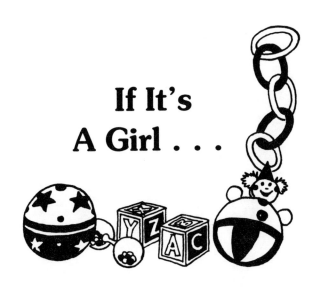

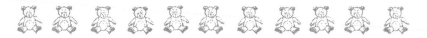

Abarrane (fem. **Abraham**) Basque. from Heb. "Father of many."
Abame
Abebi Nig. "She came after asking."
Abelia (fem. **Abel**) Fr. from Heb. "Sigh."
Abella, Abelle

Abellona (fem. **Apollo**) Dan. In Greek myth, Apollo is the sun god. See **Apolline**.

Abia Arab. "Great."

Abida Arab. "She who worships"; Heb. "My father knows."

Abigail Heb. "My father is joyful." Biblical name adopted by the Puritans and popular through the 18th century. After a hundred years of obscurity, it was revived with the trend toward old-fashioned names beginning in the 1970s. Abigail Adams, wife of President John Adams, advice columnist Abigail Van Buren.
Abagael, Abagail, Abagale, Abagil, Abaigeal, Abbe, Abbey, Abbi, Abbie, Abbigael, Abbigail, Abbigale, Abby, Abbye, Abbygael, Abbygail, Abbygale, Abigael, Abigal, Abigale, Abigall, Abigil, Abigayle, Gael, Gail, Gaila, Gayel, Gayle

Abijah Heb. "God is my father."
Abisha, Abishah

Abir Arab. "Scent."

Abital Heb. "My father is dew." Currently popular in Israel.
Avital

Abra (fem. **Abraham**) Heb. "Father of many"; Arab. "example, lesson." King Solomon's favorite concubine was named Abra.
Abame, Abarrane, Abrahana

Acacia Gr. Name of a blossoming tree that symbolized resurrection. Uncommon even in Greece, though the derivatives like Casey occur often in the U.S.
Cacia, Cacie, Casey, Casia, Cassie, Cassy, Kacey, Kacie, Kasey, Kasi, Kassja, Kassy

Acadia Place name: The French settlers of Nova Scotia called it Acadia after the name of a river there. When

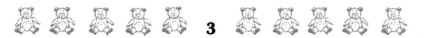

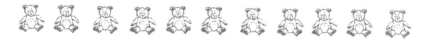

the French settlers were driven out by the English in the 18th century, many of them settled in Louisiana and became known as "Cajuns."

Accalia Lat. In myth, the name of the human foster mother of Romulus and Remus, the twins who founded Rome. Legend has it that after their abandonment as infants, they were initially suckled by a she-wolf, whose name is not known. Accalia was her replacement.

Aceline (fem. **Acelin**) Fr. "Highborn."
Asceline

Acima (fem. **Acim**) Heb. "The Lord will judge."
Acimah, Achima, Achimah

Ada Ger. "Noble, nobility." Originated as a short form of names like Adelaide, and popular in the last quarter of the 19th century, though infrequently used now.
Adan, Adda, Addi, Addie, Addiah, Addy, Adey, Adi, Adia, Adiah, Adie, Aida, Aidah

Adah Heb. "Ornament, adornment." Biblical name. Unusual, but brought to prominence in the 19th century by American actress Adah Isaacs Mencken.

Adalia Heb. "God is my refuge"; OG. "Noble one." See also **Adelaide**.
Adal, Adala, Adalee, Adali, Adalie, Adalley, Addal, Addala

Adamina (fem. **Adam**) Heb. "Child of the red earth." In the Bible God created Adam out of the "red earth" and breathed life into him. This unusual feminine version of the name is Scottish in origin.
Ada, Adamine, Adaminna, Addie, Mina, Minna

Adara Gk. "beauty"; Arab. "virgin."
Adra

Addula Teut. "Noble cheer."

Adelaide OG. "Noble, nobility." First popular in England after the reign of William IV and Queen Adelaide. The city of Adelaide, Australia, was named for her.
Addala, Addalla, Addey, Addi, Addie, Addy, Adel, Adela, Adelaida, Adelais, Adele, Adelheid, Adelina, Adeline, Adelice, Adelicia, Adelis, Adelle, Adey, Adi, Ado, Ady, Aline, Aliosha, Alline, Alyosha, Del, Della, Delle, Delli, Delly, Edeline, Eline, Heidi, Lady, Laidey

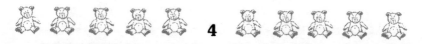

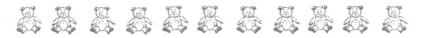

Adele OG. "Noble, nobility." See **Adelaide**. Nutritionist Adelle Davis; writer Adela Rogers St. John.
Adelia, Adell, Adella, Adellah, Adelle

Adelinda Teut. "Noble, sweet." Com. form **Adele** and **Linda**.
Adele, Adeline, Adelinde, Linda

Adeline OG. "Noble, nobility." See **Adelaide**. Adelina enjoyed a burst of popularity during the career of operatic soprano Adelina Patti, in the late 19th century.
Adalina, Adaline, Adallina, Adelina, Adelind, Adella,
Adellah, Ahdella, Aline, Dahlina, Dalina, Daline, Dallina,
Delina, Deline, Dellina, Delly, Delyne, Edelie, Lina

Adena Heb. "Decoration."
Adene, Adina, Adinah, Denah, Dina, Dinah

Adelpha Gr. "Beloved sister."

Adeola Nig. "Crown."
Adola, Dola

Adiba Arab. "Cultured, refined."
Adibah

Adiella Heb. "The Lord's adornment."

Adima Teut. "Noble, renowned."

Adin Heb. Meaning unclear: possibly "delicate and slender." Appears in the Old Testament as a male name.
Adina, Adeana

Adira Heb. "Noble, powerful."

Adiva Arab. "Agreeable, gentle."

Adlai Arab. Heb. "Just." More familiar to us as a man's name made famous by U.S. Senator Adlai Stevenson.

Adolpha (fem. **Adolph**) Ger. "Noble wolf."

Adoncia Sp. "Sweet."
Doncia

Adonia (fem. **Adonis**) Gr. In Greek myth Adonis was a young man so beautiful that Aphrodite, goddess of love, became enamored of him. The name Adonis has come to epitomize male beauty.

Adora Lat. "Adored."
Adorabelle, Adoray, Adorée, Adoré, Adoria, Adorlee,
Dora, Dori, Dorie, Dorri, Dorrie, Dorry, Dory

Adra Arab. "Virgin."
Adara

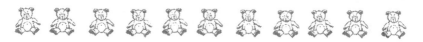

Adrian Lat. Place name: Adria was a North Italian city. First popular in the 1950s in Britain, and more common as a man's name. Hollywood costume designer Adrian (*Queen Christina, The Philadelphia Story*) and 12th-century Pope Adrian IV (the only English pope) both predate its use as a girl's name. Fashion designer Adrienne Vittadini.
Adrea, Adreea, Adria, Adriah, Adriana, Adrianah, Adriane, Adrianna, Adriannah, Adrianne, Adrie, Adrien, Adriena, Adrienah, Adrienne, Hadria, Hadrienne

Afra Arab. "color of earth"; Heb. "young deer."
Affera, Affery, Affra, Aphra

Afraima Arab. Heb. "Fertile."

Africa Gael. "Pleasant." Also, of course, a place name, and readily associated with the continent.
Affrica, Affricah, Affrika, Affrikah, Africah, Afrika, Afrikah, Aifric, Apirka, Apirkah

Afton OE. Place name: There is a town called Afton in southern Scotland. Like so many place names that have become first names, this one was first a name for boys.
Affton

Agapi Gk. "Love, affection."
Agape, Agappe

Agate OF. A semiprecious stone. Can be considered either one of the jewel names so popular in the 19th century, or a variant of Agatha. The agate, though not a particularly beautiful stone, was once believed to have numerous magical and curative powers.

Agatha Gk. "Good." Saint Agatha was a 3rd-century virgin martyr, and her name was popular in the early years of the Christian Church, but not again until the late 19th century. It now has an unfashionable ring, but some of the international variants are pretty. Writer Agatha Christie.
Ag, Agace, Agacia, Agafia, Agafon, Agapet, Agapit, Agata, Agathe, Agathi, Agatta, Aggi, Aggie, Aggy, Aggye, Agi, Agie, Agota, Agotha, Agueda, Agy, Agye

Agave Gk. "Illustrious, noble."

Aglaia Gk. In Greek myth, one of the three Graces, epit-

omizing brilliance. Thalia (blossoming) is still sometimes used; Euphrosyne (joy) is obsolete.

Agnes Gk. "Pure, virginal." Another early Christian saint's name. She was a virgin martyr, and her emblem in art is a lamb. Very popular in England between the 12th and 16th centuries, Agnes is uncommon now, perhaps because of its connotations of homeliness. Choreographer Agnes De Mille; actress Agnes Moorhead; writer Anais Nin.

Ag, Agafi, Agafia, Agafon, Aggi, Aggie, Aggye, Aghna, Agi, Agie, Agna, Agnah, Agnella, Agnellah, Agnelle, Agnese, Agnesse, Agneta, Agnetta, Agnettah, Agnola, Agnolah, Agot, Agota, Agote, Agoti, Agy, Agye, Aigneis, Aina, Ainah, Anais, Annais, Anneyce, Annis, Annisa, Annisah, Annise, Ina, Inah, Ines, Inessa, Inez, Nessa, Nessah, Nesi, Nessie, Nessy, Nesta, Nestah, Nevsa, Nevesah, Neysa, Oona, Oonagh, Oonah, Una, Unah, Ynes, Ynez

Agnola It. "Angel." Also variant of **Agnes**.
Agnolla, Agnolle

Agrafina Rus. "Born feet first." See **Agrippa**.

Agrippa Lat. "Born feet first." The name of a 1st-century Roman Emperor, the son of Herod. A man's name possibly transferred to female use because of the "-a" ending.
Agrafina, Agrippina, Agrippine

Agrippina Lat. Sister of the corrupt Roman Emperor Caligula and mother of the equally unsavory Roman Emperor Nero, who had her murdered. Not a common name, for obvious reasons.

Ahava Heb. "Loved one."
Ahuva, Ahuda

Aibhlin Ir. Gael. form of **Evelyn** or **Helen**.

Aida Arab. "Reward, present." Name of an immensely popular opera by Giuseppe Verdi.

Aidan Ir. Gael. "fire." Saint Aidan was a 7th-century Irish monk. The name is more common for men than for women.
Adan, Aden, Aiden

Aiko Jap. "Little loved one."

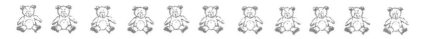

Ailbhe Ir. "Noble, bright."
Alva, Alvy, Elva, Elvy

Aileen Irish variant of **Helen**. Gk. "Light." This form has been most popular in Scotland.
Aila, Ailee, Ailene, Ailey, Ailli, Ailie, Aleen, Alene, Aline, Alleen, Allene, Alline, Eileen, Eleen, Elleen, Ellene, Ileana, Ileane, Ileanna, Ilene, Iliana, Iliane, Ilianna, Illeanne, Illene, Leana, Leanah, Leanna, Leannah, Lena, Lenah, Liana, Lianna, Liannah, Lina, Linah

Ailith OE. "Seasoned warrior."
Aldith

Ailsa Scot. The name has two possible sources. As a homonym for Elsa, a diminutive of Elizabeth, it means "pledge from God." An alternate source is the Scottish island Ailsa Craig.
Ailis, Ailse, Elsa, Elsha, Elshe

Aimée Fr. "Beloved." See **Amy**. Evangelist Aimée Semple McPherson.
Aimie, Aimey, Amey, Amie

Aina Scan. "Forever."

Aine Celt. "Happiness."

Ainsley Scot. Gael. Place name: "One's own meadow." A last name converted to a first name, used by both sexes.
Ainslee, Ainsleigh, Ainslie, Ansley, Aynslee, Aynsley, Aynslie

Airlea Gk. "Ethereal."
Airlia

Aisha Arab. "woman"; Swahili. "life." Aisha was the favored wife of Mohammed, hence the name's current popularity among Muslim families.
Aeesha, Aeeshah, Aesha, Aeshah, Aiesha, Aieshah, Aishah, Aisia, Aisiah, Asha, Ashah, Ashia, Ashiah, Asia, Asiah, Ayeesa, Ayeesah, Ayeesha, Ayeeshah, Ayeisa, Ayeisah, Ayeisha, Ayeishah, Ayisa, Ayisah, Ayisha, Ayishah, Ieasha, Ieashah, Ieashia, Ieashiah, Iesha, Ieshah, Ieesha, Ieeshah, Ieeshia, Ieeshiah, Yiesha, Yieshah

Aislinn Ir. Gael. "Dream."
Aisling, Ashling, Isleen

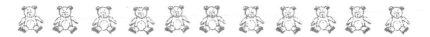

Aithne (fem. **Aidan**) Ir. Gael. "Fire." Not to be confused, despite its sound, with the name of the Sicilian volcano.
  Aine, Aithnea, Eithne, Ena, Ethnah, Ethnea, Ethnee
Aiyana NAm. Ind. "Forever flowering."
Akela Haw. "Noble." A form of **Adele**.
Akilina Gk. Rus. "Eagle."
  Acquilina, Aquilina
Akiva Heb. "Protect, shelter."
  Kiba, Kibah, Kiva, Kivah, Kivi
Alaia Arab. "Sublime."
Alaine (fem. **Alan**) Fr. from Gael. Possible meaning "rock" or "comely." Not actually used in France, where it would be very easily confused with Hélène.
  Alaina, Alayna, Alayne, Aleine, Alenne, Allaine, Allayne, Alleine, Alenne, Aleyne
Alala Gk. In Greek mythology, the sister of Ares, the god of war.
Alamea Haw. "Ripe, precious."
Alanna (fem. **Alan**) Gael. Meaning "rock" or "comely." Also a possible derivative of Elaine (OF. "bright, shining") or Helen (Gk. "light"). Actress Lana Turner.
  Alaina, Alaine, Alana, Alane, Alannah, Alayne, Aléne, Aleyna, Aleyne, Alleen, Allena, Allene, Allyna, Alleynah, Alleyne, Allina, Allinah, Allyn, Lana, Lanah, Lanna, Lannah, Aleyna, Aleynah
Alaqua NAm. In. "Sweet gum tree."
Alarice (fem. **Alaric**) OG. "Noble king." Alaric was a king of the Visigoths who sacked Rome.
  Alarica
Alastair Scot. form of **Alexander**. Gk. "Man's defender." More generally used as a man's name.
  Alasdair
Alaula Haw. "Light of daybreak."
Alba Lat. "White." See **Albinia**.
  Albane, Albina, Albine, Albinia, Albinka, Alva
Alberga Lat. "White"; OG. "noble." Also closely related to the French and Italian word for "inn."
  Alberge
Alberta OE. "Noble shining." Rare and old-fashioned now, it was most widely used during the lifetime of

Queen Victoria's Prince Consort, Albert. Also the name of a western Canadian province, and a very popular strain of peach.

Alberthine, Albertina, Albertine, Ali, Alli, Allie, Ally, Auberta, Auberte, Aubertha, Auberthe, Aubine, Berrie, Berry, Bert, Berta, Berte, Berti, Bertie, Berty, Elberta, Elbertha, Elberthina, Elberthine, Elbertina, Elbertine

Albinia (fem. **Alban, Albin**) Lat. "White, fair."
Alba, Albina, Alva, Alvina, Aubine

Albreda (fem. **Aubrey**) OG. "Counsel from the elves."

Alcestis Gk. In Euripides' play of the same name, Alcestis descends to Hades in place of her husband, and is then rescued by Hercules.

Alcina Gk. In Greek myth, a sorceress who rules over a magical island. When she tired of her lovers, Alcina turned them into animals, trees, or stones.
Alcine, Alcinia, Allcine, Allcinia, Alseena, Alsina, Alsinia, Alsyna, Alzina

Alda (fem. **Aldo, Otto**) OG. "Old, prosperous."
Aldabella, Aldea, Aldina, Aldine, Aleda, Alida

Aldara Gk. "Winged gift."

Aldis OE. "Battle-seasoned."
Aldith, Ailith

Aldonza Sp. "Sweet."

Aleeza Heb. "Joy."
Aleezah, Alieza, Aliezah, Aliza, Alizah, Alitza

Alegria Sp. "Happiness, joy." For related names, see Hilary, Felicity, Bliss. A charming choice for a much-wanted child.
Allegria

Alena Rus. var. **Helen**. Gk. "Light."

Alesia Gk. "Help, aid."

Aleta Gk. "Footloose."
Aletta, Alette, Alletta, Allette, Lettee, Lettie, Letty

Alethea Gk. "Truth." Unusual name that first appeared in Britain in the 17th century.
Alathia, Aleethia, Aleta, Aletea, Aletha, Alethia, Aletta, Alette, Alithea, Alithia

Alexandra (fem. **Alexander**) Gk. "Man's defender." Became very popular in Britain after the Prince of Wales

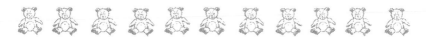

(later Edward VII) married the Danish Princess Alexandra. Still used in the English royal family and its many branches. Ballet dancer Alexandra Danilova; fashion designer Zandra Rhodes.

Alastrina, Alastriona, Alejanda, Alejandra, Alejandrina, Aleka, Aleki, Alesandare, Alesandere, Alessanda, Alessandra, Alessandre, Alessandrina, Alessandrine, Alessia, Alex, Alexa, Alexandere, Alexanderia, Alexanderina, Alexanderine, Alexandre, Alexandrea, Alexandreana, Alexandrena, Alexandrene, Alexandretta, Alexandria, Alexandrina, Alexandrine, Alexea, Alexena, Alexene, Alexia, Alexina, Alexine, Alexis, Ali, Aliki, Alissandre, Alissandrine, Alista, Alix, Alla, Allejandra, Allejandrina, Allessa, Allessandra, Alle, Allexa, Allexandra, Allexandrina, Allexina, Allexine, Alli, Allie, Allix, Ally, Anda, Cesya, Elena, Ellena, Lesy, Lesya, Lexi, Lexie, Lexine, Lissandre, Lissandrine, Sanda, Sande, Sandi, Sandie, Sandra, Sandrina, Sandrine, Sandy, Sandye, Sanndra, Sasha, Sashenka, Shura, Shurochka, Sohndra, Sondra, Xandra, Zahndra, Zanda, Zanndra, Zohndra, Zondra

Alexis Gk. "Helper." Usually thought of as a short form of Alexandra, though it has a different etymological root. Actress Alexis Smith; TV character Alexis Carrington.

Alessa, Alessi, Alexa, Alexi, Alexia, Lexi, Lexie, Lexy

Alfonsine (fem. **Alfonso**) OG. "Noble and ready for battle."

Alfonsia, Alonza, Alphonsine

Alfreda (fem. **Alfred**) OE. "Elf power." Actress Alfre Woodard.

Alfi, Alfie, Alfre, Alfredah, Alfredda, Alfreeda, Alfri, Alfried, Alfrieda, Alfryda, Alfy, Allfie, Allfreda, Allfredah, Allfredda, Allfrie, Allfrieda, Allfry, Allfryda, Allfy, Elfie, Elfre, Elfrea, Elfredah, Elfredda, Elfreeda, Elfrida, Elfrieda, Elfryda, Elfrydah, Ellfreda, Ellfredah, Ellfredda, Ellfreeda, Ellfrida, Ellfrieda, Ellfryda, Ellfrydah, Elva, Elvah, Freda, Freddi, Freddie, Freddy, Fredi, Fredy, Freeda, Freedah, Frieda, Friedah, Fryda, Frydah

Alice OG. "Noble, nobility." See **Adelaide**. An old

standby name since the Middle Ages that became enormously popular after the 1865 publication of Lewis Carroll's *Alice's Adventures in Wonderland*. Its popularity
waned in the 1930s, and it now has a pleasantly old-
fashioned air. Ballerina Alicia Markova; writer Alice
Walker; actresses Ali McGraw, Ally Sheedy.

**Adelice, Ailis, Ala, Aleceea, Alecia, Aleetheea, Aleethia,
Ali, Alica, Alicah, Alicea, Alicen, Alicia, Alidée, Alie,
Alika, Alikah, Aliki, Alis, Alisa, Alisah, Alisann, Alisanne,
Alisha, Alison, Alissa, Alisz, Alitheea, Alitia, Aliz, Alla,
Allecia, Alleece, Alleeceea, Alles, Alless, Alli, Allice,
Allicea, Allie, Allis, Allison, Allissa, Allisun, Allisunne,
Allsun, Ally, Allyce, Allyceea, Allys, Allyse, Allysia,
Allysiah, Allyson, Allyssa, Allysson, Alyce, Alyceea, Alys,
Alyse, Alysia, Alyson, Alyss, Alyssa, Elissa, Elli, Ellie,
Ellissa, Ellsa, Elsa, Illyssa, Ilysa, Ilysah, Ilyssa, Ilysse,
Leece, Leese, Licha, Lichah, Lissa, Lyssa**

Alida Lat. "Small winged one."
**Adela, Adelina, Adelita, Adellyna, Adellyta, Adelyna,
Adelyta, Alaida, Alda, Aldina, Aldine, Aldona, Aldonna,
Aldyne, Aleda, Aleta, Aletta, Alette, Alidah, Alidia, Alita,
Allda, Alldina, Alldine, Alldona, Alldonna, Alldyne,
Alleda, Allida, Allidah, Allidia, Allidiah, Allyda, Allydah,
Alyda, Alydah, Dela, Della, Dila, Dilla, Elida, Elita, Leda,
Ledah, Lida, Lidah, Lita, Lyda, Lydah, Oleda, Oleta,
Oletta, Olette**

Alima Arab. "Cultured."

Alina Slavic. Var. **Helen**. Gk. "Light."
**Aleen, Aleena, Alena, Alenah, Alene, Aline, Alleen,
Allena, Allene, Alline, Allyna, Allynah, Allyne, Alyna,
Alynah, Alyne, Leena, Leenah, Lena, Lenah, Lina, Linah,
Lyna, Lynah**

Alisa Heb. "Great happiness."
**Alisah, Alissa, Alissah, Aliza, Allisa, Allisah, Allissa,
Allissah, Allysa, Allysah, Alyssa, Alyssah**

Alison Dim. Alice. OG. "Noble, nobility."
**Aili, Alisann, Alisanne, Alisoun, Alisun, Allcen, Allcenne,
Allicen, Allicenne, Allie, Allisann, Allisanne, Allison,
Allisoun, Allsun, Ally, Allysann, Allysanne, Allyson,
Allysoun, Alysan, Alysann, Alysanne, Alyson, Alysoun**

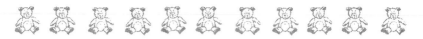

Alix OG. "Noble." See **Alexandra**.
   Alex, Alexa, Alexis, Aliki, Alissandre, Alissandrine, Lissandre

Aliya Arab. "Highborn."
   Aliyah, Aliye

Allegra It. "Joyous." The musical term "allegro" means "quickly, with a happy air." Ballerina Allegra Kent.
   Alegra, Legra, Leggra

Allena (fem. **Allen, Alan**) Ir. Possible meaning "rock" or "comely." See **Alanna**.
   Alana, Alanna, Alena, Alene, Allene, Alleyne, Allynn, Allynne, Allynn, Alynne

Allyriane Fr. from Gk. "Lyre." The lyre was a stringed instrument, a predecessor of today's harp or guitar.

Alma Lat. "giving nurture"; It. "soul"; Arab. "learned." Also the name of a river in the Crimea where a famous 19th-century battle was fought, bringing it into prominence as a first name. The more common usage, of course, is "alma mater" for a college or university.
   Almah, Allma

Almarine OG. "Work ruler."
   Almeria

Almeda Lat. "Goal-directed, ambitious."
   Allmeda, Allmedah, Allmeta, Allmetah, Allmida, Allmidah, Allmita, Allmitah, Almedah, Almeta, Almetah, Almida, Almidah, Almita, Almitah, Maelle

Almera (fem. **Elmer**) Arab. "Aristocratic lady."
   Allmeera, Allmeria, Almeera, Almeeria, Almeria, Almire, Almirah, Almyra, Ellmera, Ellmeria, Elmeera, Elmeeria, Elmera, Elmeria, Elmira, Elmyra, Elmyrah, Mera, Meera, Mira, Mirah, Myra, Myrah

Almodine Lat. "Precious stone."

Aloha Haw. "Love, kindness, affection." The familiar Hawaiian greeting.

Aloisia (fem. **Aloysius**) OG. "Famous fighter."
   Aloysia

Alona Heb. "Oak tree."
   Allona, Allonia, Alonia

Alonsa (fem. **Alonso**) Sp./OG. "Ready for battle."
   Alonza

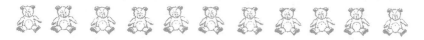

Alpha Gk. First letter of Greek alphabet, corresponding to *A*. Appropriate for a first daughter.
　Alfa
Alphonsine (fem. **Alphonse**) Fr. from OG. "Ready for battle."
Alta Lat. "Elevated."
　Allta
Altair Arab. "Bird."
Althea Gk. "With healing power." Tennis star Althea Gibson.
　Altha, Althaia, Altheda, Althia, Eltha, Elthea, Thea
Altheda Gk. "Like a blossom."
Alura OE. "Godlike adviser."
　Alurea, Allura
Alva Sp. "Blond, fair-skinned." See **Alba, Albina**. Better-known as a man's name, as in Thomas Alva Edison.
　Alba, Albina, Albine, Albinia, Alvah
Alvar OE. "Army of elves." Also used as a man's name, but very unusual.
Alverdine OE. "Counsel from the elves." A rare feminine variant of Alfred. Alfreda is more common.
Alvina (fem. **Alvin**) OE. "Noble friend" or "elf-friend."
　**Alveena, Alveene, Alveenia, Alvine, Alvineea, Alvinia,
　Alwinna, Alwyna, Alwyne, Elveena, Elvena, Elvene,
　Elvenia, Elvina, Elvine, Elvinia, Vina, Vinni, Vinnie,
　Vinny**
Alvita Lat. "Lively."
Alysia Gk. "Entrancing."
Alyssa Gk. "Rational." Also the name of a bright yellow flower, alyssum, and its use may have been influenced by the 19th-century vogue for flower names. Also see the variants of Alice.
　Alissa, Allissa, Alysa, Ilyssa, Lyssa
Alzena Arab. "Woman."
　Alzeena, Alzina
Amabel Lat. "Lovable, amiable." Somewhat popular in the 19th century.
　Ama, Amabelle, Belle, Mab, Mabel
Amada Lat. "Loved one."

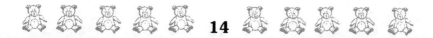

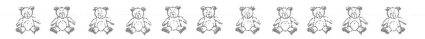

Amadea (fem. **Amadeus**) Lat. "God's beloved." Amadeus was Mozart's middle name, given great prominence by Peter Shaffer's play and the subsequent film.
Amadée, Amédee

Amadore It. "Gift of love."
Amadora

Amal Arab. "Hope."
Amahl, Amahla, Amala

Amalida OG. "Hardworking woman." See **Amelia**.

Amana Heb. "Loyal, true."

Amanda Lat. "Much-loved." Regularly used since the 17th century, and ever more popular with the 1990s turn to nostalgic-sounding names. Actress Amanda Plummer.
Amandi, Amandie, Amandine, Amandy, Amata, Manda, Mandaline, Mandee, Mandi, Mandie, Mandy

Amara Gk. "Lovely forever."
Amargo, Amargoe, Amargot, Amarinda, Amarra, Amarrinda, Mara, Marra

Amarantha Gk. "Deathless." Also the name of both a mythical and a real plant. The mythical one was supposed to be immortal.
Amarande, Amaranta, Amarante

Amaris Heb. "Pledged by God."
Amariah

Amaryllis Gk. "Fresh." Also the name of a flower. Used in 18th-century poetry to refer to an unspoiled country beauty like an idealized shepherdess.

Amber OF. Name of the gold-brown semiprecious stone. Jewel names were popular in the 19th century, but Amber came to prominence again in the 1960s, prompted by the Kathleen Winsor novel and film, *Forever Amber*.
Ambar, Amberetta, Amberly, Ambur

Ambika Hindi "Mother." Also one of many names for the goddess Sakti, who reigns over power and destruction.

Ambrosine (fem. **Ambrose**) Gk. "Ever-living." Like other names with an "-ine" ending, this one has a French air.
Ambrosia, Ambrosina, Ambrosinetta, Ambrosinette, Ambrosiya, Ambrozetta, Ambrozia, Ambrozine

Amelia OG. "Industrious." See **Emily**. An 18th-century Princess Amelia brought the name to Britain, where it

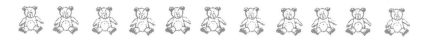

was popular in the 19th century. Dress reformer Amelia
Bloomer; aviatrix Amelia Earhart.

**Aimiliona, Amalea, Amalee, Amaleta, Amalia, Amalie,
Amalija, Amalina, Amaline, Amalita, Amaliya, Amalya,
Amalyna, Amalyne, Amalyta, Amelie, Amelina, Ameline,
Amelita, Ameliya, Amelyna, Amelyne, Amelyta, Amilia,
Amy, Em, Emelie, Emelina, Emeline, Emelita, Emma,
Emmeline, Emmie, Emmy, Mali, Malia, Malika, Meline,
Millie, Milly**

Amelinda Lat./Sp. Com. form "beloved" and "pretty."

Amethyst Gk. "Precious wine-colored jewel." An unusual
jewel name, though appropriate for a February baby,
since amethyst is that month's birthstone.

Amica Lat. "Friend." Very unusual. Closely related to
Spanish *amiga* or Italian *amica*, the everyday words for
"friend" in those languages.

Amice

Amilia Lat. "Amiable." Also possible variant spelling for
Amelia.

Amina Arab. "Honest, trustworthy." Mother of the
prophet Mohammed.

Aminah

Aminta Lat. "Protector." Aminta was the heroine of a
well-known pastoral play of the Renaissance, but her
name was not much used in real life.

Amynta, Minta, Minty

Amira Arab. "Highborn girl." Currently popular in the
Arabic-speaking countries.

**Ameera, Ameerah, Amera, Amerah, Amirah, Amyra,
Amyrah, Meera, Meerah, Mera, Merah, Mira, Mirah**

Amisa Heb. "Companion, friend."

Amissa

Amita Heb. "truth"; It. "friendship." See **Amica, Amy.**

Amitola NAm. Ind. "Rainbow."

Amity Lat. "Friendship, harmony."

Amitie

Amor Sp. "Love."

Amorette Fr. "Little love."

Amy Lat. "Loved." In spite of the prominence given the
name by Louisa May Alcott's *Little Women* (one of whom

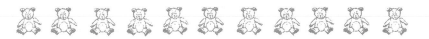

is named Amy), it didn't become a favorite until the 1950s. Poet Amy Lowell; evangelist Aimée Semple Mc-Pherson; singer Amy Grant.

Aimée, Aimie, Amada, Amata, Amé, Amecia, Ami, Amia, Amiah, Amice, Amie, Amii, Amye, Esma, Esmé

Anastasia Gk. "Resurrection." Indelibly associated with the daughter of Czar Nicholas II who supposedly escaped death when her family was assassinated during the Russian Revolution. The 1956 film starring Ingrid Bergman popularized her story, but the name is still something of a mouthful. Short forms like Stacey are much more common. Actress Nastassja Kinski.

Ana, Anastaise, Anastase, Anastasie, Anastasija, Anastasiya, Anastassia, Anastay, Anasztaizia, Anasztasia, Anestassia, Anstass, Anstice, Asia, Nastassia, Nastassiya, Nastassja, Nastassya, Nastya, Stace, Stacey, Stacia, Stacie, Stacy, Stasiya, Stasja, Stasya, Tasenka, Tasia, Tasiya, Tasja, Tasya

Anatola Gk. "From the east." Anatolia is a region of Turkey.

Ancelote Fr. Feminine form of Lancelot, the famous knight of the Round Table.

Andrea (fem. **Andrew**) Gk. "A man's woman." Little-used, even in its most common form, in English-speaking countries.

Aindrea, Andee, Andere, Anderea, Andi, Andie, Andra, Andre, Andreana, Andreas, Andrée, Andrel, Andresa, Andrewena, Andrewina, Andri, Andria, Andriana, Andy, Aundrea, Ohndrea, Ohndreea, Ohndria, Ondrea, Ondreea, Ondria, Onndrea, Onndreea, Onndria

Andromeda Gk. In Greek myth, the beautiful daughter of Cassiopeia (now famous as a constellation), she was chained to a rock as a sacrifice to a sea monster until Perseus rescued her. She, too, became a star. Also the name of a spring-blooming shrub.

Anemone Gk. "Breath." In Greek myth, Anemone was the name of a nymph who was turned into a flower, which is also called a windflower.

Ann-Aymone, Anne-Aymone

Angela Gk. "Messenger from God, angel." Angel was

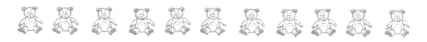

originally used as a name for men, and in Latin countries Angelo is still popular. Angela came into frequent use in the early 20th century. Actresses Angela Lansbury, Angie Dickinson.

Aingeal, Ange, Angel, Angele, Angeleta, Angelica, Angelika, Angeliki, Angelina, Angeline, Angelique, Angelita, Angelle, Angellina, Angie, Angil, Angiola, Angy, Angyola, Anjel, Anjela, Anjelica, Anjelika, Anngela, Anngil, Anngilla, Anngiola, Annjela, Annijilla, Gelya

Angelica Lat. "Angelic." See **Angela**. Actress Anjelica Huston.

Angelika, Angelique, Angyalka, Anjelica, Anjelika

Anisah Arab. "Friendly, congenial."

Annissa

Anita Sp. form of **Ann**. Most common in 1950s, possibly because of the popularity of Swedish actress Anita Ekberg. Writers Anita Loos, Anita Brookner.

Anitra, Annita, Annitra, Annitta

Ann Anglicization of **Hannah**. Heb. "Grace." One of the most frequently used names for girls until the mid–19th century, when it became less popular. When Elizabeth II of England named her daughter Anne in 1950, it became more prominent, but is still more common as a middle name (Betty Ann, etc.). Though the name Ann may seem plain to many, its numerous derivatives offer plenty of variety. Saint Anne (mother of the Virgin Mary); Anne Boleyn, Queen of England; ballerina Anna Pavlova; Wild West sharpshooter Annie Oakley; actresses Anouk Aimée, Anne Bancroft; writer Ayn Rand; diarist Anne Frank.

Aine, Ana, Anci, Anechka, Anet, Anett, Anette, Ania, Anica, Anika, Aniko, Anissa, Anita, Anitra, Anka, Anke, Anki, Anna, Annabel, Annabella, Annabelle, Annaelle, Annelle, Annelore, Annetta, Annette, Anni, Annice, Annick, Annie, Annimae, Annina, Annis, Annise, Annora, Annus, Annuska, Anny, Anona, Anouche, Anouk, Anoushka, Anouska, Anushka, Anuska, Anya, Anyoushka, Anyshka, Anyu, Asya, Ayn, Hajna, Hana, Hanja, Hanka, Hanna, Hannah, Hanneke, Hannelore,

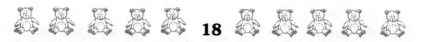

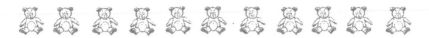

Hanni, Hannie, Hanny, Nan, Nana, Nance, Nancee,
Nancey, Nanci, Nancie, Nancy, Nanete, Nanette, Nanice,
Nanine, Nanni, Nannie, Nanny, Nanon, Nanor, Neti,
Nettia, Nettie, Netty, Nina, Ninette, Ninon, Ninor, Nita,
Nona, Nonie

Annabel Possibly com. form **Anna** and **Belle**: "graceful"
and "beautiful." Also mutation of Amabel. Most famous
bearer was Edgar Allan Poe's Annabel Lee, in the poem
of the same name.
**Anabel, Anabella, Anabelle, Annabal, Annabelinda,
Annabell, Annabella, Annabelle**

Annamaria Com. form **Ann** and **Mary**. Annemarie is the
most popular variation, especially since the 1950s. The
reverse form, Marianne, is also frequently used. The
popularity of the pairing may originate in Roman Catholic veneration of Saint Anne and Saint Mary, mother
and daughter.
Annamarie, Annemarie, Annmaria

Annelise Com. form **Ann** and **Lise**.
**Analeisa, Analiesa, Analiese, Analise, Anelisa, Anelise,
Annaleisa, Annalie, Annaliesa, Annaliese, Annalise,
Annelie, Anneliese, Annelisa, Annelise, Annissa**

Annemae Com. form. **Ann** and **May**
Annamae, Annamay, Annemie

Annette Dim. **Ann**. Most baby boomers will always associate this name with Mouseketeer Annette Funicello.
Anet, Anett, Anetta

Annis Gk. "Finished, completed." See also variants of
Ann. Also easily confused by the ear with Agnes, a point
prospective parents might keep in mind.
Anissa, Annes, Annice, Annys

Annora Lat. "Honor." A phonetic version of Honora.
Anora, Anorah, Onora, Nora, Norah

Annunciata Lat. Allusion to the Annunciation, when the
Virgin Mary learned she would be Jesus' mother. Some-
times given to a girl born in March, the logical month
for such an announcement.
**Anonciada, Annunziate, Anunciacion, Anunciata,
Anunziata**

Annot Heb./Scot. "Light."

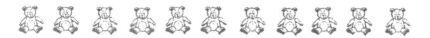

Anonna Lat. Name of the Roman goddess of the annual harvest. An appropriate name for an October or November baby.
Anona, Nona

Anselma (fem. **Anselm**) OG. "Godly helmet." The short forms are much more common.
Selma, Zelma

Ansonia (fem. **Anson**) Unclear origin and meaning. Possibly "son of Ann," though "son of the divine" seems more likely.

Anthea Gk. "Flowerlike." Used by English 17th-century poets to symbolize spring, but occurring infrequently in real life.
Annthea, Anthe, Antia, Thia

Anthemia Gk. "In bloom." From the same Greek root as Anthea.
Antheemia, Anthemya, Anthymia

Antje Ger. form of **Ann**. Heb. "Grace." Currently popular in Germany.

Antigone Gk. In myth, the daughter of Oedipus.

Antoinette (fem. **Anthony**) Lat. "Beyond price, invaluable." Also a diminutive of **Ann**. Irresistibly associated with the ill-fated French Queen Marie Antoinette.
Antonetta, Antonia, Antonie, Antonietta, Antonina, Antonine, Netta, Netti, Nettie, Netty, Toinette, Toni, Tonia, Tonie, Tony, Tonye

Antonia Lat. "Beyond price, invaluable." Also a diminutive of **Ann**. Willa Cather novel *My Antonia;* English writer Antonia Fraser.
Antoinette, Antonetta, Antonie, Antonietta, Antonina, Netta, Nettie, Netty, Toinette, Tonechka, Tonette, Toni, Tonia, Tonie, Tony, Tonya

Anwen Welsh. "Very fair."
Anwyn

Anwar Arab. "Rays of light." Most familiar as a man's name borne by Egyptian President Anwar Sadat.

Aphra Heb. "Dust." The English Puritans actually used both Dust and Ashes as first names in the 17th century.
Affery, Afra

Apolline (fem. **Apollo**) Gk. The god of the sun in Greek

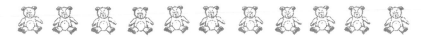

mythology. Saint Apollonia was an early Christian martyr, now the patron saint of teeth. In art she is often
portrayed with a pair of tongs and an outsized molar.

**Abbeline, Abbelina, Appoline, Appolinia, Apollinia,
Apollonia, Apollyne, Appolonia**

Aponi NAm. Ind. "Butterfly."

April Lat. "Opening up." First used as a name in the 20th
century, and naturally popular for a girl born in that
month. Curiously, only the months April, May, and June
are used for names, with **June** the most popular.

**Aprilete, Averel, Averell, Averil, Averill, Averyl, Averyll,
Averylle, Avril, Avrill**

Aquilina (fem. **Aquilino**) Sp. "Like an eagle."

Ara Arab. "Brings rain."

Ari, Aria, Arria

Arabella Lat. "Answered prayer." Unusual name that occurs most frequently in England.

**Ara, Arabel, Arabela, Arabele, Arabelle, Arbela, Arbell,
Arbella, Arbelle, Bel, Bella, Belle, Orabel, Orabella,
Orabelle, Orbel, Orbella, Orbelle**

Arachne Gk. In myth, a young maiden who challenged
the goddess Athena to a weaving contest and was turned
into a spider for her presumption.

Araminta Com. form **Arabella** and **Aminta**. Invented by
an 18th-century English playwright, and very unusual.

Arcadia Gk. Originally the place name of a region in
Greece which eventually came to stand for the home of
simple pastoral happiness.

Arcadie

Arcelia Sp. "Treasure chest."

Arda Heb. "Bronze."

Ardah, Ardath

Ardelle Lat. "Burning with enthusiasm." See **Arden**.

**Arda, Ardeen, Ardelia, Ardelis, Ardella, Ardene, Ardia,
Ardine, Ardis, Ardra**

Arden Lat. "Burning with enthusiasm." The Forest of Arden in Shakespeare's *As You Like It* was a magically
beautiful place. Most famous in modern times as the surnames of cosmetics queen Elizabeth Arden and actress
Eve Arden.

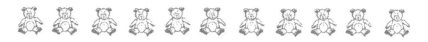

Ardeen, Ardena, Ardenia, Ardin

Arella Heb. "Messenger from God, angel."
Arela

Arete Gk. "Woman of virtue." Singer Aretha Franklin has put an indelible stamp on her version of this name.
Areta, Aretha, Arethusa, Aretina, Aretta, Arette, Oreta, Oretha, Oretta, Orette, Retha

Argenta Lat. "Silvery."

Aria It. "A melody." In the classical operatic form, arias are solos performed by the leading characters.

Ariadne Gk. The mythological daughter of Cretan King Minos, who gave Theseus a thread to guide him out of the mazelike prison known as the Labyrinth. Theseus married, then abandoned, her. Also the subject and title of a Richard Strauss opera.
Arene, Ariadna, Ariana, Ariane, Arianie, Arianna, Arianne, Aryana, Aryane, Aryanie, Aryanna, Aryanne

Ariana Welsh "Like silver."
Ariane

Ariel Heb. "Lioness of God." In Shakespeare's *The Tempest*, Ariel is a sprite who can disappear at will. The name has the connotation of something otherworldly, and though Shakespeare's Ariel is male, the name is used mostly for girls.
Aeriel, Aeriela, Aeriell, Ariela, Ariella, Arielle, Ariellel

Arista Gk. "The best."

Arlene (Derivation unclear. Possibly dim. **Charles**) OE. "man"; possibly fem. **Arlen**, related to Gael. "pledge." The name first appeared in the mid–19th century, and was popular by the 1930s. Actresses Arlene Francis, Arlene Dahl.
Arla, Arlana, Arlee, Arleen, Arlen, Arlena, Arleta, Arlette, Arleyne, Arlie, Arliene, Arlina, Arlinda, Arline, Arluene, Arly, Arlyn, Arlyne, Arlynn, Lena, Lene, Lina

Arlette Fr. From **Charles**. OE "Man."
Arlet, Arletta

Arlise (fem. **Arliss**) Heb. "Pledge."
Arlyss

Armida Lat. "Little armed one."

Armina (fem. **Armand**) OG. "Fighting maid."

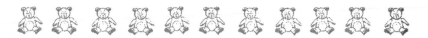

Armantine, Armine, Arminie, Armyne, Erminia, Erminie, Ermyne

Arnalda (fem. **Arnold**) OG. "Eagle-strength."

Arnina (fem. **Aaron**) Heb. "On high."

Arona

Artemisia Gk./Sp. "Perfect." Also a version of Artemas, a man's name that occurs in the Bible.

Artemesia

Arthuretta (fem. **Arthur**) Celt. Possibly "bear" or "rock." A 19th-century version of the man's name that was very popular until about 1920. The women's versions never really caught on.

Arthurina, Arthurine, Artice, Artina, Artis, Artrice

Asencion Sp. Literally ascension, marking Christ's ascension into heaven, which is commemorated 40 days after Easter.

Asuncion

Ashanti Af. Area in West Africa where many American slaves came from. Used, more often for girls, in modern American black families.

Ashanta, Ashante, Ashantee, Ashaunta, Ashaunte, Ashauntee, Ashaunti, Ashuntae

Ashira Heb. "Rich."

Ashley OE. Place name: "Ash-tree meadow." Originally a surname that migrated to first-name status, possibly helped along by Ashley Wilkes in Margaret Mitchell's *Gone With the Wind*. Though originally used for boys, it is now tremendously popular for girls, having reached top-ten stature in the 1980s.

Ashely, Ashla, Ashlan, Ashlee, Ashleigh, Ashlen, Ashli, Ashlie, Ashly

Asia Name of the continent. The feminine "-ia" ending lends itself to adaptation as a girl's name.

Asima Arab. "Guardian."

Aspasia Gk. "Welcoming." The famous Athenian statesman Pericles had a mistress named Aspasia, who was famous for her beauty and wit. Surprisingly the name enjoyed mild popularity in the straitlaced 19th century. Almost unknown now.

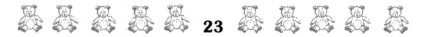

Asphodel Gk. "Lily." Flower name, albeit an unusual one. The asphodel is a member of the lily family.

Asta Gk. "Like a star." Also short form of Anastasia, Astrid, Augusta, etc. The most famous Asta is probably the terrier owned by Nick and Nora Charles in the famous *Thin Man* movies of the 1930s.
Astera, Asteria, Astra, Estella, Esther, Estrella, Etoile, Hadassah, Hester, Stella

Astra Lat. "Starlike, of the stars." First appeared in the 1940s, though other "star names," like Estella, have been around longer.
Asta, Astera, Asteria, Astraea, Astrea, Astria

Astraea Gk. The goddess of justice in classical mythology. When she retired from the earth, according to legend, she became the constellation Virgo. A clever name for a girl born under that sign.

Astrid ONorse. "Beautiful like a god." Unusual in English-speaking countries, but occurs in the royal families of Norway and Belgium. Astrud Gilberto, Brazilian singer.
Assi, Astra, Astrud, Astryr, Atti

Asuncion Sp. Marking the Virgin Mary's ascent into Heaven, which is commemorated on August 15.
Asencion

Atalanta (fem. **Atlas**) Gk. "Immovable." In Greek myth, Atalanta was an extremely athletic young maiden who refused to marry any man who couldn't beat her in a foot race. In the end, she was defeated by a ruse involving three golden apples.
Atlanta, Atlante

Atara Heb. "Diadem."
Atera, Ateret

Athalia Heb. "The Lord is exalted." In the Old Testament, Athalia was wife of the King of Judah. She murdered 42 princes to win the throne for herself, and after a reign of six years, was ultimately killed by a mob.
Atalee, Atalia, Atalie, Athalee, Athalie, Attalie

Athanasia (fem. **Athanasius**) Gk. "Immortal."

Athena Gk. The goddess of wisdom in Greek myth. She was a virgin goddess who sprang fully armed from Zeus's head, and Homer, in the *Odyssey*, frequently re-

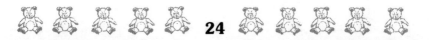

fers to her as "gray-eyed Athena." A daunting name to live up to.

Athenais, Athene, Athie, Attie

Atifa Arab. "Empathy, affection."

Aubrey OF. "Elf ruler." Originally a man's name that arrived in England with the Norman Conquest. For a girl, the ear will readily confuse it with Audrey.

Aubary, Aubery, Aubree, Aubrette, Aubrie, Aubry, Aubury

Auda OF. "Prosperous."

Aud, Aude

Audrey OE. "Noble strength." Also the root, via Saint Audrey, for the word "tawdry." (In England gaudy necklaces used to be sold at Saint Audrey's Fair.) Most popular in the 1920s and 1930s, now out of fashion. Actress Audrey Hepburn.

Audi, Audie, Audra, Audre, Audree, Audreen, Audria, Audrie, Audry, Audrye

Audris OG. "Lucky."

Augusta (fem. **Augustus**) Lat. "Worthy of respect." Imported to England by the German mother of George III. Though common enough in the 18th and 19th centuries, it is little used now. P. G. Wodehouse's foppish hero Bertie Wooster had a terrifying Aunt Augusta, and she may be responsible for the slightly intimidating connotations of the name.

Auguste, Augustina, Augustine, Augustyna, Augustyne, Austina, Austine, Austyna, Austyne, Gus, Gussie, Gusta, Tina

Aura Gk. "Soft breeze"; Lat. "gold." Most familiar now, perhaps, in its psychic sense.

Aure, Aurea, Auria

Aurelia Lat. "Gold." Originally a name used by Roman clans, it resurfaced as a first name in the 19th century, but is seldom seen now.

Aranka, Aural, Auralia, Aurea, Aurel, Aureliana, Aurelie, Aurita, Ora, Oralia, Orel, Orelee, Orelia

Auriel Lat. Dim. of "golden." Not to be confused with Ariel. A name used for slaves in the Roman Empire, possibly as a descriptive term. The 19th-century penchant

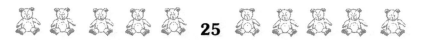

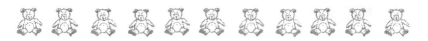

for unusual names brought it back to occasional use, but it is rare now.

Aureola, Aureole, Auriol, Oriel, Oriole

Aurora Lat. "Dawn." Aurora was the Roman goddess of sunrise. Used by 19th-century poets such as Byron and Browning, but never common.

Aurore, Ora, Rora, Rory, Zora, Zorica

Austine (fem. **Austin** or **Augustine**) Lat. "Worthy of respect."

Autumn Season name, only recently used as a first name.

Ava Lat. "Like a bird." May have originated as a form of Eva. Actress Ava Gardner.

Avis

Avalon Celt. "Island of apples." In Celtic myth, Avalon is an island paradise. In Arthurian legend, it is the island where King Arthur took refuge after his final defeat, and whence he will reappear.

Ave Lat. "Hail."

Avena Lat. "Field of oats."

Avichayil Heb. "Strong father."

Abichail, Avigail

Aviva Heb. "Springlike, fresh, dewy."

Avivah, Avivi, Avivit, Viva, Auvit

Avril A French version of April, the month name. Also possibly a version of the name of a 7th-century saint, Everild.

Averel, Averell, Averil, Averill, Averyl

Axelle (fem. **Axel**) OG. "Father of peace."

Aya Heb. "Bird."

Ayanna Recently invented name that may be considered an elaboration of Anna, or of the typically feminine "-ana" ending. Probably popular because it sounds pretty.

Aiyana, Aiyanna, Ayana, Ayania, Ayannia, Iana, Ianna

Ayesha Per. "Small one."

Aza Arab. "Comfort."

Azalea Lat. "Dry earth." More familiar to us as the name of the shrub that produces brilliantly pink blooms in the spring.

Azalia

Azelia Heb. "Aided by God."

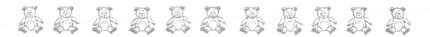

Aziza Heb. "mighty"; Arab. "precious."

Azuba Meaning unknown. Biblical name, used occasionally from the 17th through 19th centuries.
Azubah, Zuba, Zubah

Azura OF. "Azure, sky blue." A good attribute name for a blue-eyed baby.
Azor, Azora, Azure, Azzura, Azzurra

Babe Dim. **Barbara**. Gk. "Foreign." Also short for "baby," as in "See ya, babe." Socialite Babe Paley.

Babette Fr. Dim. **Barbara**. Gk. "Foreign."

Baila Sp. "Dance."
Beyla, Byla

Bailey OE. "Law enforcer, bailiff." A surname that metamorphosed into a first name in the 19th century, though uncommon. Used more often for boys than for girls.
Bailee, Baily

Balbina Lat. "Little stutterer."
Balbine

Bambi It. "Child." Short for *bambino*. Of course, the most famous Bambi is Walt Disney's cartoon deer, who happens to be male.
Bambie, Bamby

Baptista Lat. "One who baptizes."
Baptiste, Batista, Battista, Bautista

Bara Heb. "To select."
Bari, Barra

Barbara Gk. "Foreign." The adjective was originally applied to anyone who did not speak Greek; it has the same root as "barbarian." The early Christian martyr Saint Barbara was imprisoned in a tower by her father; she is patroness of engineers and architects. The name had its greatest popularity in the 19th-20th centuries, peaking around 1925, when in the U.S. it was second only to Mary. Use since then has dropped off dramati-

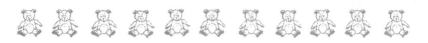

cally, and in one 1989 poll it didn't even make the top 100. Many people may associate this name with the popular doll Barbie. Actress Barbara Stanwyck; singer Barbra Streisand; writer Barbara Tuchman; First Lady Barbara Bush.

Bab, Baba, Babara, Babb, Babbett, Babbette, Babbie, Babe, Babett, Babette, Babita, Babs, Baibin, Bairbre, Barb, Barbary, Barbe, Barbee, Barbette, Barbey, Barbi, Barbie, Barbra, Barbro, Barby, Basha, Basia, Baubie, Bauby, Berbera, Berberia, Berberya, Berbya, Bobbe, Bobbee, Bobbi, Bobbie, Bobby, Bonni, Bonnie, Bonny, Varvara, Varina

Barrie A place name (Barry Islands, Wales) turned into a surname turned into a first name used by both sexes. Possibly influenced by the fame of Sir James Barrie, author of *Peter Pan*, since it first appeared as a given name during the height of his renown. It can also be considered a more feminine version of Barry.

Bari, Barri

Bartha OG. "Shining, brilliant." Variant of Bertha.

Barta

Basha Pol. "Stranger." From the same root as Barbara.

Basia

Basilia (fem. **Basil**) Gk. "Royal, regal." Common in the Middle Ages, but very unusual now.

Baseele, Baseelia, Baseelle, Bazeele, Bazeelia, Bazeelle, Basile, Basilie, Basille, Bazile, Bazille, Bazilia

Bathilda OG. "Woman warrior." Saint Bathild was a young English girl who became queen of the Franks in the 7th century. She was apparently canonized for opposing the then-flourishing slave trade, and also for founding a convent.

Bathild, Bathilde, Berthilda, Berthilde, Bertilda, Bertilde

Bathsheba Heb. "Daughter of the oath." Biblical name: Bathsheba was the mistress and later the wife of King David. Surprisingly (given her history), the name was used often by the Puritans. Now rare.

Bathseva, Bathshua, Batsheba, Batsheva, Batshua, Bethsabee, Sheba

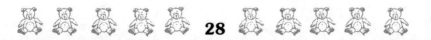

Bathshira Arab. "Seventh girl-child." Unlikely to be appropriate in this age of small families.

Batya Heb. "God's daughter."
Bitya

Beata Lat. "Blessed." First word of the Latin version of the famous "beatitudes" section of the biblical Sermon on the Mount: "Blessed are the poor in spirit . . ." A popular name in Northern Europe.
Beate

Beatrice Lat. "Bringer of gladness." The original form, Beatrix, was often found in the Middle Ages in England, then forgotten until its Victorian revival as Beatrice. Its popularity was no doubt boosted by Queen Victoria's naming one of her daughters Beatrice. It fell out of fashion after the 1920s, but may become popular again following the Duke and Duchess of York's use of it for their elder daughter. Heroine of Dante's *Divine Comedy* and of Shakespeare's *Much Ado About Nothing;* entertainer Beatrice Lillie; writer Beatrix Potter; actress Bea Arthur; Queen Beatrix of the Netherlands.
Bea, Beatrisa, Beatrix, Bebe, Bee, Beea, Beeatrice, Beeatris, Beeatrisa, Beeatriss, Beeatrissa, Beeatrix, Beitris, Beitriss, Trix, Trixi, Trixie, Trixy

Bebba Heb. "God's pledge."

Becky Dim. **Rebecca**. Heb. "Noose." Often used as an independent first name. Becky Sharp, heroine of William Thackeray's novel *Vanity Fair.*

Beda OE. "Battle maid."

Bedelia Ir. variant of **Bridget** (Ir. Gael. "Strength, power") by way of **Biddy**.
Bedeelia, Bidelia

Bee Dim. **Beatrice**. Lat. "Bringer of gladness." Also the name of an obscure 7th-century English saint. There is an English village called Saint Bees.

Behira Heb. "Shining, bright."

Belinda Unclear origin; possibly com. form **Belle** and **Linda**. Since the name first occurs in 18th-century English poet Alexander Pope's *The Rape of the Lock*, that derivation seems unlikely. It may be related to the Old

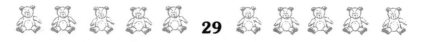

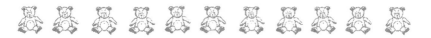

German for "dragon." Has upper-class English conno-
tations.
**Bel, Belle, Bellinda, Bellynda, Belynda, Linda, Lindie,
Lindy**

Belita Sp. "Little beauty."

Bell Dim. Isabel. Heb. "Pledged to God." Also, surname
used as a first name.

Bella Lat. "Beautiful." Dim. Isabella. Heb. "Pledged to
God." Used as early as the Middle Ages, but not popular
until the 18th century. Politician Bella Abzug.
Bell, Belle, Bellette

Bellanca It. "Blond."
Bianca, Blanca

Belle Fr. "Beautiful." Enjoyed a brief fad in the 1870s, but
almost unheard-of since then. Author Belva Plain.
Belinda, Bell, Bella, Bellina, Belva, Belvia, Billie, Billy

Bellona Lat. "Goddess of battle."

Bena (fem. Ben) Heb. "Wise."

Benedicta (fem. Benedict) Lat. "Blessed." Extremely rare.
Benita is the more common form.
**Benedetta, Bénédicte, Benedikta, Benetta, Benita,
Benoite, Bennie, Dixie**

Benigna Lat. "Kindly, benevolent."

Benita Sp. Var. Benedicta. More common than Benedicta,
but very unusual in English-speaking countries.
**Bendite, Benedetta, Benedicta, Benedikta, Benetta,
Benni, Bennie, Benny, Benoite, Binnie, Binny**

Bentley OE. "Meadow of ben (grass)." Place name become surname become first name, more common for
boys. Irresistibly linked in most minds with the luxurious English cars.
Bentlea, Bentlee, Bentleigh, Bently

Bera Teut. "Bear."

Berdine OG. "Bright or glowing maiden."

Berengaria OE. "Maiden of the bear-spear." The wife of
English King Richard the Lion-Heart.

Berit Scan. "Gorgeous, splendid, magnificent." Currently
popular in Sweden.
Beret

Bernadette (fem. Bernard) Fr. "Bear/courageous." Made

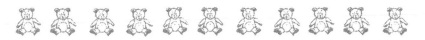

famous by Saint Bernadette of Lourdes, a miller's daughter who in 1858 repeatedly saw visions of the Virgin Mary. By the time she was canonized in 1933, Lourdes had become a world-famous destination for pilgrims. The name was popular among Catholic families especially after the 1943 movie *Song of Bernadette*, but is now unusual in English-speaking countries. Actress Bernadette Peters.

Berna, Bernadeena, Bernadene, Bernadett, Bernadetta, Bernadina, Bernadine, Bernadyna, Bernardina, Bernardine, Bernee, Berneta, Bernetta, Bernette, Bernie, Bernita, Berny

Bernice Gk. "She who brings victory." From the same root as Veronica. The name appears in the New Testament and first occurred in Britain in the 16th century, but its only real popularity came at the end of the 19th century. Little used today.

Barri, Barrie, Barry, Beranice, Beraniece, Beranyce, Bereniece, Berenice, Berenyce, Berneece, Bernelle, Bernetta, Bernette, Bernee, Berni, Bernie, Berniece, Berny, Bernyce, Berri, Berrie, Berry, Bunni, Bunnie, Bunny, Nixie, Veronica, Veronika, Veronike, Veronique

Berry Nature name. Also diminutive of Bernice, Bernadette, etc. Flower names enjoyed a vogue, especially in Britain, in the 1880s. Berry is also used for men, in that case more often as a transferred surname or a diminutive for Bernard.

Bertha OG. "Bright." Also related to the name of a Teutonic goddess. Very popular in the late 19th century, but almost unheard of since 1920. This disuse may be explained by the fact that a German cannon used in World War I was nicknamed "Big Bertha" after Bertha Krupp, daughter of the family that manufactured the weapon.

Berrta, Berrte, Berrti, Berrtina, Berrty, Berta, Berte, Berthe, Berti, Bertie, Bertina, Bertine, Bertuska, Berty, Bird, Birdie, Birdy

Bertilde OG. "Bright warrior maiden."
Bertina Ger. "Bright, shining." Dim. **Bertha.**
Bertrade OE. "Bright adviser."
Berura Heb. "Pure."

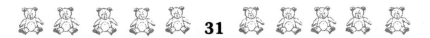

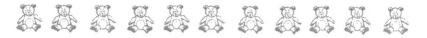

Beruria Heb. "God-selected."

Beryl Gk. "Pale green gemstone." The beryl was considered a token of good luck. The name first appeared with the fashion for jewel names in the late 19th century. Its popularity peaked in the 1920s, and it is now rare. Author Beryl Markham.
Berri, Berrie, Berry, Beryle

Beta Gk. Second letter of the Greek alphabet. Also a middle-European variant of Beth.

Beth Heb. "House." Dim. **Elizabeth** (Heb. "pledged to God"), **Bethany**. In Louisa May Alcott's *Little Women*, Beth is the sweet, gentle sister who dies young.

Bethany Biblical: the name of the village near Jerusalem where Lazarus lived. In some cases a variant on the combined form Beth-Ann.
Bethanie, Bethanne, Bethannie, Bethanny

Bethel Heb. "House of God." Another biblical place name: the spot where Abraham built an altar. Unusual as a first name.
Bethell, Bethuel, Bethuna, Bethune

Bethesda Heb. "House of mercy." Bethesda pool in Jerusalem was supposed to have healing powers after being stirred by an angel.

Bethia Heb. "Daughter of Jehovah." Popular in the eras, such as the 17th century, when Old Testament names have been intensively used.
Betia, Bithia

Bettina Dim. **Elizabeth**. Heb. "Pledged to God." Spanish or Italian in origin, and briefly popular in the sixties.
Betina, Bettine

Betty Dim. **Elizabeth**. Heb. "Pledged to God." A nickname with great popularity in its own right. It first became common in the 18th century, and after a spell of disuse, by the 1920s was one of the top names in every English-speaking country. Now it appears most often in combination with other names: Betty Lou, Betty Ann, etc. Actresses Betty Grable and Bette Davis; singer Bette Midler; First Lady Betty Ford.
Bett, Betta, Bette, Betti, Bettie, Bettina, Bettine

Beulah Heb. "Married." Also used to refer to Israel, and

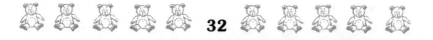

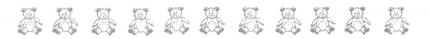

in John Bunyan's *Pilgrim's Progress*, Beulah is the promised land. It first became a girl's name in the late 16th century. References to "Beulah land" appear in American spirituals.
Beula

Beverly OE. Place name: "Beaver-stream." Originally an English place name and a surname, then used for both sexes as a first name. Probably still most famous as a place name, referring to Beverly Hills. The English spelling is usually Beverley. Singer Beverly Sills.
Bev, Beverle, Beverlee, Beverley, Beverlie, Beverlye, Bevlyn, Bevverlie, Bevverly, Bevvy, Buffy, Verlee, Verlie, Verly, Verlye

Bevin Ir. Gael. "Singer." More commonly a man's name, although Ireland's famous 11th-century king Brian Boru had a daughter with the name.
Bevan

Bianca It. "White." The meek younger daughter in Shakespeare's *Taming of the Shrew,* and subject of a song in the spin-off musical *Kiss Me Kate.* The most famous Bianca in recent times is former Rolling Stone wife Bianca Jagger.
Blanca, Blancha

Bibi Arab. "Lady."
Bebe, Beebee

Bibiana Sp. Var. **Vivian**. Lat. "Alive."
Bibiane

Bienvenida Sp. "Welcome."

Billie OE. Dim. **Wilhelmina**. OG. "Will-helmet." Feminine use of what is generally considered a man's name; more popular in the South, though uncommon now. Singer Billie Holliday; actress Billie Burke; tennis player Billie Jean King.
Billi, Billy, Willa

Bina Heb. "Knowledge, perception." Also dim. **Albina, Sabina**, etc.
Binah, Buna

Bird Eng. Unusual nature name.
Birdey, Birdie, Byrd, Byrdie

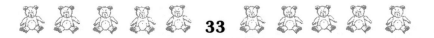

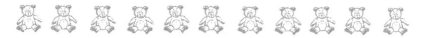

Birgit Nor. "Splendid." Var. **Bridget**.
  Birgitt, Birgitta, Birgitte
Bithron Heb. "Daughter of song."
Blaine Ir. Gael. "Slender." Surname now used as a first name, more usually for boys. Cropped up as a first name in the 1930s.
  Blane, Blayne
Blair Scot. Gael. Place name referring to a plain or flat area. Surname now used as a first name, again more common for boys. Like many similarly transferred names, Blair was used for girls in greater numbers starting in the early 1980s.
  Blaire
Blaise Lat. "One who stutters." Used for both sexes, though more common for men. The alternate spelling of Blaze probably refers to fire instead. French philosopher Blaise Pascal.
  Blaize, Blase, Blasia, Blaze
Blake OE. Paradoxically, could mean either "pale-skinned" or "dark." Surname used as a first name for either sex, but more common for boys.
  Blakelee, Blakeley, Blakely, Blakenee, Blakeney, Blakeny
Blanche Fr. "White, pale." Very popular in America at the end of the 19th century, but unusual now.
  Bellanca, Bianca, Blanca, Blanch, Blanka, Blinny
Blanchefleur Fr. "White flower."
Blanda Lat. "Smooth, seductive." Saint Blandina was a 2nd-century martyr, a slave girl who was gored to death by a bull.
  Blandina, Blandine
Blasia Var. **Blaise**. Lat. "One who stutters."
Blessing OE. "Consecration."
Blima Heb. "Blossom."
  Blimah, Blime
Bliss OE. "Intense happiness."
  Blisse, Blyss
Blodwen Welsh. "White flower." Literal translation into Welsh of Blanchefleur. Little used outside Wales.
  Blodwyn

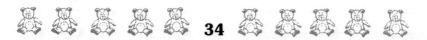

Blondelle Fr. "Little pale one."
Blondell, Blondie, Blondy

Blossom OE. "Flowerlike." Generic flower name, used mostly at the turn of the 20th century.

Bluebell Flower name popular in the 19th century, though when it became the typical name for a cow (like Rover for a dog), it dropped out of human use.

Blythe OE. "Happy, carefree." Made famous by the opening lines of Shelley's poem "To a Skylark" ("Hail to thee, blithe spirit!") and Noel Coward's play *Blithe Spirit*. Actress Blythe Danner.
Blithe

Bo Chinese. "Precious." More often used as a masculine diminutive for names like **Robert**. Bo Derek, actress.

Boadicea Name of a heroic queen of early Britain, who led a massive army against Roman invaders. Has rather intimidating connotations.

Bobbie Dim. **Roberta**. OE. "Bright renown." Like Billie, a feminine version of a man's nickname, often used in combination with a monosyllabic second name, and more common in the South. Also derives from Barbara. Gk. "Stranger." Author Bobbie Ann Mason.

Bogdana Pol. "Gift from God."
Bogna, Bohdana

Bolade Nig. "The coming of honor."

Bolanile Nig. "This house's riches."

Bonfilia It. "Good daughter."

Bonita Sp. "Pretty." Popular in the early 1940s, but unusual now.
Bo, Bonie, Bonnie, Bonny, Nita

Bonnie Scot. "Good, fair of face." The Scots adopted the French word *bonne*, meaning "good." Its most common use as an adjective is the fond nickname "Bonnie Prince Charlie." The old nursery rhyme claims that "the child who is born on the Sabbath Day/Is bonny and blithe and good and gay," which makes this an appropriate name for a Sunday's child.
Bonne, Bonnebell, Bonnee, Bonni, Bonnibel, Bonnibell, Bonnibelle, Bonny, Bunni, Bunnie, Bunny

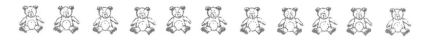

Borbala Hung. "Foreigner." Var. **Barbara**.
Bora, Boriska, Borka, Borsala, Borsca

Bradley OE. Place name: "Broad field." Surname now used as a first name for either sex, though more common for boys. Little seen outside America.
Bradlea, Bradlee, Bradleigh, Bradly

Brandy Name of a liquor. In the early 1980s, one of the most popular names for American girls, reaching the top ten in some surveys.
Brandais, Brande, Brandea, Brandee, Brandi, Brandice, Brandie, Brandye, Branndais, Brannde, Branndea, Branndi, Branndie

Brenda (fem. **Brendan**) OE. "Burning." One source translates the Irish as "stinking hair," though the origin may also be a Norse word for "sword." Brenda was originally a Scottish name and was particularly fashionable in the 1940s. Actress Brenda Vaccaro; comic strip heroine Brenda Starr.
Bren, Brenn, Brennda, Brenndah

Brenna Ir. Gael. "Raven; black-haired." Also dim. **Brendan**.
Bren, Brenn, Brenne, Brennah

Brett Lat. "From Britain." Surname transferred to first name. Still more common for boys, but may be boosted by the huge popularity of Brittany in the late 1980s.
Brette, Britt

Briana (fem. **Brian**) Ir. Gael. Meaning obscure, possibly "strong" or "hill."
Brana, Breana, Breanne, Breeann, Breeanna, Breeanne, Breena, Bria, Brianna, Brianne, Brina, Briney, Brinn, Brinna, Briny, Bryana, Bryann, Bryanna, Bryanne, Bryn, Bryna, Brynne

Brice Obscure origin, possibly OE. "Noble" or Celt. "swift." Originally a surname.
Bryce

Bridget Ir. Gael. "Strength, power." May also derive from the name of a goddess of ancient Ireland. Very popular name in Ireland from the 18th century to the 1950s, so much so that in the late 19th century in the U.S. the stock

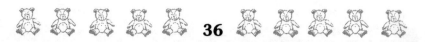

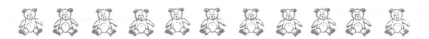

figure of the Irish housemaid (in plays, cartoons, etc.) was frequently called Bridget. Saint Brigid of Kildare, patroness of Ireland; opera star Birgit Nilsson; actresses Brigitte Bardot, Brigitte Nielsen.

Beret, Berett, Berget, Bergett, Bergette, Biddie, Biddy, Birget, Birgett, Birgit, Birgitt, Birgitta, Birgitte, Birkita, Birkitta, Birkitte, Birte, Bitta, Breeda, Bride, Bridee, Bridey, Bridgett, Bridgette, Bridgit, Bridgitt, Bridgitta, Bridgitte, Bridie, Bridy, Brietta, Briget, Brigett, Brighid, Brigid, Brigida, Brigit, Brigitt, Brigitta, Brigitte, Brijet, Brijit, Brijitte, Brita, Britt, Britta, Britte, Brydie, Brydget, Brydgit, Brydgitta, Brydgitte, Brydjette, Brydjitt, Bryget, Brygette, Brygid, Brygit, Brygitte, Bryjet, Bryjit

Brie Fr. Place name for a region in France most famous for the production of its cheese.

Bree, Briette

Brier Fr. "Heather." Unusual botanical name. Though the personal name derives from the French term for heather, the word in English usually describes a wild rose with small, prickly thorns. In some versions of "The Sleeping Beauty," Prince Charming has to cut through a hedge of briers to reach the princess.

Briar

Brina (fem. **Brian**) Slavic. "defender."

Bryn, Bryna, Brynn, Brynna, Brynne

Brit Celt. "Spotted, freckled." Also a diminutive of Brittany.

Britannia Lat. "Britain." Personification of Britain or the British Empire. She first appeared on a coin in the 2nd century A.D. For zealous Anglophiles.

Brites Port. "Power."

Brittany Lat. "From England." According to one 1989 survey, the third most fashionable name for American girls, behind Sarah and Katherine. It may derive some of its popularity from associations with England, which held tremendous glamor in the 1980s in America.

Brett, Brit, Briteny, Britney, Britni, Britny, Britt, Britta, Brittan, Brittaney, Brittani, Britteny, Brittnee, Brittney, Brittni, Brittny

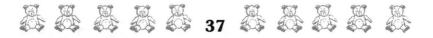

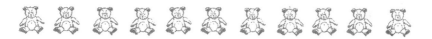

Bronwyn Welsh. "Fair breast." Use of Welsh-language names such as Bronwyn, Blodwyn, and the like may be related to periodic surges of separatist or nationalistic feeling in Wales.
Bronnie, Bronny, Bronwen, Bronya

Brooke OE. Place name: "Small stream." Also a surname, and used for either sex, though more commonly for girls. Actresses Brooke Adams, Brooke Shields.
Brook, Brookie, Brooks, Brooky

Brucie (fem. **Bruce**) OF. "Thicket of brushwood." The man's name was first common in Scotland, after a 14th-century king. The feminine variant is little used.
Brucina, Brucine

Bruna (fem. **Bruno**) It. "Brown-skinned, brown-haired."

Brunella OF. "Little one with brown hair."
Brunelle, Brunetta, Brunette

Brunhilda OG. "Armor-wearing fighting maid." Heroine of the Siegfried legend popularized in the Ring cycle of operas by Richard Wagner. Brunhilda is one of the Val-kyrie, maidens who ride into battle. The name naturally has connotations of great physical strength.
Brinhild, Brinhilda, Brinhilde, Brunhild, Brunhilde, Brunnhilda, Brunnhilde, Brynhild, Brynhilda, Brynhilde, Brynnhild, Brynnhilda, Brynnhilde, Hilda, Hilde, Hildi, Hildie, Hildy

Bryony Botanical name. Bryony is a vine native to Europe that has large leaves and small flowers.
Bryonie, Briony

Bryn Welsh. "Mount." Another place name converted to a Christian name in the 20th century.
Brynn, Brynna, Brynne

Buena Sp. "Good, excellent."

Bunny Nickname deriving from a number of *B* names such as Barbara or Bernice. Has come to be a child's name for a rabbit, of course. Likely to be associated with the famous Playboy Bunnies, the now defunct mid–20th-century emblem of a slightly licentious good time.
Bunni, Bunnie

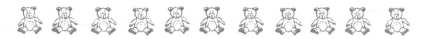

Cadence Lat. "With rhythm."
Cadena, Cadenza, Kadena, Kadence, Kadenza
Cady OE. Last name of uncertain meaning. It may have been successfully adopted as a girl's first name because of its resemblance to other popular girls' names like Katie.
Cade, Cadee, Cadey, Cadi, Cadie, Cadye, Kade, Kadee, Kadi, Kadie, Kady, Kadye
Cai Viet. "Feminine."
Caitlin Ir. See **Catherine**.
Caitilin, Caitlan, Caitlann, Caitlinn, Caitlyn, Caitlynn, Catlin, Catlinn, Kaitlan, Kaitlann, Kaitlin, Kaitlinn, Kaitlyn, Kaitlynn
Cala Arab. "Castle, fortress."
Calandra Gk. "Lark."
Cal, Calandre, Calandria, Calendre, Callee, Calley, Calli, Callie, Cally, Kalandra
Calantha Gk. "Lovely flower."
Cal, Calanthe, Callee, Calley, Calli, Callie, Cally, Kalantha
Caledonia Lat. "From Scotland." Place name adapted to first name, probably because of its typically feminine "-ia" ending. The Caledonian Canal runs through Northern Scotland, while New Caledonia consists of a group of tiny islands in the South Pacific.
Calida Sp. "Heated, with warmth."
Calla, Calli, Callida
Calla Gk. "Beautiful." Also the name of a flower, though the calla lily, with its smooth, sculptured lines, was not fashionable at the same time as the general vogue for flower names.
Callidora Gk. "Gift of beauty."
Calligenia Gk. "Daughter of beauty." A subtle compliment to the baby's mother.
Calliope Gk. Muse of epic poetry. See **Clio**. Also the name of a musical instrument typically seen at circuses and carnivals.
Callia, Callyope, Kalliope
Callista Gk. "Most beautiful."

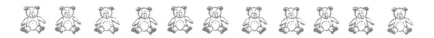

Cala, Calesta, Calista, Calla, Callesta, Calli, Callie, Cally, Callysta, Calysta, Kala, Kalesta, Kalista, Kalla, Kallesta, Kalli, Kallie, Kallista, Kally, Kallysta

Callula Lat. "Small beauty."

Caltha Lat. "Golden flower."

Calvina (fem. **Calvin**) Lat. "Hairless." Very unusual.
Calvine

Calypso Gk. "She who hides." In Greek myth the nymph Calypso held Odysseus captive for seven years. The name is also applied to the distinctive music of the West Indies.

Cameo It. from Middle French. "Skin." A stone or shell (frequently pinkish), carved with a picture, often a tiny portrait. Cameos have been very popular as jewelry at various periods, most recently the Victorian era.
Cammeo

Camelia Flower name first used in the 1930s. Its root is actually distinct from the more common Camille.
Camellia

Camille Lat. Meaning unclear, though some sources trace it to the young girls who assisted at pagan religious ceremonies. The heroine of Alexandre Dumas's famous story "The Lady with the Camellias" was actually named Marguerite, but through a translation became known as Camille. The name has been used consistently since the 19th century, usually in the form Camilla. Camille has been more common in the U.S., and some sources predict it will be popular in France during the upcoming decade.
Cam, Cama, Camala, Cami, Camila, Camile, Camilla, Cammi, Cammie, Cammilla, Cammille, Cammy, Cammylle, Camyla, Camylla, Camylle, Kamila, Kamilka, Kamilla, Kamille, Kamyla, Milla, Mille, Millee, Milli, Millie, Milly

Candace Possibly Lat. "Brilliantly white." Historically the name was the ancient title of the queens of Ethiopia before the 4th century. Not much used until the mid–20th century. Actress Candice Bergen.
Candee, Candi, Candie, Candis, Candiss, Candy, Dace,

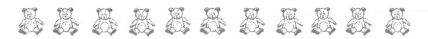

Dacee, Dacey, Dacie, Dacy, Kandace, Kandice, Kandiss, Kandy

Candida Lat. "White." Popular in the early Christian era, then very rare until this century, when it has been used occasionally.
Candi, Candide, Candie, Candy

Candra Lat. "Glowing."

Cantara Arab. "Little bridge."

Caprice It. "Ruled by whim."

Capucine Fr. "Cowl." French form of an Italian word for a cloak with a deep collar, characteristic of a certain order of Franciscan monks. A French actress who worked in Hollywood in the 1960s gave the name some exposure in the U.S., but it is rare.

Cara Lat. "Darling." Began to be fashionable from the 1970s onward.
Caralie, Carina, Carine, Carrie, Carry, Kara, Karina, Karine, Karrie, Karry

Carey Welsh. Place name: "Near the castle." A name used for both men and women. In this form it is a transferred surname, but, especially for women, it may be considered a diminutive of Caroline.

Carina It. "Dear little one." Dim. **Cara.** Often used in Italy in the exclamation *"Che carina!"* meaning, "How darling!" or even "How cute!"
Careena, Caren, Carena, Carin, Carine, Karena, Karina, Karine

Carinthia Place name: an idyllic region of southern Austria.

Carissa Gk. "Grace." See **Charis.** Also possibly another variation of Cara.
Caresa, Caressa, Carisa, Charissa, Karisa, Karissa

Carita Lat. "Beloved." Also possibly derived from the Latin word for charity, *caritas.* Occasionally used in the last hundred years.
Caritta, Karita

Carla (fem. **Carl**) Dim. **Caroline.** OG. "Man." A European-sounding version of the many names that derive from **Charles.**
Carlla, Karla, Karlla

Carlie (fem. **Charles**) Dim. **Caroline, Charlotte**. OG. "Man." The form Carleen (or Carlene) was primarily a product of the 1960s; this shorter version is now more popular. Singer Carly Simon.
Carlee, Carleen, Carlene, Carley, Carli, Carline, Carlita, Carly, Carlye, Carlyne, Carlyta, Karlee, Karlene, Karli, Karlie, Karline, Karlita, Karly, Karlyta

Carlin Gael. "Little champion."
Carling

Carmel Heb. "Garden." Biblical place name: Mount Carmel is in Israel, and is often referred to as a kind of paradise. The name has been used by Catholic families for some hundred years, though the form Carmen is much more common.
Carma, Carmela, Carmelina, Carmelita, Carmie, Carmina, Carmine, Carmy, Lina, Lita, Melina, Melita, Mina

Carmen Lat. "Song." A derivation of **Carmel**. One of the titles of the Virgin Mary is Santa Maria del Carmen (meaning Saint Mary of Mount Carmel), and this form of the name honors her. The most famous Carmen, of course, is the ill-fated heroine of Bizet's opera.
Carma, Carmelia, Carmelina, Carmelita, Carmencita, Carmia, Carmie, Carmina, Carmine, Carmita, Carmyna, Carmyta, Charmaine, Karmen, Karmia, Karmina, Karmita, Lita, Mina

Carna Lat. "Horn." See **Cornelia**.
Carniela, Carniella, Carnyella, Karniela, Karniella, Karnyella

Carnation Lat. "Becoming flesh." Unusual flower name.

Carol (fem. **Carl, Charles**) OG. "Man." Originally a short form of Caroline, not an adoption of "Christmas carol." It first appeared about a hundred years ago, and by mid–20th century was enormously popular, possibly influenced by the career of actress Carole Lombard. It is sometimes paired with a monosyllabic second name, most commonly Ann, as in Carol-Ann. The popularity of the name peaked in the mid-sixties, and it is now out of style. Actresses Carol Burnett, Carol Channing; skater Carol Heiss.

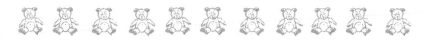

Carel, Carey, Cari, Carla, Carleen, Carlene, Carley, Carlin, Carlina, Carline, Carlita, Carlota, Carlotta, Carly, Carlyn, Carlynn, Carlynne, Caro, Carola, Carole, Carolena, Carolin, Carolina, Carolinda, Caroline, Caroll, Carolyn, Carolynn, Carolynne, Carri, Carrie, Carroll, Carrolyn, Carry, Cary, Caryl, Caryll, Charla, Charleen, Charlena, Charlene, Charlotta, Charmain, Charmaine, Charmian, Charmion, Charyl, Cheryl, Cherlyn, Ina, Karel, Kari, Karla, Karleen, Karli, Karlie, Karlina, Karlinka, Karlote, Karlotta, Karole, Karolina, Karyl, Karyll, Karryl, Karryll, Kerril, Kerryl, Keryl, Lola, Loleta, Lolita, Lotta, Lotte, Lotti, Lottie, Sharleen, Sharlene, Sharline, Sharmain, Sharmian

Caroline (fem. dim. **Carl, Charles**) OG. "Man." A rather stately diminutive with royal connotations. The name was brought to England by George II's queen and was popular until the end of the 19th century. It is now enjoying a revival. Princess Caroline of Monaco; fashion designers Carolina Herrera, Carolyne Roehm.

Caraleen, Caraleena, Caraline, Caralyn, Caralyne, Caralynn, Carla, Carleen, Carleena, Carlen, Carlene, Carley, Carlin, Carlina, Carlita, Carlota, Carlotta, Carly, Carlyn, Carlyna, Carlyne, Carlynn, Carlynne, Carol, Carola, Carole, Carolin, Carolina, Carolyne, Carolynn, Carolynne, Carri, Carrie, Caroll, Carollyn, Cary, Charla, Charleen, Charleena, Charlena, Charlene, Charline, Charlyne, Ina, Karaleen, Karaleena, Karalina, Karaline, Karalyn, Karalynna, Karalynne, Karla, Karleen, Karlen, Karlena, Karlene, Karli, Karlie, Karlina, Karlinka, Karolina, Karoline, Karolinka, Karolyn, Karolyna, Karolyne, Karolynn, Karolynne, Leena, Lina, Sharla, Sharleen, Sharlena, Sharlene, Sharline, Sharlyne

Carys Welsh. "Love." A Welsh name dating from the 1960s.

Casey Ir. Gael. "Watchful." Made famous by the song about the engineer of the Cannon Ball Express, Casey Jones. Used for both boys and girls. Can be considered a diminutive of Acacia.

Cacey, Cacie, Caisee, Caisey, Caisi, Caisie, Casee, Casi,

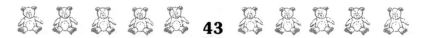

Casie, Caycee, Caycey, Cayci, Caycie, Caysee, Caysey, Caysi, Caysie, Kacey, Kacie, Kacy, Kacyee, Kasey, Kaycee, Kaycey, Kayci, Kaycie, Kaysee, Kaysey, Kaysi, Kaysie, Kaysy, Kaysyee

Casilda Lat. "Dwelling place."

Cassandra Gk. Perhaps a version of **Alexander**. In Greek myth, she was the daughter of King Priam of Troy. Apollo gave her the gift of foresight but, because she spurned his advances, decreed that her prophecies would never be believed. In vain she warned the besieged Trojans against accepting the gift of a gigantic wooden horse presented by their Greek enemy; it was full of Greek soldiers, who took the city captive. The name now indicates someone who is always prophesying doom and gloom.

Casandera, Casandra, Cass, Cassandre, Cassandry, Cassaundra, Cassi, Cassie, Cassondra, Cassy, Kasandera, Kassandra, Kassi, Kassie, Kassy, Sande, Sandee, Sandera, Sandi, Sandie, Sandy, Saundra, Sohndra, Sondra, Zandra

Cassia Gk. "Cinnamon."

Cassidy Ir. "Clever." Surname transferred to male first name transferred to girl's name.

Catherine Gk. "Pure." One of the oldest recorded names, with roots in Greek antiquity. Almost every Western country has its own form of the name, and phonetic variations are endless. It has been borne by such illustrious women as Saint Catherine of Alexandria, the early martyr who was tortured on a spiked wheel; Empress Catherine the Great of Russia; and three of Henry VIII's six wives. It is currently very popular in England and France, and was one of the top ten American girls' names in the 1980s. Actresses Catherine Oxenberg, Catherine Deneuve.

Cait, Caitey, Caitie, Caitlin, Caitlinn, Caitrin, Caitrine, Caitrinn, Caitriona, Caitrionagh, Caity, Caren, Cari, Carin, Caron, Caronne, Carren, Carri, Carrin, Carron, Caryn, Carynn, Cass, Cassey, Cassi, Cassie, Cassy, Cat, Cataleen, Cataleena, Catalin, Catalina, Cataline, Catarina, Catarine, Cate, Cateline, Caterina, Catey,

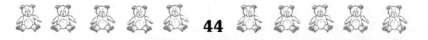

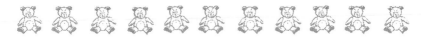

Catha, Cathaleen, Cathaline, Catharin, Catharina,
Catharine, Catharyna, Catharyne, Cathe, Cathee,
Cathelin, Cathelina, Cathelle, Catherin, Catherina,
Catherinn, Catheryn, Cathi, Cathie, Cathirin, Cathiryn,
Cathleen, Cathlene, Cathline, Cathlyne, Cathrine,
Cathrinn, Cathryn, Cathrynn, Cathy, Cathye, Cathyleen,
Cati, Catia, Catie, Catina, Catlaina, Catreena, Catrin,
Catrina, Catrine, Catriona, Catrionagh, Catryna, Caty,
Cay, Caye, Ekaterina, Kait, Kaitey, Kaitie, Kaitlin,
Kaitlinne, Kaitrin, Kaitrine, Kaitrinna, Kaitriona,
Kaitrionagh, Kaity, Karen, Karena, Kari, Karin, Karon,
Karri, Karrin, Karyn, Karynn, Kasia, Kasienka, Kasja,
Kaska, Kass, Kassey, Kassia, Kassy, Kasya, Kat, Kata,
Kataleen, Katalin, Katalina, Katarina, Katchen, Kate,
Katee, Katell, Katelle, Katenka, Katerina, Katerinka,
Katey, Katinka, Katha, Katharine, Katharyn, Katharyne,
Kathee, Kathelina, Katheline, Katherin, Katherina,
Katherine, Katheryn, Katherynn, Kathi, Kathie,
Kathileen, Kathiryn, Kathleen, Kathlene, Kathleyn,
Kathline, Kathyleen, Kathrine, Kathrinna, Kathryn,
Kathryne, Kathy, Kathyrine, Kati, Katica, Katie, Katina,
Katka, Katla, Katlaina, Katleen, Katoushka, Katrena,
Katrine, Katrina, Katriona, Katrionagh, Katryna,
Katushka, Katy, Katya, Kay, Kaye, Kit, Kittee, Kittie,
Kitty, Trina, Trine, Trinette, Yekaterin, Yekaterina

Cecilia (fem. **Cecil**) Lat. "Blind one." From a Roman clan
name. Saint Cecilia is the patroness of music. The name
was used in Roman times, then resurfaced in the Victo-
rian era, possibly given a boost by the fame of industri-
alist (and founder of Rhodesia) Cecil Rhodes. The form
Cecily was briefly popular in the 1920s, but neither name
has been used much since. Actress Cicely Tyson.
Ceceley, Cecely, Cecil, Cecile, Ceciley, Ceciliane,
Cecilija, Cecilla, Cecily, Cecilyann, Cecyl, Cecyle,
Cecylia, Ceil, Cele, Celia, Celie, Cesia, Cesya, Cicely,
Cicily, Cile, Cilka, Cilia, Cilla, Cilly, Cissie, Kikelia,
Kikylia, Sacilia, Sasilia, Sasilie, Seelia, Seelie, Seely,
Sesilia, Sessaley, Sesseelya, Sessile, Sessilly, Sessily,
Sile, Sileas, Sisely, Siselya, Siseel, Sisile, Sisiliya,
Sissela, Sissie, Sissy

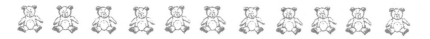

Celandine Gk. Botanical name: a yellow-blossomed wild-flower.

Celena Gk. Goddess of the moon, later identified with Artemis. A version of the more common Selina, although neither name is very common.
Cela, Celeena, Celina, Celinka, Cesia, Cesya, Salena, Salina, Selena, Selina

Celeste Lat. "Heavenly." Unusual in any of its forms, and probably most familiar through the fame of actress Celeste Holm. Baby boomers may associate the name with Queen Celeste, wife of Jean and Laurent de Brunhoff's children's book character Babar, the Elephant.
Cela, Celesta, Celestena, Celestene, Celestia, Celestijna, Celestina, Celestine, Celestyne, Celia, Celie, Celina, Celinda, Celine, Celinka, Celka, Celyna, Saleste, Salestia, Seleste, Selestia, Selestina, Selestine, Selestyna, Selestyne, Silesta, Silestena, Silestia, Silestijna, Silestina, Silestyna, Silestyne, Tina, Tinka

Celinda Gk. Var. Celeste.
Celinde, Salinda, Salinde, Selinda, Selinde

Celosia Gk. "Aflame."

Cenobia Gk. "Power of Zeus." A Spanish form of the slightly more common Zenobia.

Cerelia Lat. "Relating to springtime." A nice name for a spring baby.
Cerella

Cerise Fr. "Cherry." See **Cherry**.
Cherise, Sherise

Cesarina (fem. **Caesar**) Lat. Probably "hairy, hirsute."
Cesarea, Cesarie, Cesarine, Kesare

Chanah Heb. "Grace." See **Hannah**.

Chandra Sanskrit "Like the moon." The greatest Hindu goddess Sakti is also known as Chandra.
Candra, Shandra

Chanel Fr. Surname of the legendary fashion designer Coco Chanel, and by extension, the name of a number of famous perfumes. Began to be used as a first name in the 1980s.
Chanelle, Channelle, Shanel, Shanell, Shanelle, Shannel, Shannelle

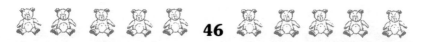

Chantal Fr. Originally a place name meaning "stony spot," but possibly also derived from the verb *chanter*, "to sing." Not uncommon in France, but unusual in the U.S.

Chantalle, Chantel, Chantelle, Chantele, Shantal, Shantalle, Shantel, Shantell, Shantelle

Charis Gk. "Grace." One of the mythological Three Graces.

Charity Lat. "Brotherly love." One of the three cardinal virtues, along with Faith and Hope. They have survived better than many of the other virtue names (Temperance, Fortitude, Humility, Chastity, Mercy, Obedience) popular among the Puritans in the 17th century.

Carissa, Carita, Chareese, Charis, Charissa, Charisse, Charita, Charitee, Charitey, Charitye, Cherri, Cherry, Sharitee, Sharitey, Sharity, Sharitye

Charlotte Fr. "Little and womanly." One of the most popular feminine forms of Charles. Like Caroline, Charlotte was popularized in England by a queen (George III's wife) and was much used from the 18th century to the beginning of the 20th. In the U.S. its use peaked in the 1870s, but with the recent return to "old-fashioned" names, it has been dusted off for a reappearance. In E. B. White's *Charlotte's Web,* the heroine of the title is a spider. Novelist Charlotte Bronte; actress Charlotte Rampling.

Carla, Carleen, Carlie, Carline, Carlota, Carlotta, Carly, Carlyne, Char, Chara, Charill, Charla, Charlaine, Charleen, Charlene, Charline, Charlotta, Charly, Charlyne, Charmain, Charmaine, Charmian, Charmion, Charo, Charyl, Cherlyn, Cheryl, Cheryll, Karla, Karleen, Karlene, Karli, Karlicka, Karlie, Karlika, Karline, Karlota, Karlotta, Karlotte, Karly, Karlyne, Lola, Loleta, Loletta, Lolita, Lolotte, Lotta, Lottchen, Lotte, Lottey, Lotti, Lottie, Lotty, Sharel, Sharil, Sharla, Sharlaine, Sharleen, Sharlene, Sharline, Sharmain, Sharmayne, Sharmian, Sharmion, Sharyl, Sheri, Sherie, Sherrie, Sherry, Sherye, Sheryl

Charmaine From a Latin clan name; also possibly related

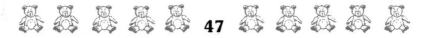

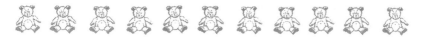

to Carmen and Caroline. Enjoyed bursts of popularity in the 1920s and 1950s.

Charmain, Charmane, Charmayne, Charmian, Charmion, Charmyan, Charmyn, Sharmain, Sharman, Sharmane, Sharmayne, Sharmian, Sharmion, Sharmyn

Charmian Gk. "Joy." A distinctly separate name from Charmaine, though they are often confused. Because of its Greek origin, Charmian should be pronounced with a hard *C*, but it rarely is.

Charmiane, Charmyan

Chasidah Heb. "Devout woman."

Chastity Lat. "Purity." A virtue name that has, for obvious reasons, fallen out of favor, though Cher used it for her daughter.

Chava Heb. "Life."

Chabah, Chaya, Chayka, Eva, Hava, Haya, Kaija

Chaviva Heb. "Beloved."

Eva

Chelsea OE. "Port or landing place." Place name; possibly owes some of its appeal to British pop culture of the late 1960s.

Chelsee, Chelsey, Chelsie, Chelsy

Chephzibah Heb. "My delight is in her." See **Hepzibah**.

Cher Fr. "Beloved." For most people, inseparable from the singer and actress who uses this name alone, without a surname. Somewhat popular in the late 1960s and early 1970s.

Chere, Cherée, Cherey, Cheri, Cherice, Cherie, Cherise, Cherish, Cherrie, Cherry, Chery, Cherye, Cherylee, Cherylie, Sher, Sherelle, Sherey, Sheri, Sherice, Sherie, Sherry, Sheryll

Cherry OF. "Cherry." The 19th-century vogue for botanical names did not usually extend to fruit, so when Cherry occurs, it is most likely a variant of Charity.

Chere, Cheree, Cherey, Cherida, Cherise, Cherita, Cherrey, Cherri, Cherrie

Cheryl familiar form of **Charlotte** or **Cherry**. A 20th-century development that first became popular in the 1940s, and increased in use into the 1960s. Like most 30-year-old fashions, it is now quite dated.

Charil, Charyl, Cheriann, Cherianne, Cherryl, Cheryll, Cherylle, Cherilynn, Sharil, Sharyl, Sharyll, Sheral, Sherianne, Sheril, Sherill, Sheryl

Cherilyn Form of **Cheryl**. Names that are modern developments seem more susceptible to widely variable spellings, as this one is.

Charalin, Charalyn, Charalynne, Charelin, Charelyn, Charelynn, Charilyn, Charilynn, Cheralin, Cheralyn, Cherilin, Cherilynn, Cherilynne, Cherralyn, Cherrilin, Cherrilyn, Cherrylene, Cherrylin, Cherryline, Cherrylyn, Cherylin, Cheryline, Cheryllyn, Cherylyn, Sharalin, Sharalyn, Sharelyn, Sharelynne, Sharilynn, Sheralin, Sheralynne, Sherilin, Sherralin, Sherrilyn, Sherrylene, Sherryline, Sherrylyn, Sherylin, Sherylyn

Chesna Slavic. "Peaceful."

Chessa, Chessy

Chiara It. "Light." See **Claire**.

Chiquita Sp. "Little one." Most parents will probably associate this name with the heavily advertised Chiquita banana.

Chickie, Chicky, Chiquin

Chloe Gk. "Young green shoot." Appears in the Bible, and as a name in literature, especially in the tale of Daphnis and Chloe, set to music by Ravel. Since the late seventies, it has been gaining popularity in England.

Chloé, Clo, Cloe

Chloris Gk. "Pale." Another name from Greek mythology, though an obscure one. Actress Cloris Leachman.

Cloris

Cholena Delaware Indian. "Bird."

Christabel Lat./Fr. "Fair Christian." Use has been primarily literary, as in Samuel Taylor Coleridge's poem of the same name, in which the heroine is an example of innocent purity. Used occasionally in Britain.

Christabella, Christabelle, Christobel, Chrystabel, Chrystabelle, Chrystobel, Cristabel, Cristabella, Cristabelle, Crystabel, Crystabella

Christina (fem. Christian) Gk. "Anointed, Christian." Christian was used for women in medieval times, but by the 18th century Christina was the more common form.

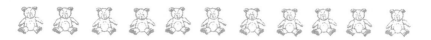

It was superseded in the 1930s by the French form Christine, which was very popular in the fifties and sixties, but the cycle of fashion has now brought Christina back. Christiane is currently very popular in Germany. Queen Cristina of Sweden; poet Christina Rossetti; tennis star Chris Evert; model Christie Brinkley.

Chris, Chrissie, Chrissy, Chrissta, Chrisstan, Chrissten, Chrissti, Chrisstie, Chrissty, Christa, Christan, Christeen, Christel, Christen, Christi, Christian, Christiana, Christiane, Christianna, Christie, Christin, Christine, Christinn, Christy, Christyna, Chrystal, Chrystalle, Chrystee, Chrystel, Chrystelle, Chrystle, Cris, Crissey, Crissie, Crissy, Crista, Cristal, Cristel, Cristelle, Cristen, Cristena, Cristi, Cristie, Cristin, Cristina, Cristine, Cristiona, Cristy, Crysta, Crystena, Crystene, Crystie, Crystina, Crystine, Crystyna, Khristeen, Khristena, Khristina, Khristine, Khristya, Kirsten, Kirstin, Kit, Kris, Krissy, Krista, Kristeen, Kristel, Kristen, Kristi, Kristijna, Kristin, Kristina, Kristy, Krysta, Krystka, Krystle, Stina, Teena, Teyna, Tina, Tiny

Christmas OE. Name of the holiday, used occasionally through the 19th century for Dec. 25 babies, but now more usually replaced by the French, and somewhat subtler, form, Noel.

Chryseis Lat. "Golden daughter." A very beautiful young girl named Chryseis appears in Homer's *Iliad*.
Chrysilla

Chumani Sioux. "Drops of dew."

Cinderella Fr. "Little ash-girl." The name from the fairy tale. Very rare.
Cindie, Cindy, Ella

Cindy Originally a nickname for **Cynthia** (Gk. "Goddess from Mt. Cynthos") or **Lucinda** (Lat. "Light"). Popular for children born in the fifties and sixties, but rarely used for *their* children of the eighties and nineties. Singer Cyndi Lauper.
Cindee, Cindi, Cindie, Cyndee, Cyndi, Cyndie, Cyndy, Sindee, Sindi, Sindie, Sindy, Syndi, Syndie, Syndy

Cipriana It. "From Cyprus."

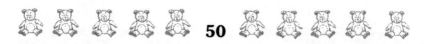

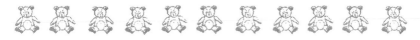

Cipriane, Ciprianna, Cypriana, Cyprienne

Claire Lat. "Bright." The original form was Clare, as in Saint Clare, 13th-century founder of a Franciscan order of nuns. In the 19th century Clara became fashionable, but since the 1960s, the French form Claire has dominated. Writer Clare Booth Luce; actresses Clara Bow, Claire Bloom.

Cheeara, Chiara, Ciara, Clair, Claire, Claireen, Clairene, Claireta, Clairette, Clairey, Clairice, Clairinda, Clairissa, Clairita, Clairy, Clarabel, Clarabelle, Clare, Clarene, Claresta, Clareta, Claretta, Clarey, Clari, Claribel, Claribella, Claribelle, Clarice, Clarie, Clarinda, Clarine, Clarissa, Clarisse, Clarita, Clarrie, Clarry, Clary, Claryce, Clayre, Clayrette, Clayrinda, Clayrissa, Clerissa, Cliara, Clorinda, Klaire, Klara, Klaretta, Klarissa, Klaryce, Klayre, Kliara, Klyara

Claramae Eng. A compound form of Clara, probably dating from the late 19th century, when May was also a popular name.

Claramay

Clarice Variant of Claire, which enjoyed a flurry of popularity around the turn of the 20th century. Clarissa is a Latinized version made famous by Samuel Richardson's 18th-century novel *Clarissa Harlowe.*

Claris, Clarise, Clarisse, Claryce, Clerissa, Clerisse, Cleryce, Clerysse, Klarice, Klarissa, Klaryce

Clarimond Lat./Ger. "Shining defender."

Claudia (fem. **Claude, Claudius**) Lat. Clan name probably meaning "lame." The name has never been very popular in English-speaking countries in any of its forms, in spite of the exposure given it by Colette's novels (*Claudine at School,* etc.) and the career of actress Claudette Colbert. It is currently used quite a bit in Germany. Actress Claudia Cardinale.

Claude, Claudelle, Claudetta, Claudette, Claudie, Claudina, Claudine, Claudey, Claudy

Clea Unknown derivation, but possibly invented by author Lawrence Durrell, for a character in his famous *Alexandria Quartet.* See also **Cleopatra, Clio.**

Clelia Lat. "Glorious." A maiden who figures in the leg-

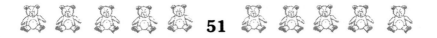

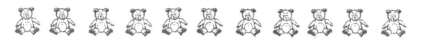

endary history of Rome. Her story was retold (in 10 volumes!) by the 17th-century French novelist Mlle. de Scudery.

Clematis Gk. "Vine or brushwood." Flower name, from the blossoming vine with white or purple blooms.

Clementia Lat. "Mild, giving mercy." Clemence and Clemency were both Puritan virtue names, but are now unheard-of. Clementia was used until the 19th century, when it was replaced by Clementina. The well-known song "My Darling Clementine" would make it hard to use that version of the name with a straight face.
Clem, Clemence, Clementia, Clementina, Clementya, Clementyna, Clementyn, Clemmie, Clemmy, Klementijna, Klementina

Cleopatra Gk. "Her father's renown." There were actually generations of Egyptian princesses of this name, but the most famous is the intriguer who enthralled both Caesar and Antony. Very rare.
Clea, Cleo

Cleva (fem. **Cleve, Clive**) Middle English. "Hill-dweller." Place name transferred to a surname and thence to a first name used for men. This feminine form is unusual.

Cliantha Gk. "Glory-flower."
Cleantha, Cleanthe, Clianthe, Kliantha, Klianthe

Clio Gk. Mythological name of the muse of history. There are nine muses, the daughters of Zeus and Mnemosyne, and each represents an art or science. Calliope (epic poetry), Terpsichore (choral song and dance), and Thalia (comedy) have survived as first names.

Clorinda Lat. Literary name coined by 16th-century Italian poet Tasso. Possibly derived from Claire or Chloe.

Clotilda Ger. "Renowned battle." Saint Clothilde was the wife of Frankish King Clovis I in the 6th century, and supposedly went into battle by his side. One of Paris's most fashionable churches is named for her.
Clothilda, Clothilde, Clotilde, Klothilda, Klothilde

Clover OE. Flower name. Perhaps because of the modest nature of the flower, the name occurred in the 19th century more commonly as a nickname.

Clymene Gk. "Renowned one." In Greek myth, most no-

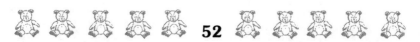

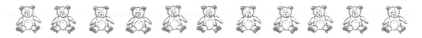

tably the daughter of Oceanus and mother of Atlas and Prometheus, though several other legendary figures also bear this name.

Clytie Gk. "Lovely one." Another mythological figure whose unrequited love for the sun god resulted in her being changed into a heliotrope, or sunflower, which turns to follow the sun's path.

Cochava Heb. "Star."

Cody OE. "Pillow." This is an example of the kind of unisex name that has been recently popular for girls in the U.S.
Codee, Codey, Codi, Codie, Kodey, Kodie, Kody

Colette Dim. **Nicole** Gk./Fr. "People of victory." Used mostly since the 1940s, though never widespread. Probably made familiar by the French writer Colette, whose last name it was.
Coletta, Collet, Collete, Collette, Nicolette

Coline (fem. **Colin**, derived from **Nicholas**) Gk. "People of victory."
Colena, Colene, Coletta, Colina, Nicoleen, Nicolene, Nicoline, Nicolyne

Colleen Ir. Gael. "Girl." In use since the 1940s in English-speaking countries *except* Ireland. A vogue in the early 1960s faded rapidly. Actress Colleen Dewhurst, writer Colleen McCullough.
Coleen, Collie, Colline, Colly, Kolleen

Columba Lat. "Dove." Saint Columba, 6th-century Irish saint, founded an influential monastery on the Scottish island of Iona, and is supposed to have exorcised the River Ness of a monster. Though the Irish Columba was a man, two other saints of that name were both women.
Collie, Colly, Colombe, Columbia, Columbine

Columbine Lat. "Dove." Columbine is also a literary character who appears in traditional Italian comedy and English pantomime as Harlequin's beloved. Also a flower name for a delicate two-colored blossom.

Comfort Fr. "To strengthen and comfort." In the Bible the Holy Ghost is referred to as the "Comforter." It was a surname in the Middle Ages, then popular among the Puritans. Almost unused since the 18th century.

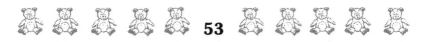

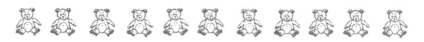

Concepcion Lat. "Conception." Used mostly in Latin American countries to honor the Immaculate Conception and, by extension, the Virgin Mary.
Cetta, Chiquin, Chita, Concetta, Concha, Concheta, Conchita

Concordia Lat. "Peace, harmony." In classical myth, Concordia was the goddess of peace succeeding a battle.

Conradine (fem. **Conrad**) OG. "Brave counsel."
Conrada, Connee, Connie, Conny

Constance Lat. "Steadfastness." Used often in the early Christian and medieval eras, then by the Puritans (usually as Constant or Constancy). After a brief revival at the beginning of this century, it lapsed back into obscurity. Singer Connie Francis.
Con, Connee, Conney, Conni, Connie, Conny, Constancia, Constancy, Constanta, Constantia, Constantija, Constantina, Constantine, Constantya, Constanz, Costanza, Konstance, Konstantija, Konstantina, Konstanze, Kosta, Kostatina, Tina

Consuelo Sp. "Consolation, comfort." Honors Santa Maria del Consuelo.
Chela, Chelo, Consolata, Consuela

Cora Gk. "Maiden." Though some sources trace the name to classical myth, its modern form was probably coined by American writer James Fenimore Cooper in *The Last of the Mohicans* (1826). It grew in popularity through the 19th century, but now its variant forms are more often used. Civil rights activist Coretta Scott King.
Corabel, Corabella, Corabelle, Corabellita, Coree, Corella, Corena, Corene, Coretta, Corey, Cori, Corie, Corilla, Corine, Corinna, Corinne, Correen, Corrella, Correlle, Correna, Correnda, Correne, Correy, Corri, Corrie, Corrina, Corrine, Corrissa, Corry, Corynna, Corynne, Coryssa, Kora, Korabell, Koreen, Korella, Koretta, Korey, Korilla, Korina, Korinne, Korry, Koryne, Korynna, Koryssa

Coral Lat. Nature name: first appeared as a name during the Victorian vogue for jewel names, usually in England.
Coralee, Coralena, Coralie, Coraline, Coraly, Coralyn, Coralyne, Koralie

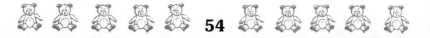

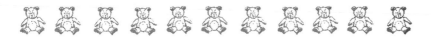

Corazon Sp. "Heart." Corazon Aquino, president of the Philippines.

Cordelia Derivation unclear, but probably related to Latin *cor* or "heart." In Shakespeare's *King Lear*, Cordelia is the youngest and only lovable daughter of the king.
Cordelie, Cordella, Cordelle, Cordey, Cordi, Cordie, Cordy, Delia, Delie, Della, Kordelia, Kordella

Corey Ir. Gael. Place name: "the hollow." Place name transferred to surname, occasionally used as a first name for either sex.
Cory, Cori, Corrie, Corry, Korie, Korry

Corinne French form of Cora, used since the 1860s.
Carinna, Carinne, Carine, Carynna, Carynne, Corenne, Corina, Corine, Corinn, Corinna, Correna, Corrianne, Corrienne, Corrine, Corrinn, Karinne, Karynna, Koreen, Korina, Korinne, Korrina

Corliss OE. "Benevolent, cheery."
Corlee, Corley, Corlie, Corly

Cornelia (fem. **Cornelius**) Lat. "Like a horn." Comes from a famous Latin clan name, and was often used in the Roman Empire. Modern use is sparing, dating from mid–19th century.
Cornalia, Corneelija, Cornela, Cornelija, Cornelya, Corelie, Cornella, Cornelle, Cornie, Korneelia, Korneelya, Kornelia, Kornelija, Kornelya, Neel, Neely, Nela, Nelia, Nell, Nella, Nellie, Nelly

Corona Sp. "Crown." A spate of English use occurred around the coronation of King Edward VII in 1902, but this sentimental homage to royalty was not repeated at subsequent coronations. Also the name of a very popular Mexican beer, which would seem to limit its further use as a given name.
Coronetta

Corvina Lat. "Like a raven."

Cosette Fr. Probably a feminine diminutive of **Nicholas**. Gk. "People of victory."
Cosetta

Cosima (fem. **Cosmo**) Gk. "Order." Very unusual in English-speaking countries.
Cosma, Cosmé, Kosma

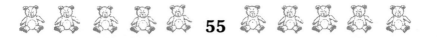

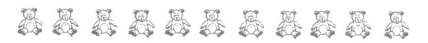

Courtney OE. "Court-dweller." Surname transferred to first name; usually feminine in U.S. Immensely popular, probably owing to upper-class connotations.
Cortland, Cortnee, Cortney, Cortny, Courtenay, Courtland, Courtnay, Courtnee, Courtny, Kortney, Kourtney, Kourtnee

Crescent OF. "Increasing, growing." Also, by extension, the shape of the crescent moon.
Crescence, Crescentia, Cressant, Cressent, Cressentia, Cressentya

Cressida Gk. Heroine of a tale that has been told by Boccaccio, Chaucer, and Shakespeare.

Crispina (fem. **Crispin**) Lat. "Curly-haired."

Cristina Lat. "Anointed, Christian." See **Christina**.

Crystal Gk. "Ice." Transferred use of the word, mostly modern, and increasing since the 1950s. Used as a man's name in Scotland, where it was a diminutive of Christopher. See **Christina**.
Christal, Christalle, Chrystal, Chrystalle, Chrystel, Chrystle, Cristal, Cristel, Cristle, Crysta, Crystel, Khristalle, Khrystle, Kristle, Krystal, Krystalle, Krystle

Csilla Hung. "Defenses."

Cyanea Gk. "Sky blue."

Cybele Gk. Asian goddess, also known in Greek myth as Rhea, and in Rome as "Great Mother of the Gods." In legend she was originally bisexual, but made female by the Olympian gods.

Cynara Gk. "Thistly plant." Made famous by the late–19th-century English poet Ernest Dowson, who is in turn largely remembered by the line "I have been faithful to thee, Cynara! in my fashion."

Cynthia Gk. "Goddess from Mount Cynthos," i.e., Artemis, the moon goddess, who was supposed to have been born there. Used as a literary name in the 17th century, and by American slave owners in the early 19th century. Enjoyed a period of popularity from the 1920s to 1950s, then was replaced by its nickname, Cindy, which is now rare. Many of the diminutives are also variants of Lucinda. Ballerina Cynthia Gregory.
Cinda, Cindee, Cindi, Cindie, Cindy, Cinnie, Cinny,

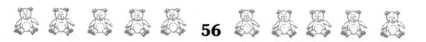

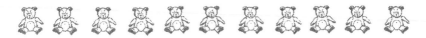

Cinthia, Cintia, Cyn, Cynda, Cyndee, Cyndia, Cyndie,
Cyndy, Cynnie, Cynthea, Cynthie, Cynthya, Kynthia,
Kynthija, Sindi, Sindy, Sindya, Sinnie, Sinny, Synda,
Syndee, Syndi, Syndy, Syntha, Synthee, Syntheea,
Synthia, Synthie, Synthya

Cypris Gk. "From the island of Cyprus."
Cipriana, Ciprienne, Cyprien, Cyprienne

Cyra (fem. Cyrus) Per. "Sun" or "throne."

Cyrilla (fem. Cyril) Lat. "Lordly."
Ciri, Cirilla, Siri, Sirilla, Syrilla

Cytherea Gk. "From the island of Cythera," i.e., Aphrodite or Venus, who is supposed to have set foot there after being born of seafoam.

D

Dacey Ir. Gael. "From the south."
Dacee, Dacia, Dacie, Dacy, Daicee, Daicy, Daisey

Dacia Lat. Place name: Dacia was a Roman province which existed where Romania is now.

Dada Nig. "Curly-haired."

Daffodil OF. Flower name for the familiar yellow blossom; an inventive name for a spring baby.

Dagmar OG. Meaning unclear, though possibly "day's glory." In Denmark Dagmar is a royal name, but it appears only rarely in English-speaking countries.

Dahlia Scan. Flower name of fairly recent vintage, first used in numbers since the 1920s. The flower itself was named in honor of the 18th-century Swedish botanist Anders Dahl.

Dai Jap. "Great."

Daisy OE. "Eye of the day." One of the most popular of the 19th-century flower names. It was often used as a nickname for Margaret, since in France the flower is called a *marguerite*. It was such a popular name that, when Henry James was writing the story of the typical

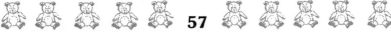

American girl in Europe, he called her *Daisy Miller*. Little used in the modern era, but this is the kind of name that nostalgia may resurrect.

Daisee, Daisey, Daisie, Dasie

Dale OE. Place name: "Valley." Originally a surname meaning "one who lives in the valley." The term "dale" is still used in parts of England. Most popular as a first name in the 1930s. Actress Dale Evans.

Daile, Dayle

Dalila Swahili. "Delicate."

Lila

Dallas Scot. Gael. Place name of a village in northeastern Scotland, used as a first name since the 19th century. Apparently unrelated to Dallas, Texas, which was named for a U.S. Vice President.

Dalmace Lat./Fr. Place name: Dalmatia is a region of northeastern Italy, extending down into coastal Yugoslavia, and the supposed origin of dalmatian dogs, white-haired with black spots.

Dalma, Dalmassa, Dalmatia

Damaris Gk. "Calf." A Damaris in the New Testament was converted by Saint Paul, and the Puritans adopted the name with enthusiasm, if not uniformity in spelling. Many variants exist, though the name is very unusual.

Damara, Damaress, Dameris, Dameryss, Damiris, Damris, Demaras, Demaris, Demarys, Mara, Mari, Maris

Damia Gk. Meaning not clear; possibly "to tame," although the Greek root is also close to the word for "spirit." The masculine form, Damian, is more often seen.

Damian, Damiana, Damiane, Damienne, Damya, Damyan, Damyana, Damyen, Damyenne

Damita Sp. "Little noblewoman."

Dana OE. "From Denmark." Also a surname, used as a boy's first name in the 19th century, but now almost exclusively a girl's name, and a specifically American one.

Danay, Dane, Danet, Danna, Dayna

Danaë Gk. A character in Greek myth, whom Zeus visited in the form of a shower of gold (a popular subject for

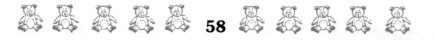

Old Master painters). The child of this union was the heroic Perseus.

Dee, Denae, Dene

Danielle (fem. **Daniel**) Heb. "God is my judge." Uncommon until the middle of the 20th century, when, following a revival of Daniel, it became more fashionable. Novelist Danielle Steele.

Danee, Danele, Danella, Danette, Daney, Dani, Danica, Danice, Danie, Daniela, Daniella, Danila, Danita,

Danitza, Danna, Danney, Danni, Danny, Dannyce, Dany, Danya, Danyelle

Daphne Gk. "Laurel tree." In Greek myth Daphne was a nymph who, attempting to flee an amorous Apollo, was turned into a laurel tree. Though used under the Roman Empire, the name disappeared until the 18th century. It came to the U.S. as a slave name, and enjoyed a brief English vogue between 1900 and 1930. Author Daphne Du Maurier.

Daffi, Daffie, Daffy, Dafne, Dafnee, Daphna, Daphney, Danfy

Dara Heb. "Nugget of wisdom." In the New Testament, a man's name, but its occasional modern use is for girls.

Darda, Daria, Darya

Daralis OE. "Beloved."

Daralice

Darby OE. Place name: "Park with deer." Derived from Derby, a surname used as a first name, almost exclusively for boys. Darby is also usually masculine.

Darb, Darbee, Darbey, Darbie, Darrbey, Darrbie, Darrby

Darcie Ir. Gael. "Dark." Also Norman place name, "from Arcy." In Britain, usually a boy's name, but in the U.S., more likely to be feminine. Ballerina Darci Kistler.

D'Arcy, Darcee, Darcey, Darcy, Darice, Darsee, Darsey

Daria (fem. **Darius**) Gk. "Rich."

Dari, Darian, Darice, Darien, Darya, Dorian, Doriane

Darlene Modern adaptation of "darling" used for a given name. First used in the late 1930s and extremely fashionable by the 1950s in the U.S. Now out of style, and unlikely to be revived soon.

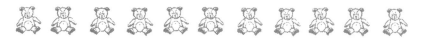

Dareen, Darelle, Darla, Darleen, Darline, Darlyne, Darrelle, Darryleen, Darrylene, Darryline

Daron (fem. **Darren**) Modern use. Darren may be a transferred Irish surname, first used widely in the 1950s as a given name. Daron can be considered a feminine form because of its similiarity to Sharon (also popular in that era).

Daryl Transferred surname, possibly originated as a French place name, like Darcy. Actress Daryl Hannah.
Darel, Darrel, Darrell, Darrelle, Darrylene, Darryline, Darryl, Darrylin, Darryline, Darrylyn, Darylin, Daryline, Darylyne

Davina (fem. **David**) Heb. "Loved one." The most commonly used feminine variant of the hugely popular masculine name.
Daveen, Daviana, Daviane, Davida, Davine, Davinia, Davita, Devina, Divina, Divinia

Dawn OE. "Dawn." Modern use of the word for a name. Aurora, the Latin term, dates back some fifteen hundred years, but Dawn first appeared in the late 1920s. Its popularity is now starting to wane.
Dawna, Dawnita, Dawnyelle, Dawnysia

Day OE. "Day." Possibly use of the word as a name, like Dawn, but more likely to be a transferred surname.

Dea Lat. "Goddess."

Deanna OE. Place name "valley" or occupational name "church leader." Feminine of Dean, which only came into use as a first name in the 1950s. Could also be considered a version of Diana. Actress Deanna Durbin.
Deana, Deann, Deanne

Deborah Heb. "Bee." One of the few significant women's names to figure in the Old Testament; in the Book of Judges, she was an important prophetess and judge. Predictably, the Puritans latched on to the name, but it was not widely used until the 1950s, possibly influenced by the career of actress Deborah Kerr. Actresses Debbie Reynolds, Debra Winger.
Deb, Debb, Debbee, Debbera, Debbey, Debbi, Debbie, Debbra, Debby, Debee, Debera, Deberah, Debi, Debor, Debora, Debra, Debrah, Debs, Devora, Devorah, Dobra

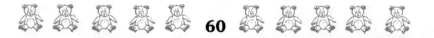

Decima Lat. "Tenth girl." Unlikely to be used in these days of small families.
Decia

Dee Welsh. "Swarthy." Dim. **Deirdre, Diana, Delia, etc.**
Dede, Dedie, DeeDee, DeeAnn, Didi

Deifilia Lat. "God's daughter."

Deirdre Ir. Possible meanings are "fear" or "raging woman." In Irish myth, Deirdre was the most beautiful woman in Ireland, whose tragically complex love life caused several deaths, including her own. The name, currently popular in Britain, has only been in use since the 1920s.
Dede, Dedra, Dee, DeeDee, Deedre, Deidra, Deidre, Deidrie, Derdre, Didi, Dierdre

Delaney Ir. Gael. "Offspring of the challenger."
Delaine, Delainey, Delainy, Delane, Delanie, Delany

Delia Gk. "From Delos." In Greek myth, the goddess Artemis was born in Delos, so Delia could be an allusion to her. It may also be a diminutive of Cordelia or Adelaide. Though it has never had a period of great popularity, it has never faded from sight either.

Delicia Lat. "Delight." Used in the Roman Empire, and occasionally since then, but never common.
Dee, DeeDee, Dela, Delice, Delise, Delisha, Della, Delyse, Delysia, Didi

Delight OF. The emotion as a name. Scarce.

Delilah Heb. "Lovelorn, seductive." In the Old Testament, mistress of Samson. The familiar story of how she cuts off his hair to sap his strength probably limits use of her name.
Dalila, Delila, Lila, Lilah

Della Short for Adelle, Adeline, Adelaide. Used as an independent name since the 1870s. Singer Della Reese.

Delores Sp. "Sorrows." Var. **Dolores**.

Delphine Gk. "Dolphin." This is a French form of a name with a complex origin. It alludes to the Greek town of Delphi, home of a famous oracle. The Greeks believed that Delphi was the earth's womb; the dolphin's shape resembles that of a pregnant woman. The larkspur flower, whose center resembles a dolphin, is also known

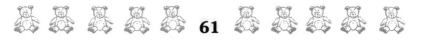

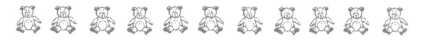

as delphinium, so in some respects this is a flower name. French actress Delphine Seyrig.

Delfin, Delfine, Delfyne, Delphina, Delphinea, Delphinia

Delta Fourth letter of the Greek alphabet, thus a name for a fourth child. May also be a place name, as in the Mississippi Delta. Actress Delta Burke.

Demetria Gk. In Greek myth, Demeter was goddess of corn, and mother of Persephone, whose abduction to Hades led to the cycle of seasons.

Demeter, Demetra, Demetris

Demelza Cornish. "Fort on the hill." First used as a given name in the 1950s, probably because of its pretty sound.

Dena OE. Place name. "Valley." Use of Dena followed the popularity of Dean in the 1950s.

Deana, Deane, Deanna, Deena, Dene, Denna, Denni, Dina

Denise (fem. **Dennis**) Fr. "Follower of Dionysius." Though there is an ancient Latin form of the name (Dionysia) this variation dates back only to the 1920s. It was very popular in the 1950s, but since the mid–1960s, has been eclipsed. Singer Deniece Williams.

Denese, Deni, Denice, Deniece, Denize, Denni, Dennie, Dennise, Denny, Denyce, Denys, Denyse, Dinnie, Dinny

Deolinda Port. "Beautiful God."

Derinda Modern name, probably formed from Derek and Linda.

Dorinda

Deryn Welsh. "Bird." Dates from the 1950s, and its popularity mirrors names like Karen and Sharon. Unusual after the 1970s.

Deren, Deron, Derrine, Derron

Desdemona Gk. "Wretchedness." In Shakespeare's *Othello*, Desdemona is the beautiful, innocent heroine, wrongly accused of adultery by her husband, who then murders her, and commits suicide in a fit of remorse. Little used, for obvious reasons.

Desmona

Desirée Fr. "Much desired." The Puritans used Desire as a given name, though its connotations in the 17th cen-

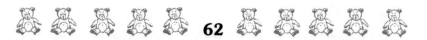

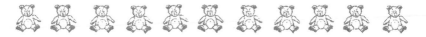

tury were religious rather than erotic. The French form is more usual today.

Desideria, Desir, Desirae, Desirat, Desiri

Desma Gk. "Binding oath."

Destinée OF. "Fate."

Detta Dim. **Benedetta.** Lat. "Blessed."

Deva Hindi. "Godlike." In Hindu myth, Deva is another name for the moon goddess.

Devi

Devin Ir. Gael. "Poet."

Deva, Devinne

Devon OE. Place name: a county in Southern England. More common for girls than for boys. Devin may also be considered a variant.

Devona, Devondra, Devonne

Dextra (fem. **Dexter**) OE. "Dyer." Lat. "Right-handed." Dexter, like most occupational names, was originally a surname. Dextra could also mean "skillful, dextrous."

Diamond Unusual jewel name, first used in the 1890s but never as common as Ruby, Emerald, etc. It is the birthstone for April.

Diana Lat. "Divine." The Roman goddess of the moon, corresponding to the Greek Artemis. Used steadily since the 16th century, though the French version Diane eclipsed it in the mid–20th century. The vogue for Diane faded after the 1960s, and the apotheosis of Lady Diana Spencer as Princess of Wales in 1980 has given Diana new charm for prospective parents, especially in Britain. French courtesan Diana de Poitiers; actresses Diahann Carroll, Dyan Cannon, Diane Keaton, Dianne Wiest.

Danne, Dayann, Dayanna, Dayanne, Deana, Deane, Deanna, Dede, Dee, DeeDee, Deana, Deane, Deann, Dena, Di, Diahann, Diahanne, Dian, Diandra, Diane, Diann, Dianna, Dianne, Didi, Dyan, Dyana, Dyane, Dyann, Dyanna, Dyanne

Dianthe Gk. "Flower of the gods."

Diandre, Diantha

Didi Var. **Diana, Deirdre.**

Didiane Fr. Feminine form of Didier, which is in turn a

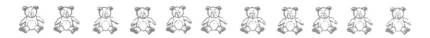

form of Desirée, through the Latin Desideratus.
Didiere

Dido Gk. In Vergil's *Aeneid,* the queen of Carthage who falls in love with the wandering Aeneas, and commits suicide when he leaves her. The name's origins are obscure: Vergil may have coined it.

Didrika (fem. **Dietrich**) OG. "People's ruler."

Dielle Fr. "God." Probably a female version of the French *dieu,* for "God." Unusual.
Diella

Digna Lat. "Worthy."
Dinya

Dilys Welsh. "Reliable." Somewhat older than many names now popular in Wales, since it dates from the mid–19th century.
Dylis, Dyllis, Dylys

Dinah Heb. "Justified." Old Testament name. In the U.S., has been popular in the South. Dina may also be considered a diminutive of names like Claudina. Actresses Dina Merrill, Dinah Shore.
Dina, Dyna, Dynah

Dionne Two possible sources: Dione, in Greek myth, is the mother of Aphrodite. The name can also be a feminine version of Dion, "follower of Dionysus." It is also a homonym for the French pronunciation of Diane. Singer Dionne Warwick.
Deonne, Dion, Diona, Dione, Dionis, Dionna

Dionysia Lat. Form of **Denise**. Gk. "Follower of Dionysus."

Dita Var. **Edith**. OE. "Prosperity/battle."

Divina It. "Divine." Also var. **Davina.** Heb. "Loved one."
Divinia

Dixie Fr. "Tenth." The term "Dixie" for the Southern states, made popular by the song, is mysterious. It might come from the Mason-Dixon line, or from Louisiana dollars printed in French with the word *dix* on them (hence, "the land of 'dixies'").
Dix, Dixee

Docila Lat. "Biddable."

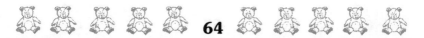

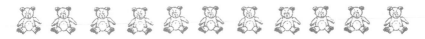

Dodie Heb. "Well loved." Familiar form of **Dora, Dorothy**. Gk. "Gift of God."
Dodee, Dodey, Dodi, Dody

Dolly Familiar form of **Dorothy**. As an independent name, it was most popular at the turn of the century, but never a favorite. First Lady Dolley Madison; country singer Dolly Parton.
Dollee, Dolley, Dollie

Dolores Sp. "Sorrows." An allusion to the Virgin Mary, Santa Maria de los Dolores. Actress Dolores del Rio.
Delora, Delores, Deloria, Deloris, Dolorcita, Dolorcitas, Dolorita, Doloritas, Lola, Lolita

Domina Lat. "Lady."

Dominique (fem. **Dominic**) Lat. "Lord." French form of a Latin name, rather fashionable in the last 25 years. Could be used for a child born on Sunday, "the Lord's day."
Domenica, Domeniga, Dominga, Domini, Dominica, Dominika, Dominizia, Domitia, Mika

Donalda Scot. Gael. "World mighty." One of many attempts to form a feminine of Donald, a Scottish name particularly popular in the first half of the 20th century.
Dona, Donaldina, Donaline, Donelda, Donetta, Donia, Donita

Donata Lat. "Given."

Donna It. "Lady." The original meaning is closer to "lady of the home." Strictly modern use as a given name, dating from the 1920s. Very popular in the 1950s, but little used now. Actress Donna Reed; swimming champion Donna Devarona; fashion designer Donna Karan.
Dona, Donella, Donelle, Donetta, Donia, Donica, Donielle, Donnell, Donni, Donnie, Donny, Ladonna

Dora Gk. "Gift." Probably originated as a diminutive of names like Theodora, and introduced as an independent name by a character in Charles Dickens's *David Copperfield*. Its heyday in the U.S. came at the turn of the century, but it is currently popular in Greece.
Dodee, Dodi, Dodie, Dody, Doralia, Doralyn, Doralynn, Doreen, Dorelia, Dorelle, Dorena, Dorene, Dorette, Dori, Dorie, Dorita, Dorrie, Dory

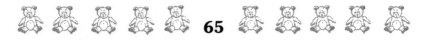

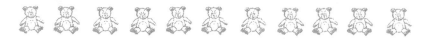

Dorcas Gk. "Gazelle." New Testament name, Greek version of Tabitha. Saint Peter raised her from the dead. Predictably, well used by the Puritans, but uncommon since.

Doré Fr. "Gilded."
Doree, Dory

Doreen Several possible origins, including Ir. Gael. "brooding," Fr. "gilded," and an elaboration of Dora. In the top ten in Britain in the 1920s, now unusual.
Dorene, Doreyn, Dorine, Doryne

Doretta Gk. "Gift from God." Variant of **Dora** or **Theodora**.

Doria Gk. Place name: "from Doris," an area in Greece. Also feminine of Dorian; var. **Dorothy, Theodora.** Gk. "Gift from God."
Dori, Dorian, Doriane, Dorianne, Dory

Dorinda Gk./Sp. Var. **Dora.** English poets in the 18th century coined a number of names with the "-inda" suffix. This one has enjoyed a small revival in this century.

Doris (Fem. **Dorian.**) Gk. Place name: "From Doris," an area in Greece. This form is more common than Doria, having been hugely popular between 1900 and the 1930s, when it subsided. Actress Doris Day; writer Doris Lessing.
Dori, Doria, Dorice, Dorisa, Dorita, Dorrie, Dorry, Dorrys, Dory, Dorys, Doryse

Dorothy Gk. "Gift of God." Theodora, never as popular, simply reverses the order of the Greek words. Has had two periods of popularity, around 1500 to 1700, and 1900 to the mid-1920s. The latter vogue may have been inspired by the heroine of Frank Baum's *The Wonderful Wizard of Oz*, published in 1900. Writers Dorothy Parker, Dorothy Sayers; actresses Dorothy Gish, Dorothy Lamour.
Dasha, Dasya, Dodie, Dody, Doe, Doll, Dolley, Dolli, Dollie, Dolly, Doortje, Dora, Doretta, Dori, Dorika, Dorinda, Dorlisa, Doro, Dorota, Dorotea, Doroteya, Dorothea, Dorothée, Dorrit, Dorthea, Dorthy, Dory, Dosha, Dosya, Dot, Dottey, Dottie, Dotty, Tea, Thea

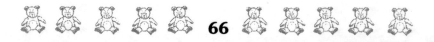

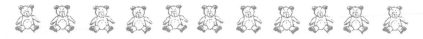

Dorrit Dim. **Dorothy**. Another example of the influence of popular culture on names, as it probably stems from Charles Dickens's novel *Little Dorrit*.
Dorita, Doritt

Dory Fr. "Gilded." Also dim. **Dorothy, Isadora.**

Douce Fr. "Sweet."

Drew Dim. **Andrew**, Gk. "Masculine." More commonly used for boys. When used as a girl's name, it is probably a transferred surname. Actress Drew Barrymore.

Drusilla Lat. Feminine version of a Roman clan name which appears in the New Testament. Very unusual nowadays.
Drewsila, Dru, Drucella, Drucie, Drucilla, Drucy, Druscilla, Drusy

Duana (fem. **Duane**) Ir. Gael. "Swarthy." Dates from the 1940s.
Duna, Dwana

Duena Sp. "Chaperone."

Dulcie Lat. "Sweet." Roman name revived for some years at the turn of the 20th century, but extremely unusual now. Cervantes used a slightly different form when he named the heroine of *Don Quixote* Dulcinea.
Delcina, Delcine, Delsine, Dulce, Dulcea, Dulci, Dulcia, Dulciana, Dulcibella, Dulcibelle, Dulcine, Dulcinea, Dulcy, Dulsea, Dulsia, Dulsiana, Dulsibell, Dulsine

Dusty (fem. **Dustin**) An English place name transferred to first name. Probably popularized in this century by English singer Dusty Springfield.

Dylana (fem. **Dylan**) Welsh. "Born from waves." Use of Dylan tends to be a tribute to the poet Dylan Thomas, and most parents today would not hesitate to use the original, masculine name for a girl.
Dylane

Dympna Ir. Gael. Saint's name of obscure origin. Many cures of epilepsy and other mental disturbances were attributed to her, and she became known as patroness of the insane. A medieval mental hospital in Belgium, in the town where her bones were discovered, is still going strong.
Dymphna

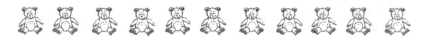

Earla (fem. **Earl**) OE. "Nobleman, leader." Several English aristocratic titles such as Duke, Earl, and Baron have been turned into proper names, a sterling example of wishful thinking. Feminine variants are more uncommon.
Earleen, Earlene, Earley, Earlie, Earline, Erlene, Erlina, Erline

Eartha OE. "Earth." Used by the Puritans in the 17th century, but obsolete since then. Singer Eartha Kitt.
Erda, Ertha, Herta, Hertha

Easter Name of the holiday, transferred to use as a Christian name predominantly in the 19th century. (Some sources trace it to a variation of Esther.) A more common Eastertide name is the French Pascale.

Eberta Teut. "Bright."

Ebony Name of the wood, which is prized for its black color. Popular since the 1970s with black families.
Ebboney, Ebbony, Ebonee, Eboney, Ebonney, Ebonni, Ebonny, Eboni, Ebonie, Ebonyi

Echo Gk. Name of a mythological nymph who was a disembodied voice. One version of her story holds that she pined away of love for Narcissus until only her voice was left.

Eda OE. "Wealthy, happy." Also possibly a variation of Edith.
Ede

Edana (fem. **Aidan**) Gael. Dim. "fire." Saint Aidan was a 7th-century Irish monk.
Aidana, Aydana

Edeline OG. "Noble, nobility." Var. **Adeline**.

Eden Heb. "Pleasure, delight." It is a short step from the Hebrew meaning of the word to its general association with Paradise. The name is used for boys as well as girls.
Eaden, Eadin, Edin

Edina OE. Possibly a form of Edwina, or a literary term meaning "from Edinburgh," the capital city of Scotland.
Edeena, Edyna

Edith OE. "Prosperity/battle." Anglo-Saxon name that continued to be used after the Norman Conquest, and

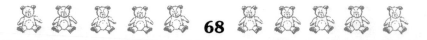

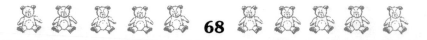

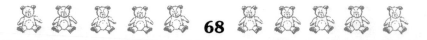

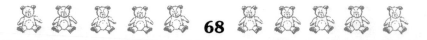

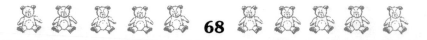

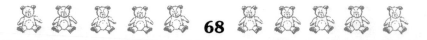

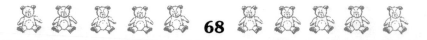

68

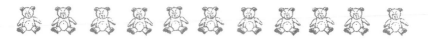

was revived along with other ancient names in the 19th century. By the 1870s it was one of the ten most popular girls' names in Britain, but has been steadily displaced since the 1930s. Writer Edith Wharton; singers Eydie Gorme and Edith Piaf; actress Dame Edith Evans.

Dita, Eadie, Eadith, Eda, Ede, Edi, Edie, Edita, Editha, Edithe, Ediva, Edy, Edyth, Edytha, Edythe, Eidith, Eidyth, Eidytha, Eyde, Eydie, Eydith

Edlyn OE. "Small noble one."

Edmonda (fem. **Edmund**) OE. "Wealthy defender." A popular, and sainted, king of the East Angles in the 9th century gave the masculine version of the name enough popularity to survive the Norman Conquest. The feminine variants are unusual.

Edma, Edmée, Edmonde, Edmunda

Edna Heb. "Pleasure, enjoyment." Perhaps arising from the same root as Eden. First used in the 18th century, but very popular in the last half of the 19th century, especially in America. Now almost unheard-of. Poet Edna St. Vincent Millay; novelist Edna Ferber.

Eddi, Eddie, Eddna, Eddnah, Eddy, Ednah

Edrea OE. "Wealthy, powerful."

Edra, Eidra, Eydra

Edris (fem. **Edric**) Anglo-Saxon. "Wealthy, powerful." The masculine version was an Old English name revived slightly in the 19th century; feminine variants are uncommon.

Edrice, Edriss, Edryce, Eidris, Eidriss, Eydris, Edrys, Idrice, Idris, Idrys

Edwardine (fem. **Edward**) OE. "Wealthy defender." Rare and slightly awkward variant of a steadily well-used masculine name.

Edwarda, Edwardeen, Edwardene, Edwardyne

Edwige Fr. from OG. "Happy battle."

Edvig, Edwig, Hedvig, Hedwig, Hedwige

Edwina (fem. **Edwin**) OE. "Wealth/friend." Feminine variant of an Anglo-Saxon name revived in the 19th century, but never hugely popular.

Edina, Edweena, Edwiena, Edwena, Edwyna

Effie Gk. "Pleasant speech." Short version of Euphemia,

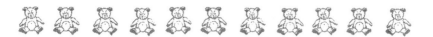

used as an independent name starting in the 1860s. Popularity faded after the 1930s.

Effi, Effy, Ephie, Eppie, Euphemia, Euphemie, Euphie

Egberta (fem. Egbert) OE. "Brilliant sword."

Egbertha, Egbertina, Egbertine, Egbertyna, Ebgertyne

Egidia Latinized feminine form of **Giles**. Gk. "Kid, young goat." Mostly Scottish use.

Eglantine OF. Poetic-sounding botanical name for the shrub also known as "sweetbrier."

Eglantyne

Eibhlin Ir. Gael. "Shining, brilliant." Form of **Evelyn**, the English phonetic version, or **Helen**. More commonly anglicized as Eileen or Aileen.

Aibhlin

Eileen Ir. "Shining, brilliant." Form of **Helen**. Irish names were fashionable in England around 1870, and by the 1920s Eileen was one of the most popular girls' names in Britain. It has never been quite as fashionable in the U.S.

Aileen, Ailene, Alene, Aline, Ayleen, Eilean, Eilleen,
Eiley, Eily, Ileana, Ileanna, Ileene, Ilene, Iliana, Ilianna,
Leana, Lena, Lianna, Lina

Eiluned Welsh. "Idol." Var. **Lynette**.

Eir ONorse. "Peacefulness/mercy."

Eira Welsh. "Snow." Mostly 20th-century use; a pretty name for a winter baby.

Eirian Welsh. "Silver." Another modern Welsh name.

Eithne Ir. "Fire." See **Aithne**, feminine version of **Aidan**.

Aine, Aithnea, Eithne, Ena, Ethnah, Ethnea,
Ethnee

Ekaterina Slavic Var. of **Catherine**. Gk. "pure."

Elaine OF. "Bright, shining, light." Form of **Helen**. In the King Arthur myths, Elaine is a maiden who desperately loves Lancelot. Tennyson's version of the tale has her dying of this love, but in an earlier telling, she actually has a son—Galahad—by Lancelot. Tennyson's poetry may have contributed to the 19th-century revival of the name. Film director Elaine May.

Alaina, Alayna, Alayne, Allaine, Elaina, Elana, Elane,

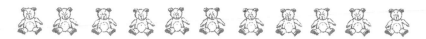

Elanna, Elayne, Ellaina, Ellaine, Ellane, Ellayne, Lainey, Layney

Elata Lat. "Lofty, elevated."

Elberta (fem. **Elbert**) OE. "Highborn/shining." Var. **Alberta**.

Eldora Sp. "Covered with gold."
Eldoree, Eldoria, Eldoris

Eleanor Possibly a form of **Helen** (Gk. "light") or from a different Greek root meaning "clemency, mercy." The queen of Henry II of England, Eleanor of Aquitaine, introduced the name to England in the 13th century, and it has been used steadily since, especially in the U.S., under the influence of much-loved First Lady Eleanor Roosevelt. Charles II's mistress Nell Gwynn; Italian actress Eleonora Duse; women's rights activist Eleanor Smeal.
Aleanor, Alenor, Aleonore, Aline, Eileen, Elaine, Eleanora, Eleanore, Elen, Elena, Elenor, Elenora, Elenore, Eleonora, Eleonore, Elianora, Elianore, Elinor, Elinore, Ella, Elladine, Elleanor, Elleanora, Elle, Ellen, Ellene, Ellenora, Ellenore, Elleonor, Elli, Ellie, Ellin, Ellinor, Ellinore, Elly, Ellyn, Elna, Elnora, Elyn, Enora, Heleanor, Heleonor, Helen, Helena, Helene, Helenora, Leanora, Lena, Lenora, Lenore, Leonora, Leonore, Leora, Lina, Nelda, Nell, Nelle, Nelley, Nelli, Nellie, Nelly, Nonnie, Nora, Norah, Norina

Electra Gk. "Shining, bright." Though the name is derived from the same roots as the word "electricity," most people will associate it with the Greek tragedies of the house of Atreus, told by Aeschylus, Euripides, Sophocles, and retold by Eugene O'Neill in the play *Mourning Becomes Electra*. All versions involve incest, murder, and vengeance.
Elektra

Elfrida OE. "Elf/power." See **Alfreda**. Uncommon.
Elfie, Elfre, Elfredah, Elfredda, Elfreeda, Elfrida, Elfrieda, Elfryda, Elfrydah, Ellfreda, Elva, Elvah, Freda, Freddi, Freddy, Freeda, Frieda, Friedah, Fryda

Elga Slavic. "Sacred." See **Olga**.
Elgiva, Helga

Eliane (fem. **Elias**) Fr. from Heb. "Jehovah is God."
Elia, Eliette, Elice, Eline, Elyette
Elidi Gk. "Gift of the sun."
Elinda Var. **Belinda**.
Eliora Heb. "The Lord is my light."
Eleora, Elleora
Elise Fr. var. **Elizabeth**. Heb. "Pledged to God."
Eliese, Elisa, Elisee, Elize, Elyse, Liese, Liesel, Lieselotte, Liesl, Lise, Lison, Lize
Elisheva Heb. "The Lord is my pledge."
Eliseva, Elisheba
Elissa Form of **Alice** or **Elizabeth**. First appeared around the 1930s.
Alissa, Allissa, Allyssa, Alyssa, Elissia, Ellissa, Elysa, Elyssa, Elyssia, Ilissa, Ilysa, Ilyssa, Lissa, Lissie, Lissy, Lyssa
Elita Lat. "The elect, chosen."
Lita
Eliza Dim. **Elizabeth**. Frequently used in its own right from the 18th century onward. Especially popular in the first decade of this century.
Elizabeth Heb. "Pledged to God." One of the 30 most popular girls' names in the U.S.; in the top 5 in Australia, Canada, and Great Britain. Used in full, it has a pleasant, old-fashioned ring, though some research attaches a "seductive" connotation to it (perhaps by association with actress Elizabeth Taylor). It is a source of endless diminutives and nicknames. Saint Elizabeth, mother of John the Baptist; poet Elizabeth Barrett Browning; Queens Elizabeth I and II of England; actresses Elizabeth Ashley, Elizabeth Montgomery; politician Elizabeth Dole; suffragette Elizabeth Cady Stanton.
Babette, Belita, Bell, Bella, Belle, Bess, Bessie, Bessy, Beth, Betsey, Betsie, Betsy, Bett, Betta, Bette, Betti, Bettina, Bettine, Betty, Bettye, Buffy, Elisa, Elisabet, Elisabeth, Elisabetta, Elise, Elissa, Eliza, Elizabet, Elizabetta, Elizabette, Elle, Elliza, Ellsa, Ellse, Ellsee, Ellsey, Ellsi, Ellspet, Ellyse, Ellyssa, Ellyza, Elsa, Else, Elsee, Elsie, Elspet, Elspeth, Elsy, Elyse, Elyssa, Elyza, Elzbieta, Helsa, Ilsa, Ilse, Isabel, Isabella, Isabelle,

Isobel, Leesa, Leeza, Lib, Libbey, Libbi, Libbie, Libby, Libbye, Lilibet, Lisa, Lisabeth, Lisbet, Lisbeth, Lisbett, Lisbetta, Lisbette, Lise, Lisette, Lissa, Lissi, Lissy, Liz, Liza, Lizabeth, Lizbeth, Lizette, Lizzi, Lizzy, Lusa, Lysa, Lysbet, Lysbeth, Lysbette, Lyssa, Lyssie, Lyza, Lyzbet, Lyzbeth, Lyzbette, Lyzette, Ylisabet, Ylisabette, Ysabel, Ysabella, Yzabelle

Elkana Heb. "God has made." More commonly used by men, and a man's name in the Old Testament.
Elkanah

Elke Ger. var. **Alice**. (OG. "Noble, nobility"). Possibly introduced to the English-speaking world by actress Elke Sommer.
Elka, Ilka

Ella OG. "All, completely." Also possibly derived from **Alice, Eleanor, Ellen**. Common in the Middle Ages and revived in America in the late 19th century, but now unusual. Singer Ella Fitzgerald.
Alla, Ela, Elladine, Elletta, Ellette, Elley, Elli, Ellie, Ellina, Elly

Ellamae Com. form **Ella** and **May**, two very popular 19th-century names.
Ellamay

Ellen Var. **Helen**. Gk. "shining, brightness." Both forms have been popular, but rarely at the same time. In America Ellen has dominated since the 1950s, but neither version is much used now. English actress Ellen Terry; American actresses Ellyn Burstyn, Ellen Barkin.
Elan, Elen, Elena, Elene, Eleni, Elenita, Elenyi, Elin, Ellan, Ellin, Ellene, Ellie, Ellon, Elly, Ellyn, Elon, Elyn

Ellice (fem. **Elias**) Gk. "The Lord is God." Also possibly variant of **Alice** or **Ellis**.
Elice

Elma Short version of names like Wilhelmina (Ger. "Will-helmet") or variant of **Alma** (Lat. "soul").

Elmina Dim. **Wilhelmina**. (OG. "will/helmet"). Mildly popular in the 19th century.
Almeena, Almena, Almina, Elmeena, Elmena

Elmira Arab. "Aristocratic lady." See **Almera**.
Allmera, Allmeera, Almeria, Almira, Almyra, Ellmera,

Ellmeria, Ellmeera, Elmeeria, Elmera, Elmeria, Elmerya, Elmyrah, Mera, Meera, Mira, Mirah, Myra, Myrah

Eloise Fr. form of **Louise**. (OG. "Renowned in battle"). Made famous in the 12th century by the love letters between Heloise and Abelard, but modern parents are more likely to think of the madcap six-year-old denizen of the New York Plaza Hotel made famous by Kay Thompson's book for children.
Aloysia, Eloisa, Elouise, Heloise

Elrica OG. "Ruler over all."

Elsa Dim. **Elizabeth**. Now rare, in spite of the lingering fame of actress Elsa Lanchester.
Else, Elsie, Elsy, Ilsa, Ilse

Elsie Var. **Elizabeth** via its Scottish form, **Elspeth**. Independently used since the 18th century, and extremely popular in the U.S. by the late 19th. After the 1920s, its use faded.
Ellsey, Ellsi, Ellsie, Elsea, Elsee, Elsey, Elsi

Elspeth Scottish var. **Elizabeth**. Unusual outside Scotland. Author Elspeth Huxley.
Elsbeth, Elsbet, Elspet, Elspie

Eluned Welsh. "Idol, image." Used mostly in Wales. The French version, Lynette, is more common in the U.S.
Elined, Eiluned, Lanet, Lanette, Linet, Linette, Luned, Lynette

Elva Ir. Meaning unclear. Phonetic anglicization of the unusual Irish name Ailbhe.
Ailbhe, Elfie, Elvia, Elvie

Elvina (fem. Elvin) OE. "Noble friend" or "elf friend."
Alveena, Alvina, Alvine, Alvinia, Elvena, Elveena, Elvene, Elvenia, Elvine, Elvinia, Vina, Vinni, Vinnie, Vinny

Elvira Sp. Meaning unclear, possibly a place name. An Elvira figures in several versions of the story of Don Juan, as well as other operas. The name seems to be used more in art than in life, however.
Ellvira, Elva, Elveera, Elvera, Elvina, Elvire, Elvyra, Elwira, Lira

Elysia Lat. From "Elysium," the mythical home of the blessed, also known as the "Elysian fields." Dates from the 1940s.

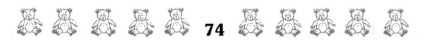

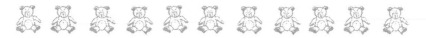

Eleese, Eliese, Elise, Elisia, Elyse, Ileesia, Ilise, Ilysa, Ilysia, Ilyse

Emeline OG. Possibly meaning "industrious." Possibly also a variant of **Emily** or **Amelia**. Norman name revived in the 18th century, now extremely rare despite its numerous variants.

Emaleen, Emalene, Emaline, Emalyn, Embline, Emblyn, Emelen, Emelyn, Emiline, Emlyn, Emmalee, Emmalene, Emmaline, Emmalyn, Emmalynne, Emmeline, Emmiline, Emylin, Emylynn

Emerald Jewel name, less common than Pearl or Ruby, and most frequently used in its Spanish form, Esmeralda. It is the birthstone for May.

Emily Lat. Clan name. In spite of the similarity of form, it has a different root from Amelia. Naturally, many of the variants are very close. A hugely popular name in the 19th century, lost status after 1900, and is now in favor again. Poet Emily Dickinson; novelist Emily Brontë; etiquette maven Emily Post.

Aimil, Amalea, Amalia, Amalie, Amelia, Amelie, Ameline, Amelita, Amy, Eimile, Em, Emalee, Emalia, Emelda, Emelea, Emelia, Emelina, Emeline, Emelita, Emely, Emelyne, Emera, Emila, Emilea, Emilee, Emiley, Emili, Emilia, Emilie, Emiline, Emilla, Emillea, Emilley, Emillie, Emilly, Emlyn, Emlynn, Emlynne, Emmalee, Emmalie, Emmaline, Emmalyn, Emmalynn, Emmalynne, Emmelee, Emmely, Emmey, Emmi, Emmie, Emmilee, Emmilie, Emmily, Emmlee, Emmy, Emmye, Emyle, Emylee, Milka

Emina Lat. "Eminent."

Emma OG. "Embracing everything." Royal name in medieval England, and hugely popular at the end of the 19th century. Brought back to notice by Emma Peel in the popular TV series "The Avengers," and is now one of the top girls' names in England. Still unusual in America, but gaining favor. Lady Emma Hamilton, Lord Nelson's mistress; Emma Bovary of *Madame Bovary*; Jane Austen's novel *Emma*; actress Emma Samms.

Em, Ema, Emelina, Emeline, Emelyne, Emmaline, Emmalyn, Emmalynn, Emmalynne, Emmeline, Emmelyn,

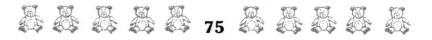

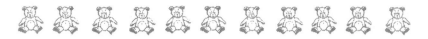

Emmelyne, Emmet, Emmett, Emmette, Emmi, Emmie, Emmot, Emmott, Emmy, Emmye

Emmanuelle (fem. **Emmanuel**) Heb. "God is among us." Fashion designer Emmanuelle Khanh.

Emanuela

Ena Short for names like Georgina, Regina, etc. Queen Victoria's granddaughter Princess Victoria Eugenie, who became queen of Spain, was known as Princess Ena.

Enid Welsh. "Life, spirit." Name from the King Arthur myths revived mildly in the early 19th century and quite popular in England by the 1920s. Never much used in America. Author Enid Bagnold.

Eanid, Enidd, Enyd, Enydd

Enrica (fem. **Henry**) It. "Home ruler."

Erica (fem. **Eric**) Scan. "Ruler forever." Though a staple in Scandinavia, it wasn't used in the English-speaking world until the late 19th century. It still has a strongly European flair. Writer Erica Jong; singer Rickie Lee Jones.

Airica, Airika, Enrica, Enrika, Eraca, Ericka, Erika, Erricka, Errika, Eyrica, Rickee, Ricki, Rickie, Ricky, Rikki, Rikky

Erin Ir. Gael. "From the island to the west." Erin is a literary name for "Ireland," hence the name's popularity among Irish-descended families. Ironically, it is not used in Ireland.

Eire, Eirin, Eirinn, Eiryn, Eirynn, Erina, Erinn, Eryn, Erynn

Erlinda Heb. "Spirited."

Erma Var. Irma. OG. "universal, complete." Enjoyed a brief period of use from around 1890 to 1940; now almost unknown. Humorist Erma Bombeck.

Ermina, Erminia, Erminie, Irma, Irminia, Irminie, Hermia, Hermine, Herminie, Hermione

Ermine OF. "Weasel." Has come to be synonymous with the trappings of royalty, since the robes of royalty are typically trimmed with the fur and tails of ermine, a variety of weasel that turns white in winter.

Ermin, Erminia

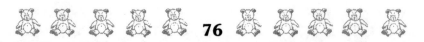

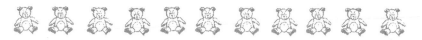

Erna Var. **Ernestine**. Also possibly derived from an Irish root meaning "to know." Modern use.
Ernaline, Ernalynn

Ernestine (fem. **Ernest**) OE. "Sincere." Use at the end of the 19th century follows Ernest's enormous popularity for boys at that period. A bit dated now, and possibly rendered silly by Lily Tomlin's inspired sketches featuring the obstructive telephone operator Ernestine.
Erna, Ernaline, Ernesta, Ernestina, Ernestyna

Erwina (fem. **Erwin**) OE. "Boar/friend."
Irwina

Esma Var. **Esmé**. Possibly short form of Esmeralda.

Esmé Fr. "Esteemed." Originally a male name brought to Scotland by a French cousin of James VI. Now used more for girls, though scarce. J. D. Salinger titled a short story "For Esmé with Love and Squalor."
Esmée

Esmeralda Sp. "Emerald." Jewel name first used in the 1880s, and more common than Emerald.
Em, Emmie, Emerald, Emerant, Emeraude, Esma, Esmaralda, Esmarelda, Esmaria, Esmie, Esmiralda, Esmiralde, Esmirelda, Ezmeralda

Esperanza Sp. "Hope."
Esperance, Esperantia

Esta Var. **Esther**.

Estelle OF. "Star." See **Astra, Esther, Stella**. French form of a name apparently coined by Charles Dickens for a character in his 1861 novel *Great Expectations*. Her name is Estella, and perhaps because she's such an unhappy creature, Estelle is the more common form of the name. Actresses Estelle Getty, Estelle Parsons.
Essie, Estel, Estele, Estell, Estella, Estrella, Estrellita, Stella, Stelle

Esther Per. "Star." More particularly, the planet Venus. Esther in the Bible was an orphan named Hadassah who became wife of King Ahasuerus under her new name. Her story is told in the Old Testament Book of Esther. In the U.S. the name reached its peak of popularity around 1900, and is now unusual. Swimming actress Esther Williams; actress Esther Rolle.

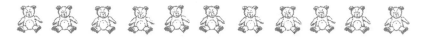

Essie, Essy, Esta, Ester, Ettey, Etti, Ettie, Etty, Hester, Hesther, Hettie, Hetty, Hittie

Etana (fem. **Ethan**) Heb. "Strength of purpose."

Ethel OE. "Noble." A short form of various old-fashioned names like Etheldreda. First appeared on its own in the 1840s, and by the 1870s was very popular. This is one 19th-century name, however, that is unlikely to be revived in the 1990s. Actresses Ethel Barrymore, Ethel Merman.

Ethelda, Ethelin, Ethelinda, Etheline, Ethelyn, Ethelynne, Ethill, Ethille, Ethyll

Etheldreda OE. "Noble power." Saint's name from the 7th century, occasionally used in Britain. Audrey is the more common modern form.

Ethelinda OG. "Noble serpent." Not a composite, but an old name revived in the 19th century, along with many variants.

Athelina, Ethelenda, Ethelene, Ethelind, Ethelinde, Etheline, Etholinda, Ethylind

Etta Feminine diminutive suffix that has attained the status of an independent name.

Ettie, Etty

Eudocia Gk. "Well thought of."

Docie, Doxie, Doxy, Eudosia, Eudoxia

Eudora Gk. "Generous gift." Unusual name from Greek mythology (Eudora was a minor goddess) that was somewhat popular at the turn of the 20th century. Writer Eudora Welty.

Dora, Dorey, Dorie, Eudore

Eugenia (fem. **Eugene**) Gk. "Wellborn." The French form, Eugenie, was made famous by Napoleon III's beautiful empress, and has persisted in the European royal houses. Recently used in Britain for the second daughter of the Duke and Duchess of York, which should bring it to greater prominence. Actresses Gena Rowlands, Geena Davis.

Eugenie, Geena, Gena, Gene, Genia, Genie, Gina, Janie, Jeena, Jenna, Jennie

Eulalia Gk. "Sweet-speaking."

Eula, Eulalee, Eulalie, Eulaylia, Eulaylie, Lallie, Lally

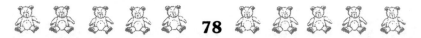

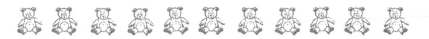

Eunice Gk. "Victorious." Biblical name: In the New Testament, Eunice is the mother of Timothy. Occasionally used in the modern era. Philanthropist Eunice Kennedy Shriver.
Euniss, Unice, Uniss

Euphemia Gk. "Favorable speech." Early Christian name borne by a 4th-century virgin martyr, but more common in its short forms through the 19th century. Rare since the 1930s.
Effam, Effie, Effy, Ephan, Ephie, Eufemia, Euphemie, Euphie, Phemie, Fanny

Eurydice Gk. In mythology, the wife of the musician Orpheus. She was poisoned by a snake, and Orpheus went to the underworld to find her. His music so charmed Hades that he was allowed to bring her back to life, if he could lead her to the upper world without looking at her. He failed, and she returned to Hades.
Euridice

Eustacia (fem. **Eustace**) Lat. "Giving fruit." The male form was used a bit in the 19th century, but the feminine form is rare.
Stacey, Stacia, Stacie, Stacy

Eva Form of **Eve**. Heb. "Life." More common in Europe. Actress Eva Gabor.

Evadne Gk. Meaning unclear, but may mean something like "enjoying good fortune."
Evadney, Evadnie, Evanne

Evangeline Gk. "Good news." Derived from the term that came to be used for the Gospels, or the four Old Testament accounts of Christ's life. First used in English by Alfred Tennyson in his 1847 poem "Evangeline."
Engie, Eva, Evangelia, Evangelina, Evangelista, Evangeliste, Eve, Vangie, Vangy

Evania Gk. "Peaceful."
Evanne, Evannie, Evanny

Eve Heb. "Life." In the form Eva, somewhat popular from the mid–19th century, usually as a shortened version of Evangeline. Eve, the French form of the name, is used steadily but not in great numbers. A clever name for the first girl in a family of boys. Actress Eve Arden.

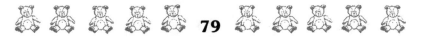

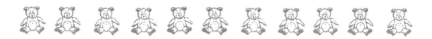

Aoiffe, Eba, Ebba, Eva, Evaleen, Evelina, Eveline, Evelyn, Evetta, Evette, Evey, Evie, Evita, Evlyn, Evonne, Evvie, Evvy, Evy

Evelina OG. or OF., possibly "hazelnut." Norman import to Britain, where it was brought to prominence by Fanny Burney's novel *Evelina*, in the 18th century. Gradually overwhelmed by Evelyn.

Eveleen, Evelene, Eveline, Evelyne

Evelyn OG. Obscure meaning, from the same root as **Evelina**. Not, as it would seem, a combination of Eve and Lynn, but originally a surname and later a boy's name. Its greatest popularity came in the first quarter of the 20th century in both Britain and the U.S.

Aveline, Evaleen, Eveleen, Evelene, Eveline, Evelyne, Evelynn, Evelynne, Evlin, Evline, Evlyn, Evlynn

Evette Fr. Variant form of **Yvette**, in turn a diminutive of **Yvonne**. Also used as a diminutive for **Eve**, though the roots are different.

Evonne Fr. Var. **Yvonne**.

Evon, Eyvonne

F

Fabia (fem. **Fabian**) Lat. clan name. Possibly meaning "one who grows beans."

Fabiana, Fabiane, Fabianna, Fabienne, Fabiola

Fabrizia It. "Works with the hands."

Fabrice, Fabricia, Fabrienne, Fabritzia

Faida Arab. "Plentiful."

Fayda

Faith Middle English. "Loyalty." One of the most common of the virtue names used by the Puritans, along with Hope and Charity. Modern use is sparing.

Fae, Faithe, Fay, Faye, Fayth, Faythe

Faline Lat. "Like a cat." Unusual spelling of a familiar term. Second-time parents may recognize this as the

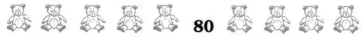

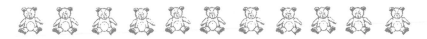

name of Bambi's girlfriend in the Disney cartoon.
Fayline, Felina, Feyline

Fallon Ir. Gael. "Descended from a ruler." Surname brought to public notice and some popularity by a character on the TV serial "Dynasty."

Fanny (dim. **Frances**) Lat. "From France." This form became extremely popular in the early 19th century and remained a favorite until around 1910, when its inexplicable adoption as a term for the buttocks extinguished it as a first name. Cookbook author Fannie Farmer.
Fan, Fannee, Fanney, Fannie

Farica (dim. **Frederica**) OG. "Peaceful ruler."

Farrah Middle English. "Lovely, pleasant." Unknown as a first name until the enormous fame of actress Farrah Fawcett.
Fara, Farah, Farra

Fatima Arab. Meaning unclear, though Fatima was Mohammed's favorite daughter. According to the Koran, she was one of only four perfect women in the world. Fatima is also the name of Bluebeard's last wife in some versions of that tale.
Fatimah, Fatma

Faustine (fem. **Faust**) Lat. "Fortunate, enjoying good luck." Two Roman empresses were called Faustina, and the name was common under the Roman Empire, but little used today.
Fausta, Fauste, Faustina

Fawn OF. "Young deer." Names for girl children have been drawn from various segments of the natural world—flowers, gems, seasons, months—but animal names, for some reason, are rarer.
Faina, Fanya, Faun, Fauna, Faunia, Fawna, Fawne, Fawnia, Fawnya

Fay OF. "Fairy." Dim. **Faith**. First used in significant numbers in the 1920s, probably inspired by the fame of actresses Fay Wray and Fay Compton. Actress Faye Dunaway.
Fae, Fay, Faye, Fee

Fayette OF. "Little fairy."

Fedora Gr. Var. **Theodora**. Gk. "gift of God." In this form,

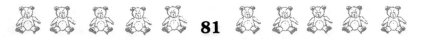

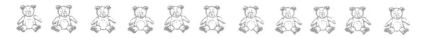

also a kind of soft felt hat with a modest brim, much favored by men until the early 1960s.

Felda OG. "From the field."

Felicia (fem. **Felix**) Lat. "Lucky." Felice was used in Britain until the early 19th century, when it was replaced by Felicia, which has since been supplanted by Felicity. None of them is very common.
Falecia, Falicia, Falisha, Falishia, Felice, Feliciana, Felicidad, Felicie, Felicienne, Felicité, Felicity, Felis, Felise, Felisha, Feliss, Felita, Feliz, Feliza, Felysse

Fenella Ir. Gael. "White shoulder." Var. **Fionnula**. This is the anglicized form.
Finella, Fynella

Fern OE. "Fern." Also, diminutive of **Fernanda**. Unusual botanical name.
Ferne

Fernanda (fem. **Ferdinand**) OG. Possibly "peace/courage" or "voyage/courage." Very rare feminine of an equally rare male name.
Anda, Ferdinanda, Ferdinande, Fern, Fernande, Fernandina, Fernandine, Nan, Nanda

Fernley OE. Place name. "Fern meadow." In Britain, has been used as a first name since the turn of the century for both sexes. Little heard in the U.S.
Fernlee, Fernleigh, Fernly

Fidelity Lat. "Loyalty." Latin form of **Faith**. In the U.S. use of the word for large financial institutions diminishes its appeal as a proper name.
Fidela, Fidele, Fidelia

Fifi Fr. Dim. **Josephine**. Heb. "Jehovah increases." The stereotypical name for a French poodle, which would seem to limit its human use.
Fifine

Filia Gk. "Friendship." Currently popular in Greece.

Filippa Var. **Philippa**. Gk. "Lover of horses."

Filomena It. Var. **Philomena**. Gk. "Loved one."

Fina Sp. Dim. **Josefina**. Heb. "Jehovah increases."

Fiona Ir. Gael. "Fair, pale." Apparently coined by an English author at the turn of the 20th century, and its pop-

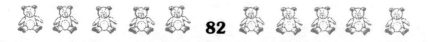

ularity in Britain has been growing since the 1930s, especially in Scotland. Rare in the U.S.

Fionna

Fionnula Ir. Gael. "White shoulder."
Fenella, Finella, Finola, Fionnuala, Nola, Nuala

Flaminia Lat. "Priest."

Flanna Ir. Gael. "Russet hair."

Flavia Lat. "Yellow hair." Originally a Latin clan name, and common enough in the Roman Empire, but never revived in an English-speaking country.
Flavie, Flaviere, Flavyere

Fleur Fr. "Flower." In John Galsworthy's *The Forsyte Saga*, one of the principal characters is called Fleur, which brought the name to some prominence. The BBC TV adaptation of the 1970s also provoked a spate of use.
Fleurette, Fleurine

Flora Lat. "Flower." The name of the Roman goddess of springtime, and of a 9th-century martyred saint. Flora Macdonald is a Scottish heroine who helped Bonnie Prince Charlie escape the English. The name was naturally popular in Scotland, and throughout England in the last half of the 19th century. Now little used.
Fiora, Fiore, Fiori, Fleur, Flo, Flor, Flore, Florella, Florelle, Floria, Florida, Florie, Florine, Floris, Florise, Florrie, Florry

Florence Lat. "In bloom." Used for both men and women until the 17th century, when it faded from sight. Modern use is almost entirely inspired by the fame of Florence Nightingale, who was actually named for the Italian city where she was born. Like many names popular in the Victorian era, it fell out of fashion by the 1930s. Athlete Florence "Flo Jo" Griffith Joyner.
Fiorentina, Fiorenza, Flo, Flor, Flora, Florance, Flore, Florencia, Florentia, Florentina, Florentyna, Florenza, Flori, Floria, Floriane, Floriana, Florie, Florina, Florinda, Florine, Floris, Florrance, Florrie, Florry, Florynce, Floss, Flossey, Flossie, Flossy

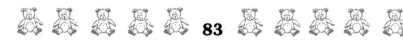

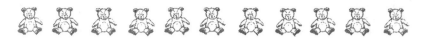

Flower OF. "Blossom."

Florida Lat. "Flowery." Spanish variant of **Florence**. Spanish explorer Ponce de Leon dubbed the southern state "Florida" for the many flowers he found there. Infrequent current use as a first name probably refers to the state.

Fortune Lat. "Good fate." Garden-variety name in the Roman Empire, revived somewhat by the Puritans but almost unknown today.
Fortuna, Fortunata

Fran (dim. **Frances**) Lat. "From France." Used as a given name on its own.
Frani, Frannee, Franni, Frannie, Franny

Frances (fem. **Francis**) Lat. "From France." Until the 17th century, Francis was used for both sexes. Spelled with an *e*, it was a very popular choice in the first quarter of the 20th century, but little used since then. Writer Fran Lebowitz, actress Fanny Brice.
Fan, Fancey, Fanchette, Fancie, Fancy, Fanechka, Fania, Fanney, Fannie, Fanny, Fanya, Fran, Francee, Franceline, Francene, Francesca, Francetta, Francette, Francey, Franchesca, Franci, Francie, Francine, Francisca, Franciska, Françoise, Francyne, Frank, Frankie, Franky, Franni, Frannie, Franny, Franzetta, Franzi, Franziska

Freda OG. "Peaceful." Dim. **Alfreda, Frederica, Winifred**. Most popular at the end of the 19th century, when Fred was fashionable for men. Artist Frida Kahloo.
Freada, Freeda, Freida, Frida, Frieda, Frydda

Fredella Com. form **Freda** and **Ella**.
Fredelle

Frederica OG. "Peaceful ruler." Following the popularity of Frederic, substantially used in the late 19th century, but now unusual. Opera singer Frederica von Stade.
Farica, Federica, Fred, Fredalena, Freddee, Freddey, Freddi, Freddie, Freddy, Fredericka, Frederickina, Frederine, Frederique, Fredi, Fredia, Fredie, Fredricia, Fredrika, Frerika, Friederike, Rica, Ricki, Rickie, Ricky, Rikki, Rikky

Freya Scan. "Highborn lady." In Norse myth, the goddess

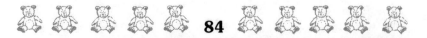

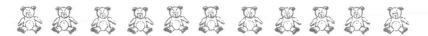

of love, corresponding perhaps to the Roman Venus. Friday is named for her.

Fraya

Fritzi (fem. **Fritz**) OG. "Peaceful ruler." German form of Frederick.

Fulvia Lat. "Blond one."

Gabrielle (fem. **Gabriel**) Heb. "Heroine of God." Used in English-speaking countries for the last 90 years, though the Italian form, Gabriella, has been popular since the 1950s. Gabriel is an archangel who appears in Christian, Jewish, and Muslim texts. Tennis star Gabriela Sabatini; fashion designer Gabrielle "Coco" Chanel.

Gabbe, Gabbi, Gabbie, Gabi, Gabriel, Gabriela, Gabriell, Gabriellia, Gabrila, Gabryel, Gabryelle, Gabryella, Gaby, Gavra, Gavrielle

Gada Heb. "Fortunate."

Gaea Gk. "The earth."

Gaia, Gaiea, Gala

Gaetana It. Place name. Gaeta is a region in southern Italy; the Gulf of Gaeta is just north of Naples.

Gaetane

Gail Heb. "My father rejoices." A diminutive of Abigail with an unusually strong life of its own, dating from around 1940, with special popularity in the 1950s in the U.S.

Gael, Gahl, Gaila, Gaile, Gaill, Gale, Gayel, Gayelle, Gayle, Gayleen, Gaylene, Gayline, Gayll, Gaylle

Galatea Gk. "White as milk." In Greek myth the sculptor Pygmalion fell in love with his ivory statue of Aphrodite, and prayed to the goddess to bring the statue to life. When his prayer was answered, he married his creation. The myth, via G. B. Shaw's play *Pygmalion*, is the source of the musical *My Fair Lady*.

Galatée

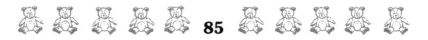

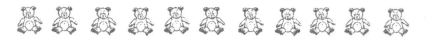

Galiena OG. "High one."
Galiana, Galianna

Galina Rus. Var. **Helen**. Gk. "Shining brightly."
Galya

Gallia Lat. "Gaul." The Latin term for the country that would later be known as France; a name used from time to time for French babies.
Gala, Galla

Galya Heb. "The Lord has redeemed."
Galia, Gallia, Gallya

Gardenia Flower name. The powerfully sweet-smelling flower is named for the 18th-century Scottish naturalist Alexander Garden, who first classified it.

Garland OF. "Garland, wreath."
Garlande

Garnet Middle English. Jewel name, appropriate for January, since it is the birthstone for that month.
Garnette

Gavrila Var. **Gabrielle**. Heb. "Heroine of God."
Gavrilla, Gavryla, Gavrylla

Gay OF. "Glad, lighthearted." A surname in the Middle Ages, used as a first name very heavily in the mid–20th century. The widespread informal use of the word to mean "homosexual" has limited its current use as a name.
Gae, Gai, Gaye

Gaynor Welsh. Var. **Guinevere**. Used primarily in Britain.
Gaenor, Gayna, Gayner

Gazella Lat. "Gazelle." Unusual use of the animal name as a given name. Gazelles are traditionally thought of as very graceful creatures.
Gazelle

Gemini Gk. "Twin." Appropriate for either a child born under the sign of Gemini, or for one of a pair of twins.
Gemella, Gemelle, Gemina

Gemma It. "Precious stone." Did not, curiously, come into fashion with other jewel names in the late 19th century, but is popular now. Probably helped along by the 1940 canonization of an Italian Saint Gemma, an ordinary young woman whose religious life included manifesta-

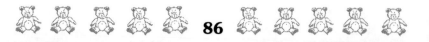

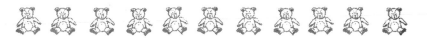

tions of the stigmata, or the marks of Christ's wounds.
Jemma

Gene Dim. **Eugenia** Gk. "wellborn" or var. **Jean**. (Heb. "the Lord is gracious") More common for boys; actress Gene Tierney may have pioneered use of this spelling for girls.
Genie

Geneva OF. "Juniper tree." There is considerable confusion about the sources of a constellation of names that include Geneva, Ginevra, and Genevieve. Use of Geneva may refer to the Swiss city; on the other hand, it may also be reference to the juniper tree, whose old Dutch name was *genever* (hence "gin," which is flavored with juniper berries). Various forms of Genevieve also overlap.
Gena, Genever, Genevra, Genevre, Genoveva, Ginebra, Ginevra, Ginevre, Janeva, Janevra

Genevieve A name whose origin is unclear, but sources suggest possibly OG. "white wave" or Celt. "race of women." Saint Genevieve, the patroness of Paris, was a 5th-century virgin who defended Paris against the depredations of Attila the Hun, among others. Use in English-speaking countries has tended to simmer along at a low level. Actress Genevieve Bujold.
Gena, Genavieve, Geneva, Geneveeve, Genivieve, Gennie, Genny, Genovera, Genoveva, Gina, Janeva, Jenevieve, Jennie, Jenny

Georgette Fr. from Lat. "Farmer." The French form of George, in mild use since the 1940s. A purposely wrinkled fabric called georgette was named after its French creator. Author Georgette Heyer.
Georgetta

Georgia (fem. **George**) Lat. "Farmer." The preferred feminine of George in the U.S. A farmer in Connecticut is reputed to have named each of his ten daughters for a state, and presumably Georgia was one of the eldest, along with Virginia and Carolina. Painter Georgia O'Keefe.
George, Georgeann, Georgeanne, Georgeina, Georgena, Georgene, Georgetta, Georgette, Georgiana, Georgianna, Georgianne, Georgie, Georgienne,

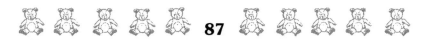

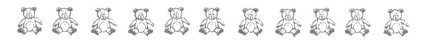

Georgina, Georgine, Georgyann, Georgyanne,
Georgyana, Giorgia, Giorgina, Giorgyna, Jorgina
Georgina (fem. **George**) Lat. "farmer." The form cur-
rently most common in England, replacing Georgiana,
which has also been much used.
Georgeina, Georgena, Georgene, Georgiana,
Georgianna, Georgianne, Georgienne, Georgine,
Georgyana, Giorgina
Geraldine (fem. **Gerald**) OG./Fr. "Spear ruler." Though
the form was coined in the 16th century, its real popu-
larity followed the fashion for Gerald, in the mid–19th
century through the 1950s. Actress Geraldine Chaplin;
politician Geraldine Ferraro.
Deena, Dina, Dyna, Geralda, Geraldeen, Geraldene,
Geraldina, Geralyn, Geralynne, Geri, Gerianna,
Gerianne, Gerilynn, Gerri, Gerrilyn, Gerroldine, Gerry,
Giralda, Jeraldeen, Jeraldene, Jeraldine, Jeralee, Jere,
Jeri, Jerilene, Jerrie, Jerrileen, Jerroldeen, Jerry
Geranium Flower name, though the name of the flower
itself derives from the Greek for "crane."
Gerda ONorse. "Shelter."
Garda
Germaine Fr. "From Germany." Use today is likely to re-
flect admiration for the famous author and feminist Ger-
maine Greer.
Germain, Germana, Germane, Germayn, Germayne,
Jermain, Jermaine, Jermane, Jermayn, Jermayne
Gertrude OG. "Strength of a spear." An old name (there
was a 7th-century Saint Gertrude) revived to immense
popularity with the late 19th-century fashion for the an-
tique. Became so common that it suffered the corre-
sponding fall from favor, and is now resoundingly out
of style. Writer Gertrude Stein; actress Gertrude
Lawrence.
Geltruda, Gerda, Gert, Gerta, Gerte, Gerti, Gertie,
Gertina, Gertraud, Gertrud, Gertruda, Gerty, Traudl,
Trude, Trudi, Trudie, Trudy
Ghaliya Arab. "Sweet-smelling."
Ghislaine Fr. Unusual name of unclear origin and mean-
ing.

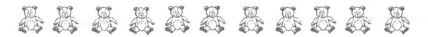

Ghita It. Dim. **Margherita**. Gk. "Pearl."

Giacinta It. "Hyacinth."
Jacinta

Gianina (fem. **John**) It. from Heb. "God is gracious." The age-old favorite boy's name has spawned endless variants, both masculine and feminine.
Gianetta, Giannina, Giannine, Ginetta, Ginette, Ginnette, Janine, Jeannine

Gilberte (fem. **Gilbert**) OG. "Shining pledge." French variant of a Norman name that was fairly popular in the north of Britain.
Berta, Bertie, Berty, Gigi, Gilberta, Gilbertina, Gilbertine, Gill, Gillie, Gilly

Gilda OE. "Gilded." More scholarly sources trace Gilda to Ermengilda, a now obsolete Anglo-Saxon name. Actress Gilda Radner.

Gillian Lat. "Youthful." Anglicization of **Juliana**. A standard name in the Middle Ages in England, and revived for about 40 years in this century, but fading since the sixties. Never widespread in the U.S., though its diminutive, Jill, had quite a fashionable spell.
Gilian, Gill, Gillan, Gillianne, Gillie, Gillyanne, Jillian, Jillianne, Jillyan

Gina Dim. **Regina, Angelina**, etc. Also could be considered a feminization of **Gene**, or a variant of **Jean**. Independent use dates from the 1920s, concentrated in the 1950s. Actresses Gina Lollobrigida, Geena Davis, Gena Rowlands.
Geena, Geina, Gena, Ginna, Jena, Jeena

Ginger Lat. "Ginger." Also can be a diminutive of **Virginia**. (Lat. "Virgin") Not to be confused with the usual botanical names, for it depends almost completely on the fame of actress Ginger Rogers, whose given name was Virginia.
Gingie

Ginny Dim. **Virginia**. (Lat. "Virgin").

Giovanna (fem. **John**) It. from Heb. "God is gracious."

Giselle OG. "Pledge/hostage." Use may reflect a fondness for the famous 19th-century ballet in which the heroine is a peasant girl betrayed by a noble suitor.

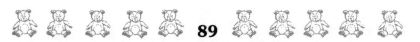

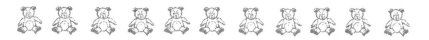

Ghisele, Ghisella, Gisela, Gisele, Gisella, Giza, Gizela, Gizella

Gitana Sp. "Gypsy."
Gitane, Gitanna

Gitta Dim. **Brigitte**. Ir. Gael. "Strength, power."
Gitte

Giulia (fem. **Giulio**) It. from Lat. "Youthful."
Giula, Giuliana, Giulietta, Julia, Juliana, Julie, Juliet, Julietta, Juliette

Giuseppina (fem. **Giuseppe**) It. from Heb. "The Lord adds."
Josefina

Giustinia (fem. **Justin**) It. from Lat. "Just, fair."
Giustina

Gladys Welsh. Var. **Claudia**. Lat. "Lame." Suddenly glamorous in the late 19th century, and used in several Edwardian romantic novels, which further heightened its appeal. By the 1930s, beginning to be dated, and now rare. Singer Gladys Knight.
Glad, Gladdis, Gladdys, Gladi, Gladyss, Gwladys, Gwyladyss

Glenda Welsh. "Fair and good." Mildly popular from the 1930s to the 1960s. Actress Glenda Jackson.

Glenna (fem. **Glenn**) Ir. Gael. "Glen." A glen is a narrow valley between hills. Actress Glenn Close.
Glenda, Gleneen, Glenene, Glenine, Glen, Glenn, Glenne, Glennene, Glennie

Glenys Welsh. "Holy."
Glenice, Glenis, Glennice, Glennis, Glennys

Gloria Lat. "Glory." Apparently coined by playwright George Bernard Shaw, in 1898's *You Never Can Tell*; the form Gloriana had earlier been used to refer in flattering fashion to Queen Elizabeth I. The exposure given the name by actress Gloria Swanson was probably crucial to its popularity from the 1920s through the 1960s. Now a bit passé. Writer Gloria Steinem.
Gloree, Glori, Glorie, Gloriana, Gloriane, Glorie, Glorria, Glory

Glynis Welsh. "Small glen." Related to **Glenn** and its vari-

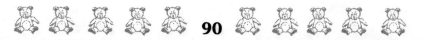

ants. Popular in the middle of the 20th century, but mostly in Britain. Actress Glynis Johns.

Glinnis, Glinyce, Glinys, Glinyss, Glynnis

Godiva OE. "God's gift." The famous story runs that in the 11th century Lady Godiva rode through the town of Coventry naked, covered only by her long hair. Her motive (generally forgotten) was a pact with her husband, the Earl of Mercia, who relieved the townsfolk of certain taxes after her ride.

Golda OE. "Gold." Use is generally tribute to the late Israeli Prime Minister Golda Meir. Actress Goldie Hawn.

Goldarina, Goldarine, Goldi, Goldie, Goldina, Goldy, Goldia

Grace Lat. "Grace." Originally had nothing to do with physical grace, but rather with divine favor and mercy. Used in that sense by the Puritans, and taken to America, where it was very fashionable at the turn of the century. Periods of popularity followed in England (in the twenties) and Scotland (through the fifties). Little used now, but ripe for revival. Actress and princess Grace Kelly; singer Grace Jones.

Engracia, Gracee, Gracey, Gracia, Graciana, Gracie, Grata, Gratia, Gratiana, Grayce, Grazia, Graziella, Graziosa, Grazyna

Grainne Ir. Gael. "Love." Popular in Ireland.

Grainnia, Grania

Greer Scot. Dim. **Gregory**. Lat. "Alert, watchful." Given fame by actress Greer Garson, whose mother's maiden name it was.

Grier

Gregoria (fem. **Gregory**) Lat. "Alert, watchful."

Greta Ger. Dim. **Margaret**. Gk. "Pearl." Most used during the 1930s, clearly inspired by Greta Garbo.

Greeta, Gretal, Gretchen, Grete, Gretel, Grethel, Gretna, Gretta, Grette, Grietje, Gryta

Gretchen Ger. Dim. **Margaret**. Gk. "Pearl." Used on its own in English-speaking countries in this century.

Griselda OG. "Gray fighting maid." In a famous tale told by both Boccaccio and Chaucer, "Patient Griselda" is a meek wife who submits to numerous trials devised by

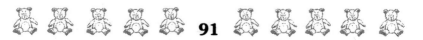

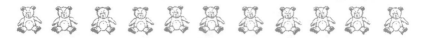

her husband. The name has long since been eclipsed by
its short form, Zelda.

**Chriselda, Griseldis, Grishelda, Grishilde, Grissel, Grizel,
Grizelda, Gryselde, Gryzelde, Selda, Zelda**

Gudrun Scan. "Battle."

Gudren, Gudrin, Gudrinn, Gudruna

Guida It. "Guide."

Guinevere Welsh. "White and smooth, soft." The name of
King Arthur's ill-fated queen. The most common form
today is Jennifer.

**Gaenna, Gaynor, Genevieve, Genna, Gennie, Gennifer,
Genny, Ginevra, Guenever, Guenevere, Gueniveer,
Guenna, Guennola, Guinever, Guinna,
Gwen, Gweniver, Gwenn, Gwennie, Gwennola,
Gwennora, Gwennore, Gwenny, Gwenora, Gwenore,
Gwyn, Gwynn, Gwynna, Gwynne, Janifer, Jen, Jeni,
Jenifer, Jennee, Jenni, Jennie, Jennifer, Jenny, Wendee,
Wendie, Wendy, Win, Winne, Winnie, Winny**

Gulielma (fem. **Wilhelm**) It. from OG. "will-helmet."

Gunhilda ONorse. "Battle-maid."

Gunhilde, Gunilda, Gunilla, Gunnhilda

Gustava (fem. **Gustav**) Swed. "Staff of the gods."

Gustha

Gwenda Welsh. "Fair and good." Rare since the 1960s,
even in Wales.

Gwendolyn Welsh. "Fair bow." In some legends, Merlin
the magician has a wife named Gwendolyn. The old
Welsh name was revived in the late 19th century, and is
now rare, though its diminutive, Wendy, lingers on.

**Guendolen, Guenna, Gwen, Gwenda, Gwendaline,
Gwendolen, Gwendolene, Gwendolin, Gwendoline,
Gwendolynne, Gwenna, Gwenette, Gwenndolen, Gwenni,
Gwennie, Gwenny, Gwenyth, Gwyn, Gwyneth, Gwynn,
Gwynna, Gwynne, Wendi, Wendie, Wendy, Win, Winne,
Wynne**

Gwladys Welsh. Var. **Gladys.**

Gwyneth Welsh. "Happiness." Most popular in Wales
and Britain in the 1930s and 1940s, but never a strong
name in America.

Gweneth, Gwenith, Gwenyth, Gwineth, Gwinyth,

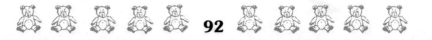

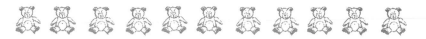

Gwynith, Gwynna, Gwynne, Gwynneth, Winnie, Winny, Wynne, Wynnie

Gwynn Welsh. "Fair, blessed." Also dim. **Gwendolyn** or **Gwyneth**.

Gwynne

Gypsy OE. The tribe of Romany was originally called "gypsy" because it was thought that they had originated in Egypt. Use of the name, as in the case of Gypsy Rose Lee, is more often as a nickname.

Gipsy

Habibah Arab. "loved one."

Hadria Lat. Place name. "From Adria." Var. **Adrian**.

Hadria, Hadrianna, Hadrien, Hadrienne

Hagar Heb. "Forsaken." In the Old Testament, Hagar is the handmaid of Abraham's wife, who is sent away when she becomes pregnant by Abraham. Though the Puritans tended to scour the Old Testament for feminine names, this was not one they popularized, and its sparing use has dwindled further since early in the 20th century.

Haggar

Haidée Gk. "Modest." The name was brought to public knowledge by Byron, who used it in his poem "Don Juan." It has never really caught on.

Halcyone Gk. "Kingfisher." In ancient myth, the kingfisher laid its eggs on the sea, and they lay on the water for the two weeks preceding the winter solstice. During this time the waves were always calm, hence the expression "halcyon days" to mean a time of tranquil happiness.

Haldana ONorse. "Half-Danish." The name takes on a certain significance when you consider that in ancient Britain, the Danes were fierce and frequent invaders.

Haldane

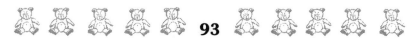

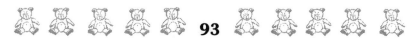

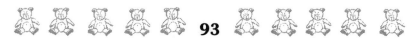

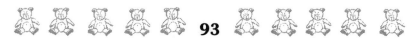

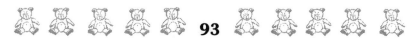

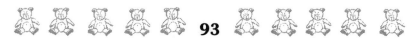

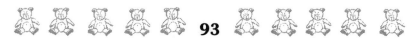

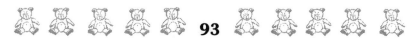

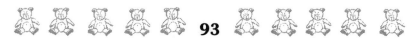

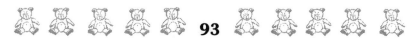

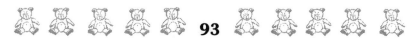

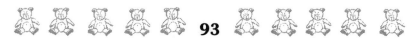

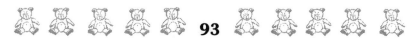

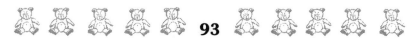

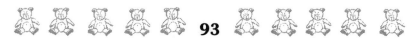

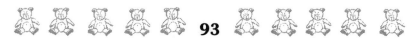

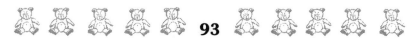

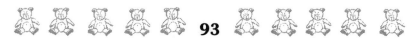

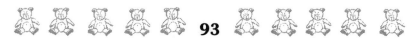

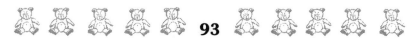

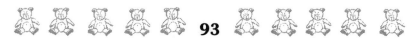

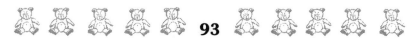

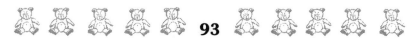

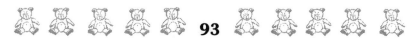

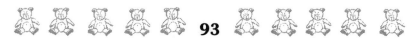

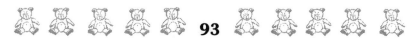

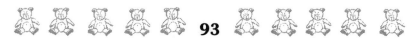

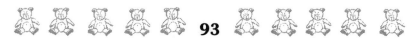

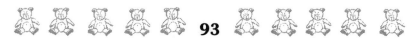

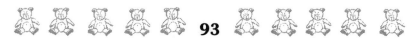

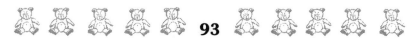

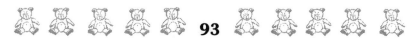

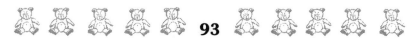

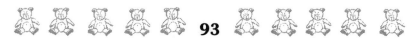

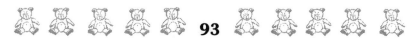

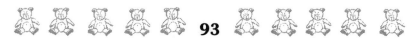

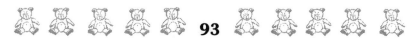

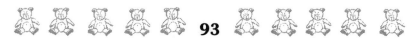

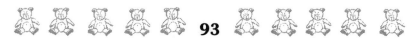

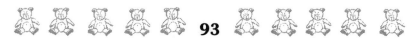

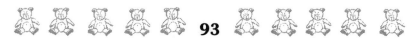

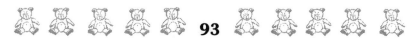

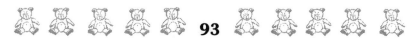

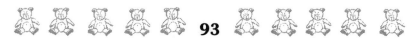

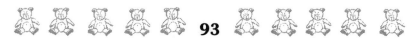

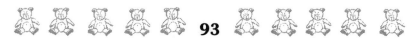

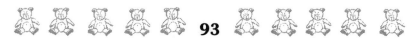

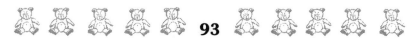

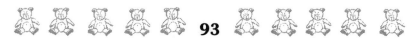

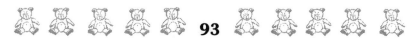

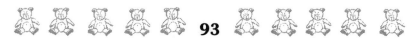

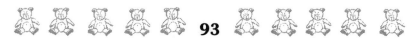

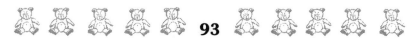

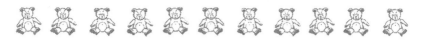

Halfrida OG. "Peaceful heroine" or "peaceful home."

Halimah Arab. "Gentle, soft-spoken."

Halimeda Gk. "Thinking of the sea."
Halette, Hali, Hallie, Meda, Medie

Hana Jap. "Flower." Fashion designer Hanae Mori.
Hanae, Hanako

Hannah Heb. "Grace." In the Old Testament **Hannah** is the mother of the prophet Samuel. The name was steadily popular from around 1600 through the 19th century, peaking around 1800. It is now emerging from disuse, though the European forms of the name—Ann, Anne, Anna, etc.—remain far more common.
Ann, Anna, Anne, Annie, Hana, Hanna, Hanne, Hannele, Hannelore, Hannie, Hanny, Honna, Nan, Nanney, Nannie, Nanny

Happy Eng. "Cheerful, lighthearted." Though it was common enough in the 19th century, Felicity or Hilary are now more likely to be used, though Happy occurs as a nickname.

Haralda ONorse. "Army ruler" or "army power." This form was coined during the great 19th-century popularity of Harold, but (as with many feminine variants, like Arthuretta) never really caught on.
Halley, Hallie, Hally, Haroldene

Harley OE. Place name. "The long field." Familiar to most people as half of the name of a great motorcycle, the Harley-Davidson.
Arlea, Arlee, Arleigh, Arley, Harlea, Harlee, Harleigh, Harly

Harmony Lat. "Harmony."
Harmonia, Harmonie

Harriet (fem. **Henry**) OG. "Ruler of the home or estate." An informal version of Henrietta, very popular in the 18th and 19th centuries, and after nearly 100 years of obscurity, ready for a revival. Many people may think of the children's book *Harriet the Spy*. Author Harriet Beecher Stowe.
Harrie, Harrietta, Harriett, Harrietta, Harriette, Harriot, Harriott, Hatsie, Hatsy, Hattie, Hatty

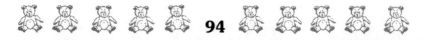

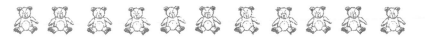

Hayfa Arab. "Slender, well-shaped."
Haifa

Hayley OE. Place name. "Hay meadow." Made famous by actress Hayley Mills.
Hailea, Hailee, Haileigh, Haily, Haleigh, Halie, Hally, Haylea, Haylee, Hayleigh, Hayley

Hazel OE. Tree name. The late–19th-century vogue for botanical names tended to concentrate on flowers rather than trees; Hazel is an exception.
Hazal, Hazell, Hazelle

Heather Middle English. Flower name. Introduced with other botanical names in the late 19th century, but really took off in the late 20th century, especially in the U.S., where its association with Scotland may lend it an upper-class aura.

Hebe Gk. "Youth." In Greek legend, Hebe was the goddess of youth and also cupbearer to the gods. Her name was used mostly in the late 19th century.

Hedda OG. "Warfare." The more common anglicized version of **Hedwig**. Mid–20th-century gossip queen Hedda Hopper.
Heda, Heddi, Heddie, Hedi, Hedvig, Hedvige, Hedwig, Hedwiga, Hedy, Hetta

Hedwig OG. "Warfare, struggle, strife." Almost unknown in English-speaking countries. Actress Hedy Lamarr (née Hedwig Kiesler).
Hadvig, Hadwig, Hedvig, Hedviga, Hedvige, Hedwiga, Hedwige, Hedy

Hedy Gk. "Delightful, sweet."
Hedia Hedyla

Heidi Dim. var. **Adelaide**. OG. "Noble, nobility." Made popular by Johanna Spyri's famous novel of 1881, first in German-speaking countries, later in the U.S. Its surge of popularity in the 1970s may have been influenced by a highly publicized TV production of the late 1960s.
Heida

Helen Gk. "Light." The most famous Helen is probably Helen of Troy, the daughter of Zeus by Leda. Her beauty was, in some versions, the root cause of the Trojan War; hers was "the face that launched a thousand ships." The

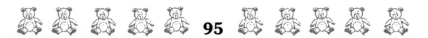

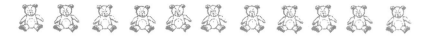

name has been understandably popular through the ages, and has spawned many variants, of which Ellen is the most popular. Writer Helen Keller; actress Helen Hayes; publisher Helen Gurley Brown; singer Helen Reddy.

Aileen, Ailene, Aleanor, Alene, Aline, Eileen, Elaina, Elaine, Elana, Elayne, Eleanor, Eleanore, Elena, Eleni, Elenora, Elenore, Eleonora, Elianora, Elinor, Ella, Elladine, Elleanora, Elle, Ellee, Ellen, Ellenora, Ellette, Ellie, Ellin, Elliner, Ellinor, Elly, Ellyn, Galina, Halina, Heleanor, Helenore, Helena, Hélène, Hellen, Hellena, Hellene, Hellenor, Ileana, Ilene, Ilona, Jelena, Lana, Leanora, Lena, Lenore, Leonora, Leonore, Leora, Lienor, Lina, Nelda, Nell, Nellette, Nelliana, Nellie, Nelly, Nonnie, Nora, Yelena

Helga OG. "Holy, sacred." Var. **Olga**.

Helice Gk. "Spiral." An unusual name that comes from the same Greek root as helix, or double helix, the shape of the DNA molecule.

Helike

Helma OG. "Helmet." See **Wilhelmina**.

Hillma, Hilma

Heloise Fr. Var. **Louise**. OG. "Renowned in war." The 12th-century French philosopher Pierre Abelard fell in love with and seduced his student Heloise. Her uncle and guardian had him emasculated, even though he married Heloise. She became a nun, he a monk.

Aloysia, Eloisa, Eloise, Heloisa, Lois

Helsa Dan. Var. **Elizabeth**. Heb. "Consecrated to God."

Henrietta (fem. Henry) OG. "Ruler of the house." More formal version of Harriet briefly popular at the turn of the century.

Enrichetta, Enrichette, Enriqueta, Etta, Ettie, Etty, Hatsie, Hatsy, Hattie, Hatty, Hendrika, Henia, Henie, Henka, Hennie, Henrie, Henrieta, Henriette, Henrika, Henryetta, Hetti, Hettie, Yetta, Yettie

Hepzibah Heb. "My delight is in her." Old Testament name widely used by the Puritans, but by the 20th century it had almost died out, in part because of its lack of euphony.

Eppie, Hepsie, Hepsibah, Hephzibah

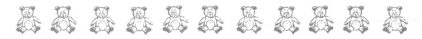

Hera Gk. "Queen." In Greek myth, Hera was the wife (and sister) of Zeus, ruler of the gods. She is usually portrayed as a jealous woman who persecutes her husband's mistresses.

Hermione Gk. "Earthly." Very rare. Actress Hermione Gingold.
Erma, Hermia, Hermina, Hermine, Herminia

Hermosa Sp. "Beautiful."

Hertha OE. "Earth." The name of the German or Scandinavian Earth Mother.
Eartha, Erda, Ertha, Herta

Hesper Gk. "Evening or evening star." The Greeks referred to Italy as Hesperia, since the sun set and the evening star rose there.
Hespera, Hesperia

Hester Gk. "Star." Var. **Esther**. The most famous Hester is probably the adulteress in Hawthorne's *The Scarlet Letter*, Hester Prynne.
Hesther, Hestia, Hettie, Hetty

Hibernia Lat. Place name for Ireland.

Hibiscus Lat. Botanical name for the plant colloquially known as the marsh mallow.

Hilary Gk. "Cheerful, happy." The name comes from the same root as the word "hilarious." There were a 4th-century saint and a 5th-century pope named Hilary, and the name was used for boys until the 17th century. The late–19th-century revival, though, made it generally a girl's name, which was especially fashionable in the 1950s.
Hilaria, Hilarie, Hillary, Hillery, Hilliary

Hilda OG. "Battle woman." One of the Valkyrie of Teutonic legend was named Hilda. A medieval name with a Victorian revival that lasted through the 1930s. Now unusual.
Hilde, Hildie, Hildy

Hildegarde OG. "Battle stronghold." Rare in English-speaking countries.
Helle, Hilda, Hildagard, Hildagarde, Hilde, Hildegard, Hildegaard, Hildegunn, Hille

Hildemar OG. "Battle-renowned."

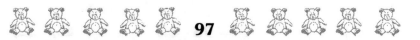

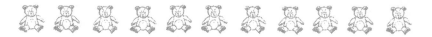

Hildreth OG. "Battle counselor." Briefly used at the turn of the 20th century in Britain.
   Hildred
Hilma Dim. **Wilhelmina.** OG. "Will-helmet."
   Halma, Helma
Hinda Heb. "Doe, female deer."
   Hynda
Hippolyta Gk. Meaning not entirely clear, but alludes to horses. Very unusual.
Holda OG. "Hidden."
   Holde, Holle, Hulda
Hollis OE. Place name. "Near the holly bushes." The usual transference of a masculine to a feminine name may be accelerated in this case because Hollis sounds like Holly.
Holly OE. Botanical name. First used at the turn of the 20th century and newly popular in the 1960s. Obviously a seasonal favorite most intensively used in December.
   Holley, Hollie
Honey OE. The word used as a name. May be as a diminutive of **Honora,** but is more likely to be a transference of the endearment.
Honora Lat. "Woman of honor." As Honour, used by the Puritans (along with other abstract concepts like Constance). Honoria was more common in the 18th century. No version of the name is widely used now.
   Honor, Honorah, Honorata, Honoria, Honorine, Honour, Nora, Norah, Norine, Norry
Hope OE. "Hope." One of the three cardinal virtues, along with Faith and Charity, and probably the one that has survived best, particularly in the U.S.
Horatia Lat. Clan name, possibly meaning "timekeeper." The name was coined by the 18th-century admiral Lord Horatio Nelson, for his daughter.
   Horacia
Hortense Lat. Clan name. A related word means "of the garden." Hortensia is the French term for the hydrangea shrub.
   Hortensia, Hortenspa, Ortensia
Huberta (fem. **Hubert**) OG. "Brilliant mind."

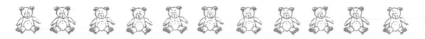

Huette (fem. **Hugh**) OG. "Mind, intellect." A feminization of a name that has never had a particular vogue.
Huetta, Hugette, Hughette, Hughina

Hulda OG. "Loved one." Or Heb. "mole." Very unusual, in Scandinavian or English-speaking countries.
Huldah, Huldie

Hyacinth Gk. Flower name. There was a 3rd-century saint of this name, which was used for boys as well as girls. In Greek legend, Apollo loved a beautiful youth of the name; the hyacinth flower sprang up from his blood when he died.
Cinthia, Cinthie, Cinthy, Giacinta, Giacintia, Hyacintha, Hyacinthe, Hyacinthia, Hyacinthie, Hyacintia, Jacenta, Jacinda, Jacinta, Jacintha, Jackie, Jacky, Jacynth

Hypatia Gk. "Highest."

Iantha Gk. "Purple flower." Popular in the later 19th century, possibly influenced by Romantic poets earlier in the century.
Ianthe, Ianthia, Ianthina, Janthia

Ida Meaning unclear: possibly OE. "prosperous, happy" or OG. "hardworking." Very fashionable at the turn of the 20th century in America, but little used in modern times.
Idaleen, Idalene, Idalia, Idalina, Idaline, Idalya, Idalyne, Ide, Idell, Idella, Idelle, Idetta, Idette

Idina Var. **Edina**. OE. "from Edinburgh, Scotland."

Iduna ONorse. "Loving one."
Idonia, Idunna

Ieesha Var. **Aisha**. Arab. "woman"; Swahili. "life."
Ieasha, Ieashia, Ieashiah

Ignacia (fem. **Ignatius**) Meaning unclear, though some sources suggest Lat. "ardent, burning."
Ignatia, Ignazia, Iniga

Ila OF. Place name. "Island."

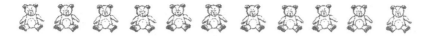

Ilana Heb. "Tree."
Elana, Ilanit

Ilene Modern variant of **Aileen**. Gk. "Light."
Ilean, Ileen, Ileene, Ilene

Iliana Gk. "Trojan." The poetic name for the ancient city of Troy was "Ilion." Ileana has been used by the Greek royal family.
Ileana, Ileane, Ileanne, Illia

Ilka Slavic. "Flattering, hardworking." Writer Ilka Chase.
Ilke, Milka

Ilona Hung. Var. **Helen**. Gk. "Light." Also carries the connotation of "beautiful," no doubt because of the legendary beauty of Helen of Troy.
Ilone, Ilonka

Ilsa Ger. Var. **Elizabeth**. Heb. "Pledged to God." Mostly limited to Germany, especially in the 19th century.
Elsa, Else, Ilse

Iluminada Sp. "Lit up."

Ima Var. **Emma**. OG. "Embracing everything."

Imelda OG./It. "All-consuming fight." A name occasionally used (especially in Catholic families, after a virgin saint) until the explosive fame of Philippine First Lady Imelda Marcos. Now it seems slated for a long period of neglect.
Imalda

Immaculada Sp. "Without stain." A reference to the Immaculate Conception.
Immaculata

Imperia Lat. "Imperial."

Imogen Lat. Some sources claim it means "last-born," while others suggest "image," while still another traces it back to "innocent." Despite Shakespeare's use of the name, it was obscure until the 20th century. Still unusual. Actress Imogene Coca.
Emogen, Emogene, Imogene, Imogenia, Imogine,
Imojean, Imojeen

Ina Lat. Suffix to make male names feminine, as in **Clementina** or **Edwina**. Used independently since the Victorian era.
Ena

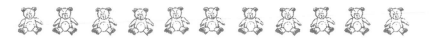

India Country name. Like any pretty geographic name, could be used by parents who have a special attachment to the country.

Inez Sp. Var. **Agnes**. Lat. "Pure." Unusual in English-speaking countries.

Ines, Inesita, Inessa, Ynes, Ynesita, Ynez

Inga Scan. "Guarded by Ing." Ing, in Norse mythology, was a powerful god of fertility and peace. His name is an element in several modern names like Ingrid and Ingmar.

Ingaberg, Ingaborg, Inge, Ingeberg, Ingeborg

Ingrid Scan. "Beautiful." The most popular of the "Ing–" names, doubtless because of the fame of Swedish actress Ingrid Bergman.

Inga, Inge, Inger, Ingmar

Inocencia Sp. "Innocence."

Inocenta, Inocentia

Ioanna Gk. Var. **Hannah**. Heb. "grace"

Iola Gk. "Cloud of dawn."

Iole

Iolanthe Gk. "Violet flower." The more common form is the Spanish variant, **Yolanda**. Gilbert and Sullivan's 1882 operetta *Iolanthe* did little to popularize this form.

Iona Gk. Place name. Island off the coast of Scotland, site of an early monastery. Use as a name is mostly Scottish.

Ione Gk. "Violet." Flower name in an exotic, little-used form. Actress Ione Skye.

Ionia, Ionie

Iphigenia Gk. "Sacrifice." In Greek myth, the daughter of Agamemnon. Her father sacrificed her to gain advantage in the Trojan war, though in most versions of the story, she is saved by Artemis.

Iphigenie, Genia

Irene Gk. "Peace." Very common under the Roman Empire, but first appeared in English-speaking countries in the mid–19th century. It caught on quickly and was very popular in the first quarter of the 20th century. Actresses Irene Dunne, Irene Worth.

Arina, Eireen, Eiren, Eirena, Eirene, Erena, Erene, Ira, Ireen, Iren, Irena, Irenea, Irénée, Irina, Irine, Iryna, Orina, Oryna, Rena, Rene, Renie, Rina, Yarina

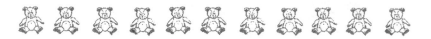

Iris Gk. "Rainbow." Also (and this is probably the source of its popularity) name of a flower. Its use was established and faded with other flower names, from around 1890 to the 1920s. Novelist Iris Murdoch.
Irisa, Irita

Irma OG. "Universal, complete." Rare now, but somewhat used in the first part of this century.
Erma, Irmina, Irmine, Irmgard, Irmgarde

Irvette (fem. **Irving**) OE. "Seafriend." Also Scot. place name. A rather awkward transformation of a name that was never immensely popular.

Isabel Sp. Var. **Elizabeth**. Heb. "pledged to God." Most fashionable in the last quarter of the 19th century. Belle and Bella are also independently used, probably because of their own attractive meaning ("beautiful") in French and Spanish. Henry James named the heroine of his *Portrait of a Lady* Isabel Archer. Actress Isabella Rossellini.
Bel, Belia, Belicia, Belita, Bell, Bella, Belle, Bellita, Ib, Ibbie, Isa, Isabeau, Isabelita, Isabell, Isabella, Isabelle, Ishbel, Isobel, Isobell, Isobella, Isobelle, Issie, Issy, Izabella, Izabelle, Izzie, Izzy, Ysabeau, Ysabel, Ysabella, Ysobel, Yzabelle

Isadora (fem. **Isidore**) Lat. "Gift of Isis." Isis was the principal goddess of ancient Egypt, and Isidore was a popular name among the ancient Greeks. The most famous Isadora was, of course, modern dance pioneer Isadora Duncan.
Isidora

Isis Egypt. The supreme goddess of ancient Egypt, Isis ruled with her brother/husband, Osiris, and her son, Horus.

Isla Name of a Scottish river, used in Britain as a first name.

Isolde Meaning unclear, though some sources offer Welsh "fair lady." In legend Isolde is an Irish princess loved by Tristan, but she marries his uncle, King Mark. There are many versions of the tale, the most famous of which is probably Wagner's opera *Tristan und Isolde*. Use of this version of the name probably reflects admiration for the opera.

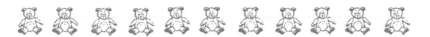

Iseult, Iseut, Isold, Isolda, Isolt, Isolte, Yseult, Yseulte, Yseut, Ysolda, Ysolde

Ita Ir. Gael. "Thirst." Name of a 6th-century Irish saint. Rare outside of Ireland.

Ivana (fem. **Ivan.**) Slavic var. **John.** Heb. "Jehovah is gracious." Most recently in the news with Ivana Trump, the ex-wife of Donald Trump.
Iva, Ivanna

Ivory Lat. Word used as name, possibly related to the vogue for jewel names in the late 19th century.
Ivoreen, Ivorine

Ivy OE. Botanical name. Most popular in the first quarter of the 20th century.
Ivee, Ivey, Ivie

Jacinda Sp. Var. **Hyacinth** Gk. Flower name. There was a 3rd-century Saint Hyacinth, and the name was used for boys as well as girls. In Greek legend, Apollo loved a beautiful youth of the name; the hyacinth flower sprang up from his blood when he died.
Giacinda, Giacintha, Giacinthia, Jacenda, Jacenta, Jacey, Jacie, Jacindia, Jacinna, Jacinta, Jacinth, Jacintha, Jacinthe, Jacinthia, Jacy, Jacynth, Jacyntha, Jacynthe, Jacynthia

Jackie Dim., usually of **Jacqueline.** Used as an independent name in the 20th century.
Jackee, Jackey, Jacki, Jacky, Jacquey, Jacqui, Jacquie

Jacobina (fem. **Jacob**) Heb. "He who supplants." James is an anglicization of Jacob, and has always been a favorite name in Scotland, which may account for the Scottish use of this feminization.
Jackee, Jackie, Jacky, Jacoba, Jacobetta, Jacobette, Jacobine

Jacqueline Fr. Dim. **Jacob.** Heb. "he who supplants." Ex-

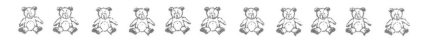

isted in Britain as early as the 17th century, but used in numbers only from the beginning of the 20th century. Grew quickly, and was quite a favorite by midcentury. In the U.S. parents may have been inspired by the glamorous First Lady Jacqueline Kennedy, who has put an indelible stamp on the name. It is, like most fashions of the early sixties, in a period of neglect. Actresses Jaclyn Smith, Jacqueline Bisset.

Jacalin, Jacalyn, Jackalin, Jackalinne, Jackelyn, Jacketta, Jackette, Jacki, Jackie, Jacklin, Jacklyn, Jacklynne, Jackqueline, Jacky, Jaclin, Jaclyn, Jacolyn, Jacqualine, Jacqualyn, Jacquelean, Jacquelin, Jacquelyn, Jacquelynne, Jacquenetta, Jacquenette, Jacquetta, Jacquette, Jacqui, Jacquine, Jaculine, Jaquelin, Jaqueline, Jaquelyn, Jaquith

Jade Sp. Jewel name, for the semiprecious green stone. Perhaps because the jewel comes from the Orient, the name has a vaguely exotic air.

Jada, Jayde

Jadwige Pol. "Safety in battle."

Jadwiga

Jael Heb. "Mountain goat." An Old Testament name that occurred from time to time in the 19th century. Now rare.

Jafit Heb. "Beautiful."

Jaffa

Jaime Sp. Var. **James**. Heb. "he who supplants." Some parents, however, may prefer to consider it as French for "I love", *J'aime*, in which case they should be prepared to insist on the "Zh–" pronunciation.

Jamesina (fem. **James**) (Heb. "he who supplants.") An old-fashioned form that has been abandoned in favor of the less formal **Jamie**, etc.

Jamie (fem. var. **James**) (Heb. "he who supplants.") Also used as a boy's name, but once a name becomes entrenched as a feminine choice, parents tend to avoid it for their male children. Jamie may be headed in this direction.

Jaime, Jaimey, Jaimi, Jaimie, Jaimy, Jamee, Jami, Jammie, Jayme, Jaymee, Jaymie

Jamila Arab. "Lovely." Currently popular among Moslem families.

Jamilah, Jamilla, Jamille, Jamillia

Jan (fem. **John**) Heb. "The Lord is gracious."

Jana, Janina, Janine, Jann, Janna

Jane (fem. **John**) Heb. "The Lord is gracious." This is the simplest current variant of John (though Joan predates it), popular since the 16th century. It has been a tried-and-true standby like Mary or Katherine, as its number of variants demonstrate. When many women at a time shared the same name, variants sprang up to differentiate them from one another, hence Janet, Janine, Janelle, etc. Author Jane Austen; actresses Jane Fonda, Jane Seymour, Jane Wyman; newsreader Jane Pauley.

Gene, Gianina, Giovanna, Iva, Ivana, Ivancka, Ivanka, Ivanna, Jaine, Jainee, Jan, Jana, Janaya, Janaye, Jandy, Janeczka, Janeen, Janel, Janela, Janella, Janelle, Janean, Janene, Janessa, Janet, Janeta, Janetta, Janette, Janey, Jania, Janica, Janice, Janie, Janina, Janine, Janique, Janis, Janise, Janit, Janka, Janna, Jannel, Jannelle, Janney, Janny, Jany, Jayne, Jaynell, Jean, Jeanette, Jeanie, Jeanne, Jeannette, Jeannine, Jenda, Jenella, Jenelle, Jenica, Jeniece, Jeni, Jenie, Jensina, Jensine, Jess, Jinna, Joana, Joanna, Johanna, Jonella, Jonelle, Joni, Jonie, Juana, Juanita, Sheena, Shene, Sinead, Vania, Vanya

Janet The currently common diminutive form of Jane is Janet, but other forms such as Janeta and Jonet preceded it. Janet was originally mostly Scots, and was very popular in the 1950s. Like most fifties favorites, it is now out of style. Actresses Janet Leigh, Janet Gaynor; singer Dame Janet Baker.

Gianetta, Janeta, Janetta, Janette, Jannet, Jannetta, Janit, Janot, Jenetta, Jenette, Jennet, Jennette, Jonette

Janice Var. **Jane.** Coined at the turn of the 20th century, in general circulation by the thirties and popular in the fifties. Like **Janet,** now out of favor. Singer Janis Joplin.

Janiece, Janique, Janis, Janiss, Jannice, Janyce

Janna Var. **Johanna.** Unusual, used mostly since the 1960s.

Jana, Janaya

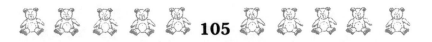

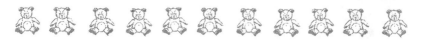

Jasmine Per. "Jasmine flower." Flower name with exotic connotations. The turn-of-the-century vogue for flower names had its source in the English upper class, but was usually confined to temperate-zone specimens. (England's Queen Mother, for instance, had sisters named Rose and Violet Hyacinth.) Jasmine became fashionable a bit later, in the 1930s.
Jasmin, Jasmina, Jassamayn, Jazan, Jazmin, Jess, Jessamine, Jessamy, Jessamyn, Jessie, Jessimine, Jessimine, Yasmeen, Yasmin, Yasmina, Yasmine

Jay Lat. "Jaybird." A medieval name that has survived in a small way, especially in the U.S., where it is given to boys and girls alike. Its use may be inspired by a great American jurist, John Jay.
Jae, Jaye, Jaylene

Jean Var. **Jane**. Scottish origin, unusual elsewhere until the turn of the 20th century; most popular in the 1930s. Now unusual. Actresses Jean Arthur, Jean Harlow.
Gene, Genie, Jeana, Jeane, Jeaneen, Jeanelle, Jeanene, Jeanette, Jeanie, Jeanine, Jeanna, Jeanne, Jeanneen, Jeannetta, Jeannette, Jeannie, Jeannine, Jenette, Jennet, Jennetta, Jennine

Jeannine (fem. **John**) Var. **Jean**. Heb. "The Lord is gracious." Modern usage, currently on the increase.
Janine, Jeanine, Jenine, Jannine, Jennine

Jelena Rus. Var. **Helen** (Gk. "light").
Yelena

Jemima Heb. "Dove." Old Testament name: Jemima was one of the three beautiful daughters of the persecuted Job. The Puritans brought the name to the U.S., where it is now probably most familiar because of the "Aunt Jemima" brand name for pancake mix and syrup.
Jamima, Jemimah, Jemmimah, Jemmie, Jemmy, Mima, Mimma

Jena Arab. "Little bird."
Jenna

Jenilee Com. form. **Jenny** and **Lee**.
Jennylee

Jennie Dim. **Janet** or **Jennifer**. Given as an independent

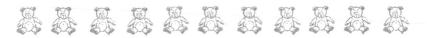

name since the 19th century. Swedish soprano Jennie Lind.

Jenney, Jenni, Jenny

Jennifer Welsh. "White and smooth, soft." The modern and most popular form of Guinevere, originally a Cornish variant. Its immense 20th-century popularity began in the 1920s and grew to a 1950s peak in Britain. In the U.S. the name reached the number one spot in the early eighties, and is now slipping down the charts. Actresses Jennifer Jones, Jennifer Jason Leigh, Jennifer O'Neill.

Genna, Genni, Gennie, Gennifer, Genniver, Genny, Jen, Jena, Jenefer, Jeni, Jenifer, Jeniffer, Jenn, Jenna, Jennee, Jenni, Jennica, Jennie, Jenniver, Jenny

Jeremia (fem. **Jeremiah**) Heb. "The Lord is exalted."

Jeree, Jeri, Jerri, Jerrie, Jerry

Jerrie OG./Fr. "Spear ruler." Dim. **Geraldine.**

Jeree, Jeri, Jerree, Jerrey, Jerri, Jerry, Jery

Jerusha Heb. "Married."

Jarusha, Jeruscha

Jessica Heb. "He sees." Coined by Shakespeare from the Old Testament Iscah or Jesca. His Jessica was the daughter of Shylock in the *Merchant of Venice.* Popular in the U.S. in the 1970s. Actresses Jessica Lange, Jessica Tandy.

Jess, Jessa, Jessalin, Jessalyn, Jesse, Jesseca, Jessey, Jessie, Jessy

Jessie Dim. **Jessica.** Also, in Scotland, a diminutive of Janet.

Jess, Jessa, Jesse, Jessey, Jessi

Jesusa Sp. Derived from Mary de Jesus, a name for the Virgin Mary.

Jette Dan. "Black as coal." Currently popular in Denmark; also used in Germany.

Jewel OF. Word used as first name. Though the vogue for jewel names occurred at the turn of the 20th century (along with the flower-name fashion), Jewel came into use a little later, in the 1930s.

Jewell, Jewelle

Jezebel Heb. "Pure, virginal." An Old Testament name that carries strong connotations: It was used as a term

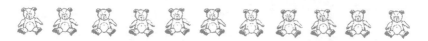

for a "painted lady" or a brazen hussy as portrayed by
Bette Davis in the film *Jezebel*.

Jessabell, Jezabel, Jezabella, Jezebelle, Jezibel, Jezybell

Jill Diminutive of **Gillian**, ultimately of **Juliana**. (Lat.
"youthful") Jill was popular before the 17th century, and
revived to widespread use after the 1920s. Actresses Jill
St. John, Jill Eikenberry, Jill Ireland; English novelist Jilly
Cooper.

**Jilian, Jillan, Jillana, Jillane, Jillayne, Jilleen, Jillene,
Jilli, Jillian, Jillianne, Jillie, Jilly, Jillyan**

Jillian Var. Gillian, Dim. Juliana. (Lat. "youthful")

**Jilian, Jiliana, Jilan, Jillana, Jillane, Jilliana, Jillianne,
Jillyan, Jillyanna, Jilliyanne**

Jimena Sp. "Heard."

Jinny Dim. **Virginia**. Var. **Jenny**. Mostly 19th-century use
in this form.

Jinnie

Jinx Lat. "Spell."

Jynx

Jo Dim. **Joan, Josephine**, etc. Often used in combination,
as in Jo Ann, Betty Jo. The second daughter in Louisa
May Alcott's *Little Women* was called Jo, short for Josephine, but the usage hasn't caught on widely.

Joakima (fem. **Joachim**) Heb. "God will judge."

Joaquina, Joaquine

Joan (fem. **John**) Heb. "The Lord is gracious." The medieval feminine version of John; Jeanne d'Arc's first
name, for instance, was translated as Joan, Jeanne's popular English equivalent. It was neglected for Jane by the
17th century. A brief intense revival occurred early in
the 20th century for a score of years, but Joan is again
widely neglected. Actresses Joan Crawford, Joan Collins;
singer Joan Baez; comedienne Joan Rivers.

Joane, Joanie, Joannie, Jone, Jonee, Joni

Joanna Var. **Jane** or **Joan**. Its 19th-century use increased
with the revival of Joan, and continued to grow until
around 1950 in the U.S. Joanne, the French form, was
hugely popular in Britain in the 1970s.

**Jo, Joana, Joann, Jo Ann, Joanne, Jo Anne, Joeann,
Johanna, Johannah**

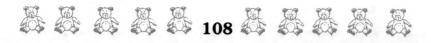

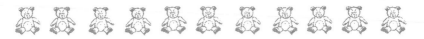

Jobeth Com. form **Jo** and **Beth**. Unusual, found mostly in the 1950s. Actress JoBeth Williams.

Joby (fem. **Job**) Heb. "Persecuted." Unusual version of an Old Testament name widely used by the Puritans and their descendants well into the 19th century.

Jobey, Jobi, Jobie, Jobina, Jobyna

Jocasta It. "Lighthearted." In spite of its pleasant meaning, the name is little used because of its history. In Greek myth, Jocasta is the mother of Oedipus; he later unwittingly marries her, unleashing a series of tragedies.

Jocelyn Derivation unclear; possibly Old German, possibly Lat. "cheerful." It was a man's name in the Middle Ages, revived as a girl's name in the early 20th century. Cellist Jocelyn DuPré.

Jocelin, Joceline, Jocelyne, Josaline, Joscelin, Josceline, Joscelyn, Joseline, Joselyn, Joselyne, Josiline, Josline, Jossline, Josselyn, Josslyn, Joycelin

Jocosa Lat. "Joking."

Giocosa

Jody Dim. **Joan, Judith**. Used mostly since the 1950s in the U.S.; in the Canadian top ten in the 1970s. Actress Jodie Foster.

Jodee, Jodey, Jodi, Jodie

Joelle (fem. **Joel**) Heb. "Jehovah is the Lord." Probably popularized by a vogue for combined forms beginning with "Jo," like Joanne and Jolene. Reached its peak in the 1960s. Actress Joely Richardson.

Joela, Joelin, Joell, Joella, Joelliane, Joellin, Joelly, Joely, Joelynn, Jowella, Jowelle

Johanna (fem. **Johann**) Ger. Var. **John**. Heb. "the Lord is gracious." A European-sounding choice among the numerous feminizations of John.

Johannah

Johnna (fem. **John**) Heb. "The Lord is gracious." May also be considered a contraction of **Johanna**.

Giana, Gianna, Johna

Joie Fr. Var. **Joy**.

Joi

Jolan Gk. "Violet flower." This is a Middle European

form of Iolanthe. The most popular form in the U.S. is Yolanda.

Jola, Jolanne, Jolanta, Jolantha

Jolene Com. form "Jo" and "lene." In the 1940s names ending in "lene" (Darlene, Marlene, etc.) began to be fashionable, and a form beginning with "Jo" was a natural result. These names are now little used.

Joeline, Joeleen, Jolean, Joleen, Jolina, Joline, Jolyn, Jolyna, Jolyne, Jolynn

Jolie Fr. "Pretty." Used mainly since the 1960s.

Jolee, Joley, Joli, Joly

Jonquil Flower name. Unlike most flower names, this one did not appear until the 1940s, and its two decades of popularity were mostly limited to Britain. The jonquil is a variety of narcissus closely related to a daffodil.

Jordan Heb. "Descend." Named after the River Jordan. First used in the Middle Ages by Crusaders returning from the Holy Land. Revived slightly in the 19th century, mostly for boys. Unusual now for either sex, but a good candidate for revival in the 1990s quest for the unusual.

Jardena, Jordain, Jordana, Jordane, Jordanna, Jordena, Jorey, Jorie, Jorry, Jourdan

Josephine (fem. **Joseph**) Heb. "Jehovah increases." Napoleon's famous Empress Josephine's real name was Marie Josephe (for the parents of Jesus), but Josephine was used as a diminutive. It did not become fashionable until the mid–19th century, and has never caught on widely in the U.S. Cabaret star Josephine Baker.

Fifi, Fifine, Fina, Guiseppina, Jo, Joette, Joey, Joline, Josée, Josefa, Josefena, Josefene, Josefina, Josefine, Josepha, Josephe, Josephene, Josephina, Josephyna, Josephyne, Josetta, Josette, Josey, Josie, Josy, Jozsa

Jovita Lat. "Made glad."

Joy Lat. "Joy." Used in the Middle Ages and sparingly by the Puritans, then revived at the turn of the 20th century. Unusual after the height of its popularity in the 1950s.

Gioia, Joi, Joie, Joya, Joyann, Joye

Joyce Lat. "Joyous." Used in the Middle Ages, but nearly died out until the early years of the 20th century, when

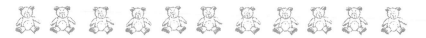

it had a spurt of immense popularity, especially in Britain. Advice columnist Dr. Joyce Brothers.
Joice, Joycelyn, Joyous

Juanita Sp. Var. **Joan**.
Janita, Juana, Juniata, Junita, Nita

Judith Heb. "Jewish." Old Testament name overlooked by the Puritans in their quest for girls' names, but fashionable from the 1920s through the 1950s. In the Apocrypha, Judith is a Jewish heroine who decapitates the Assyrian general Holofernes and shows his head to the Hebrew army, inciting them to victory. Actress Dame Judith Anderson; movie critic Judith Crist.
**Giuditta, Jodie, Jody, Judee, Judi, Judie, Juditha,
Judithe, Judit, Judita, Judite, Judy, Judye, Jutta**

Judy Dim. **Judith**. Dates back to the 18th century, but its true popularity follows that of Judith in the 20th century. Jody is another frequently used diminutive. Actress Judy Garland.
Judee, Judey, Judi, Judie, Judye

Julia (fem. **Julius**) Lat. Clan name. "Youthful." Along with Juliana, used among the early Christians, but it was rare in the Middle Ages. Since the 1700s it has gone mildly in and out of fashion without ever being a tremendous favorite. Julie, in this century, has been much more popular. Chef Julia Child.
**Giulia, Giulietta, Jiulia, Joleta, Joletta, Jolette, Julee,
Juley, Juli, Juliana, Juliane, Juliann, Julianne, Julie,
Julienne, Juliet, Julieta, Julietta, Juliette, Julina, Juline,
Julinka, Juliska, Julita, Julitta, Julyana, Julyanna,
Julyet, Julyetta, Julyette, Julyne, Yulia, Yuliya**

Juliana (fem. **Julian**) Lat. clan name. "Youthful." Appeared in the early Christian era, and medieval use contracted it to Gillian (and from there to Jill). Although a royal name in the Netherlands, it is unusual now, possibly seeming too stately. Contracted forms like Liana may eclipse it.
**Juliane, Julianna, Julianne, Julieanna, Julieanne,
Julyana, Julyane, Julyanna, Julyanne**

Julie Fr. Dim. **Julia** Lat. Clan name. "Youthful." Imported from France in the 1920s and fashionable very quickly,

especially in the 1970s. It had earlier taken root on the Continent, as evidenced by Strindberg's 1888 tragedy *Miss Julie*. Actresses Julie Andrews, Julie Harris, Julie Walters

Julee, Juley, Julienne, July

Juliet Lat. Clan name. "Youthful." Dim. **Julia**. Can scarcely be used without reference to Shakespeare's famous tragic heroine. Girls named Juliet can expect a certain amount of teasing about Romeo. Dancer Juliet Prowse.

Giulietta, Julieta, Juliett, Julietta, Juliette, Julyet, Julette

June Month used as name, dating from the 20th century but most popular in the 1950s. It is more often used than April or May, the other most common month names. Actress June Allyson.

Junella, Junelle, Junette, Junia, Juniata, Junieta, Junina, Junine

Juno Lat. "Queen of heaven." Juno was the Roman equivalent of Hera in classical mythology: Jupiter's wife, and the gods' queen. Not widely used in any era; in modern times the adjective "Junoesque" has come to be used for tall women with curvy figures, possibly because of the way Juno is often portrayed in Old Master paintings.

Justine Lat. "Fair, righteous." Justina was the original form, but the French version took over in the 1960s, probably aided by Lawrence Durrell's famous novel *Justine*. Actress Justine Bateman.

Giustina, Justa, Justene, Justie, Justina, Justinn, Justy, Justyna, Justyne

K

Kadenza Lat. "With rhythm." Modern variant of **Cadence**.

Cadenza, Kadena, Kadence

Kaitlin Var. **Caitlin**, Irish form of **Catherine** Gk. "pure." A name as popular as **Catherine** has produced endless variations over

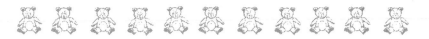

the years. In the late 20th century, the use of the initial letter *K* instead of a hard *C* gave freshness to many old favorites.

Kala Hindi. "Black/time."

Kali Sanskrit. "Energy."
Kalli

Kalila Arab. "Beloved."
Cailey, Cailie, Caylie, Kailey, Kalie, Kaly, Kaylee, Kylila

Kalliope Gk. **Calliope**, the muse of epic poetry. Many of the *C* names that come from the Greek are spelled with a *K* in their original form.
Kallyope

Kallista Gk. "Most beautiful."
Cala, Calesta, Calista, Callie, Cally, Kala, Kalesta,
Kalista, Kalli, Kallie, Kally, Kallysta

Kama Sanskrit. "Love."

Kamilah Arab. "Perfect."
Kamila, Kamilla, Kamillah

Kamilla European var. **Camille**. Some sources trace Camille to the young girls who assisted at pagan religious ceremonies.
Camilla, Cammie, Kamila, Kamilka, Kamilla, Kamille,
Kamyla, Milla, Millie

Kandace Var. **Candace**. Lat. "glowing white." Historically the name was the ancient title of the queens of Ethiopia before the 4th century. Not much used before the middle of the 20th century.
Candie, Candy, Dacie, Kandice, Kandiss, Kandy

Kara Var. **Cara**. Lat. "dear one." Principally used from the 1970s onward.
Cara, Carina, Karina, Karine, Karrah, Karrie

Karen Danish. Var. **Katherine**. Gk. "pure." Took hold in the 1930s in English-speaking countries, and blossomed to great popularity in the 1950s and 1960s. A mother who was one of four Karens in her kindergarten, however, is unlikely to use the same name for her daughter, so it is unusual today. Writer Karen Blixen (Isaak Dinesen).
Caren, Carin, Caron, Caronn, Carren, Carrin, Carron,
Carryn, Caryn, Carynn, Carynne, Kari, Karin, Karna,

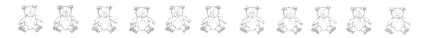

Karon, Karryn, Karyn, Kerran, Kerrin, Kerron, Kerrynn, Kerynne

Karimah Arab. "Giving."

Karla Var. **Carla**. OG. "Man." One of the endless names that derive from **Charles**. Fans of John Le Carre's novels will remember that George Smiley's Russian nemesis used the code name Karla.

Karlotta Ger. Var. **Charlotte**. Fr. from OG. "man."
Karlota

Karma Hindi. "Destiny, spiritual force." A New Age name if ever there was one.

Karolina Slavic. Var. **Caroline**. Lat. "Little and womanly."
Karaline, Karalyn, Karalynna, Karalynne, Karla, Karleen, Karlen, Karlena, Karlene, Karli, Karlie, Karlina, Karlinka, Karolina, Karoline, Karolinka, Karolyn, Karolyna, Karolyne, Karolynn, Karolynne, Leena, Lina, Lyna

Kasmira (fem. **Casimir**) Old Slavic. "Bringing peace." Very unusual.

Kassandra Var. **Cassandra**. Gk. Possibly fem. **Alexander**.

Kate Dim. **Katherine**. Long-standing independent name, especially popular in the late 19th century. Writer Kate Chopin; actresses Kate Capshaw, Kate Jackson; German artist Kaethe Kollwitz.
Cait, Caitie, Cate, Catey, Catie, Kaethe, Kait, Kaitlin, Katey, Kathe, Kati, Katie

Katherine Gk. "Pure." One of the oldest recorded names, with roots in Greek antiquity. Almost every Western country has its own form of the name, and phonetic variations are endless. It has been borne by such illustrious women as Saint Catherine of Alexandria, the early martyr who was tortured on a spiked wheel; Empress Catherine the Great of Russia; and three of Henry VIII's six wives. It is currently very popular in England and France, and was one of the top ten American girls' names in the 1980s. Actresses Catherine Oxenberg, Catherine Deneuve, Katharine Hepburn.
Cait, Caitlin, Caitlinn, Caitrin, Caitrine, Caitriona, Caitrionagh, Caity, Caren, Cari, Carin, Caron, Caronne,

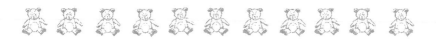

Carren, Carri, Carrin, Carron, Caryn, Carynn, Cass, Cassey, Cassi, Cassie, Cat, Cataleen, Cataleena, Catalin, Catalina, Cataline, Catarina, Catarine, Cate, Cateline, Caterina, Cathaleen, Cathaline, Catharin, Catharina, Catharine, Catharyna, Catharyne, Cathee, Cathelina, Catherine, Catherina, Catheryn, Cathie, Cathirin, Cathiryn, Cathleen, Cathline, Cathlyne, Cathrine, Cathrinn, Cathryn, Cathrynn, Cathy, Cathye, Cati, Catie, Catina, Catlaina, Catreen, Catreina, Catrin, Catrina, Catrine, Catriona, Catrionagh, Catryna, Caty, Cay, Caye, Ekaterina, Kaatje, Kait, Kaitee, Kaitie, Kaitlin, Kaitlinn, Kaitrin, Kaitrine, Kaitrinn, Kaitrinna, Kaitriona, Kaity, Karen, Karena, Kari, Karin, Karon, Karri, Karrin, Karyn, Karynn, Kasia, Kasienka, Kasja, Kaska, Kasya, Kass, Kassi, Kassia, Kassie, Kas, Kat, Kata, Kataleen, Katalin, Katalina, Katarina, Katchen, Kate, Katee, Katell, Katelle, Katenka, Katerina, Katey, Katha, Katharine, Katharyn, Kathee, Kathelina, Katheline, Katherin, Katherina, Katheryn, Katheryne, Kathi, Kathie, Kathileen, Kathirin, Kathiryn, Kathirynn, Kathleen, Kathlene, Kathleyn, Kathline, Kathlyne, Kathrene, Kathrine, Kathrinna, Kathryn, Kathryne, Kathy, Kathyrine, Kati, Katie, Katica, Katina, Katinka, Katka, Katla, Katlaina, Katleen, Katline, Katoushka, Katouska, Katrena, Katrien, Katrina, Katrine, Katriona, Katrionagh, Katryna, Katushka, Katuska, Katy, Katya, Kay, Kaye, Kit, Kittey, Kitti, Kittie, Kitty, Rina, Trina, Trinchen, Trine, Trinette, Yekaterin, Yekaterina

Kathleen Ir. Var **Katherine**. Gk. "Pure." Its use outside of Ireland began in the 1840s, and may have been influenced by the great wave of Irish emigration sparked by the potato famines of those years. U.S. popularity peaked in the 1950s. Actress Kathleen Turner.

Kaitlin, Kaitlinn, Kathelina, Katheline, Kathleyn, Kathlin, Kathline, Kathlyne, Kathyline, Katleen, Katlin, Katline, Katlyne

Kathy Diminutive, usually of **Katherine**. TV host Kathie Lee Gifford.

Kathey, Kathie

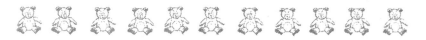

Katrina Var. **Katherine**. Gk. "Pure." Appealing for its European sound.
Catrina, Catriona, Catrionagh, Kaitrina, Kaitrona, Katreina, Katriona, Katrionagh

Kay Dim. **Katherine**. First appeared at the turn of the 20th century, but widespread in the middle of the century. Actress Kaye Ballard.
Caye, Kai, Kaye

Kayla Modern variant of **Katherine**. Gk. "Pure."
Cayla, Caylie, Kaela, Kaila, Kaylyn

Keely Ir. Var. **Kelly**. "Battle Maid."
Kealey, Kealy, Keeley, Keelia, Keighley, Keighly

Keisha Modern name, possibly formed as a short version of Lakeisha, which, in turn, may be a variant of Aisha. Arab. "woman."

Kelila Heb. "Crowned."
Kayla, Kayle, Kaylee, Kelula, Kyla, Kyle

Kelly Ir. Gael. "Battle maid." Originally a very common Irish last name, and very popular as a girl's first name from about the 1950s, peaking in the 1970s in America. Actress Kelly McGillis.
Kellee, Kelley, Kellie, Kellina

Kelsey OE. Place name, incorporating a word particle that means "island." Mostly recent usage, for boys as well as girls.
Kelcey, Kelcy, Kellsie, Kelsee, Kelseigh, Kelsy

Kendra Origin unclear: Some sources suggest OE. "knowing," while one proposes a modern combination of Ken and Sandra. Modern, in any case.
Kenna, Kinna

Kenya Place name used as first name.

Kerensa Cornish. "Love." Unusual name that has spread a bit from Cornwall since the 1970s, but still of limited popularity.
Karensa, Karenza

Kerry Ir. Place name: Kerry is a county in southwestern Ireland. Also, according to some sources, Ir. Gael. "dark-haired."
Keree, Keri, Kerrey, Kerri, Kerrie

Ketura Heb. "Incense." Old Testament name: Keturah

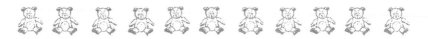

was Abraham's second wife. Revived by the Puritans and used with some steadiness through the 19th century.
Keturah

Kezia Heb. "Cassia." Cassia is the generic name for a variety of trees and shrubs, one of which produces cinnamon. One of the three daughters of Job (along with Jemima; though their existence is mentioned in the Old Testament, their names are apocryphal). The name was adopted by the Puritans and brought to the U.S. in the 18th century, when it was popular. Use has declined gradually since then.
Kazia, Keziah, Kissie, Kizzie, Kizzy

Kevyn (fem. **Kevin**) Ir. Gael. "Handsome."
Kevina

Kiana Modern name of unclear origin; one scholarly source links it to **Anna**.
Kia, Quiana, Quianna

Kim Dim. **Kimberly**. Used as an independent name from the mid–20th century, influenced by the careers of actresses Kim Novak, Kim Basinger.
Kym

Kimberly OE. Place name. The "-ly" suffix indicates a meadow. *The Facts on File Dictionary of First Names* traces the masculine use of the name to the Boer War, when many English soldiers were fighting in the South African town of Kimberley. It was used for girls after 1940 and became a great favorite in the 1960s and 1970s, now declining. Judge Kimba Wood.
Kim, Kimba, Kimber, Kimberlee, Kimberleigh,
Kimberley, Kimberlie, Kimberlyn, Kimblyn, Kimmie,
Kimmy, Kym

Kineta Gk. "Active one." From the same root as "kinetic."
Kinneret Heb. "Harp."
Kirsten Scan. Var. **Christine**. Gk. "Christian." Used generally from 1940, though the Scots had adopted this form long ago (possibly because of their geographical proximity to Scandinavia). Actress Kirstie Alley.
Keerstin, Keirstin, Kersten, Kerstin, Kiersten, Kierstin,
Kierstynn, Kirsteen, Kirsti, Kirstie, Kirstin, Kirsty,
Kirstynn, Kristyn, Krystin

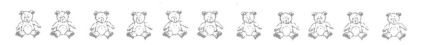

Kitty Dim. **Katherine**. Gk. "Pure." Used independently before the 16th century and during the 18th and 19th. In the intervening 200 years it was a slang term for a woman of dubious morals. Author Kitty Kelley.
Kit, Kittee, Kittey

Kizzy Var. **Keziah**. Heb. "Cassia." Adopted enthusiastically by parents after it was publicized in Alex Haley's *Roots* as a traditional African name. Spoilsport scholars, however, point out that Keziah and its variants were common slave names as early as the 18th century.
Kissie, Kizzie

Klara Hung. Var. **Clara**. Lat. "bright."
Klari, Klarice, Klarika, Klarissa, Klarisza, Klaryssa

Klaudia Pol. Var. **Claudia**. Lat. "lame."

Klementina Var. **Clementia**. Lat. "Mild, giving mercy."
Clemence, Clementine, Klementijna, Klementine, Klementyna

Klotild Hung. Var. **Clothide**. Ger. "Renowned battle."
Klothild, Klothilda, Klothilde, Klotilda

Konstanze Ger. Var. **Constance**. Lat. "Steadfastness."
Constancia, Constantina, Konstance, Konstantia, Konstantina, Kosta, Kostatina, Kostya, Tina, Stanze

Kora Gk. "Maiden." Though some sources trace the name to classical myth, its modern form was probably coined by American writer James Fenimore Cooper in *The Last of the Mohicans* (1826). It grew in popularity through the 19th century, but now its variant forms are more often used. The *K* spelling is a particularly 20th-century twist.
Cora, Corabel, Corabella, Corabelle, Corabellita, Corella, Corena, Coretta, Corey, Cori, Corilla, Corrie, Corry, Coryna, Korabell, Koree, Koreen, Korella, Korena, Korenda, Korette, Korey, Korilla, Korina, Korinna, Korinne, Korissa, Korrina, Korrine, Korynna, Koryssa

Kornelia Var. **Cornelia**. Lat. "Like a horn."
Cornelia, Kornelija, Kornelya

Kristen Com. form **Kirsten** and **Kristina**, var. **Christine**. (Gk. "anointed, Christian.") Looks Scandinavian, but isn't. Popular in the last 50 years, along with similar forms like Kristin and Kristine.

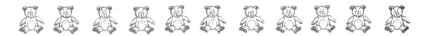

Krissie, Krissy, Krista, Kristan, Kristeen, Kristel, Kristelle, Kristi, Kristijna, Kristin, Kristina, Kristine, Kristyn, Kristyna, Krisztina, Krysta, Krystyna

Krystal Var. **Crystal**. (Gk. "ice.") Transferred use of the word, mostly modern, and increasing since the 1950s. The *K* spelling is a recent variation. Some parents may have been influenced by Krystle Carrington, a character on TV's "Dynasty."

Cristalle, Cristel, Crysta, Khristalle, Khristel, Khrystle, Khrystalle, Kristle, Krystal, Krystalle, Krystle

Kyle Scot. place name. "Narrow spit of land." Well-traveled parents may have crossed the Kyle of Lochalsh to reach the Isle of Skye. Used more often for boys than for girls.

Kynthia Gk. Var. **Cynthia**. Gk. "From Mount Cynthos."

Kyra Gk. "Lady." A contraction of the Greek title of respect. Ballerina Kyra Nichols; actress Kyra Sedgwick.

Keera, Keira, Kira, Kyria

Lacey OF. Place name of obscure meaning, used as a boy's name in the 19th century and only occasionally for either sex today.

Lacee, Lacie, Lacy

Ladonna Modern elaboration of **Donna**. It. "Lady."

Lainey Dim. **Elaine** OF. "Bright, shining, light."

Laila Arab. "Night." See **Leila**. Usually taken to indicate dark hair or a dark complexion. Actress Laila Robbins.

Lailie, Laily

Lakeisha Popular modern name made up of elements in vogue in the 1980s, the fashionable "La-" prefix attached to Aisha (Arab. "woman"). There are numerous forms, most of them phonetic variations.

Lakeesha, Lakecia, Laketia, Lakeysha, Lakicia, Lakisha, Lakitia, Lekeesha, Lekeisha, Lekisha

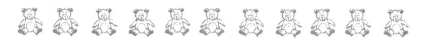

Lalage Gk. "Babbler, prattler." Extremely unusual, though it occurs in literature.
Lalia
Lallie Dim. **Lalage**. Gk. "Babbler, prattler." More common than its source, though still rare.
Lally
Lana Var. **Helen** Gk. "light." or **Alanna**. Gael. "rock" or "comely." Made famous by actress Lana Turner, but not widely used.
Lanae, Lanette, Lanna, Lanny
Lane Middle English. Place name. More common for boys than for girls, though still unusual for both. This is the kind of name that is likely to be a mother's maiden name transferred to a first name.
Laine, Layne
Lani Haw. "Sky."
Lara Unclear origin. Some sources suggest Lat. "famous"; others trace the name to the Greek **Larissa**. Today's parents may be reminded of the famous "Lara's Theme" from the 1965 film *Dr. Zhivago*.
Larina
Laraine Lat. Var. **Lorraine**.
Laraene, Larayne, Lareine, Larina, Larine
Lareina Sp. "The queen." Compares to **Leroy**. Fr. "The king." Uncommon.
Lareine, Larena
Larissa Gk. "Lighthearted." Unusual, even in times like the 18th century, when more elaborate names were the norm.
Laryssa, Lissa, Lyssa
Lark Middle English. Nature name, used since the 1950s mostly in the U.S. Larks are usually thought of as playful, lighthearted birds.
Lassie Middle English. "Little girl." "Lass" is a Scottish and Northern English term for a girl, but the association for most parents is more likely to be a highly intelligent collie as seen on a popular TV series in the 1960s and again in the 1990s.
Latanya Modern combined form: the "La-" prefix added to Tanya.

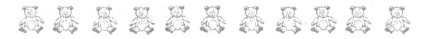

Latania, Latanja, Latonia, Latonya

Latisha Var. **Letitia**. Lat. "Happiness."

Latoya One of the most famous of the modern "La-" names, probably because of Latoya Jackson's renown. Derivation and meaning are mysterious.

Latoia, Latoyla

Latrice Modern combined form: **Patricia** Lat. "noble" with the "La-" prefix.

Latrecia, Latreece, Latreese, Latreshia, Latricia, Letreece, Letrice

Laudomia It. "Praise to the house."

Laura Lat. "Laurel." In classical times, a crown made from the leaves of the bay laurel was given to heroes or victors. Two famous Lauras are the unknown woman to whom the poet Petrarch addressed his sonnets, and the heroine of the 1940s film *Laura*. The greatest popularity of the name came at the mid to late 19th century, and it has remained quite a steady favorite ever since. A series of children's books were written by and about Laura Ingalls Wilder of *Little House on the Prairie* fame. Actress Laura Dern.

Lari, Lauralee, Laure, Laureen, Laurel, Laurella, Lauren, Laurena, Laurence, Laurene, Laurentia, Laurentine, Lauretta, Laurette, Lauri, Lauriane, Laurianne, Laurice, Lauricia, Laurie, Laurina, Laurinda, Laurine, Lollie, Lolly, Lora, Loree, Loreen, Loren, Lorena, Lorene, Lorenza, Loretta, Lorette, Lorey, Lori, Lorie, Lorinda, Lorine, Lorita, Lorna, Lorretta, Lorrette, Lorri, Lorrie, Lorry, Lory

Laurel Lat. "Laurel tree." Nature name whose popularity has coasted on the coattails of Laura, especially in the 20th century.

Laural, Lauralle, Laurell

Lauren Var. **Laura**. Introduced to the public by Lauren Bacall, and immediately popular probably because the streamlined "modern" character of the name struck a chord in the 1940s. It might be fading from sight by now, but has been given extended popularity by the influential designer Ralph Lauren (née Ralph Lefkowitz), who

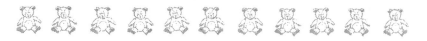

has endowed it with fashionable associations. Model Lauren Hutton.

Laurin, Lauryn, Laurynn, Loren, Lorin, Lorne, Lorren, Lorrin

Laveda Lat. "Cleansed."

Lavella, Lavelle, Lavetta, Lavette

Laverne Lat. Classical goddess of minor criminals, though the parents who made this name mildly popular in the 20th century probably didn't know that. It sounds enough like the romance languages' word for "green" (*vert, verde*) to have acquired misplaced connotations of green trees or springtime.

Laverine, Lavern, Laverna, Verne

Lavinia Lat. "Women of Rome." Classical name. Revived in the Renaissance, again used in the 18th century, rather neglected for the last 200 years.

Lavena, Lavenia, Lavina, Lavinie, Levenia, Levinia, Livinia, Lovina, Lovinia, Vinnie

Lavonne Modern combined form, probably "La-" attached to **Yvonne** OF. "yew wood." Popular somewhat earlier (1950s–1980s) than most of the other "La-" names.

Leah Heb. "Weary." Old Testament name: Leah was the wife of Jacob, married to him by a ruse in the place of her sister Rachel. Follows the typical usage pattern of the Old Testament names: revived by the Puritans, dying off gradually into this century.

Lea, Lee, Leia, Leigh

Leala OF. "Loyal."

Lealia, Lealie

Leandra (fem. **Leander**) Gk. "Lion man." A spurt of use in the 1960s and 1970s has faded.

Leanda, Leodora, Leoine, Leoline, Leonelle

Leanne Com. form **Lee** and **Ann.**

Leeann, Lee-Ann, Leigh-Anne

Leatrice Com. form **Lee** and **Beatrice.**

Leda Gk. Dim. **Letitia.** Lat. "Joy, gladness." In classical myth Leda was visited by Jupiter in the form of a swan, and produced four children, among them the beautiful Helen of Troy.

Leta, Lida

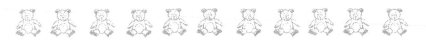

Lee OE. Place name: "Pasture or meadow." One of the few truly unisex names. Usually a name becomes exclusively feminine once it is used for girls like Ashley or Leslie. The tenacious masculine hold on Lee may have been helped by tough-guy actor Lee Marvin. U.S. use seems to have been sparked by admiration for Confederate General Robert E. Lee. Peaked in the 1950s. Actress Lee Remick; Princess Lee Radziwill.
Lea, Leigh

Leila Arab. "Night." Used by authors in the early 19th century for exotic female characters, and more widely by parents later in the century. Pronunciation of the first syllable varies, as the different spellings make clear.
Layla, Leela, Leelah, Leilah, Leilia, Lela, Lelah, Lelia, Leyla, Lila, Lilah

Leilani Haw. "Flower from heaven."

Lelia Lat. Clan name of unknown meaning, used in Britain and the U.S. in the late 19th century.
Lilia

Lemuela (fem. **Lemuel**) Heb. "Devoted to God." Feminization of a name that was mildly popular in the 19th century.

Lena Lat. Diminutive of names like **Helena, Caroline, Marlene.** Independent use dates from the mid–19th century. Actress Lena Olin; singer Lena Horne.
Lina

Lenis Lat. "Mild, soft, silky." Very rare.
Lene, Leneta, Lenice, Lenita, Lenos

Lenna (fem. **Leonard**) OG. "Lion's strength."
Lenda

Lenore Gk. "Light." Var. **Eleanor.**
Lenor, Lenora, Lenorah, Leonora, Leonore

Leoda OG. "Of the people."
Leota

Leona (fem. **Leon**) Lat. "Lion." American version; Leonie is more popular in Europe. Use since the 1940s has grown, but the notorious Leona Helmsley has probably put a stop to its popularity. Singer Leontyne Price.
Leoine, Leola, Leone, Leonelle, Leonia, Leonie, Leontine, Leontyne

Leonarda (fem. **Leonard**) OG. "Lion's strength."
Lenda, Leonarde

Leonie (fem. **Leon**) Lat. "Lion." The French form of the name, more common in Britain than **Leona**.
Leoline, Leone, Leoni, Leonine, Leontine

Leonora Gk. "Light." Var. **Eleanor**. Name used for the heroine of three major operas (*Fidelio, Il Trovatore,* and *La Favorita*), but like many literary names, uncommon in real life.
Leanor, Leanora, Leanore, Lenora, Lenore, Leonore, Nora, Norah

Leopoldine (fem. **Leopold**) OG. "Bold people."
Leopolda, Leopoldina

Leora Gk. "Light." Dim. **Eleanor**.

Leslie Scot. Gael. Place name. Some sources suggest, "the gray castle." Became a last name, then (in the 18th century) a first name used for boys and girls. Boys' use has been tied to admiration for actor Leslie Howard, and is more common in Britain. Not much used now. Actresses Leslie-Ann Down, Lesley Ann Warren.
Leslea, Leslee, Lesley, Lesli, Lesly, Lezlee, Lezley, Lezlie

Leta Lat. "Glad, joyful." Classical name mildly revived at the turn of the 20th century.

Letha Gk. "Forgetfulness." In Greek myth, a river in Hades that causes the dead to forget their lives on earth.
Leitha, Leithia, Lethe, Lethia

Letitia Lat. "Joy, gladness." In medieval England, the form was Lettice, which survived into the 20th century. (The name's resemblance to the principal ingredient of salad cannot have helped its popularity.) Current use, which is rare, is usually of the Latinized form, Letitia. Etiquette expert Letitia Baldrige.
Laetitia, Laetizia, Latashia, Latia, Latisha, Leda, Leta, Letha, Letice, Leticia, Letisha, Letizia, Letta, Lettice, Lettie, Lettitia, Letty, Tish, Tisha

Levana Lat. "To rise." In Roman mythology, the goddess of newborn babies, whose fathers accepted them as legitimate in a ceremony involving lifting the infant from the ground.
Levania, Levanna, Levona

Levina Lat. "Lightning bolt."
Lewana Heb. "Shining white one: the moon."
   Levana, Levanna, Lewanna, Livana
Lexia Dim. **Alexandra**. Gk. "Defender of mankind."
   Lexa, Lexie, Lexina, Lexine
Leya Sp. "The law."
Liana Fr. "To twine around." Liana is the name of a vine
common to tropical rain forests. Can also be a diminu-
tive of Italianate names like Ceciliana or Silviana.
   Leana, Liane, Lianna, Lianne
Liane Diminutive of French variants like Juliane, Lilliane.
Also a spelling variant of Lee-Ann.
Libby Dim. **Elizabeth**. Heb. "Pledged to God."
   Lib, Libbee, Libbey, Libbie
Liberty Middle English. "Freedom." Unusual, but occurs
in "revolutionary" times like the 1970s.
Lida Slavic. "Loved by the people."
   Lyda
Liese Dim. **Elizabeth**. Heb. "Pledged to God." Mostly
found in Germany.
   Liesa, Liesel, Liesl
Lieselotte Com. form **Liese**. Heb. "Pledged to God" and
Charlotte. Fr. "little feminine."
Lila Arab. "Night." Can be a diminutive of **Delilah**. Heb.
"lovelorn, seductive." Philanthropist Lila Acheson Wal-
lace.
   Layla, Leila, Lilah, Lyla, Lylah
Lilac Flower name. Not very common.
Lilias Scot. Var. **Lillian**. Lat. "Lily."
   Lillias
Lilibet Dim. **Elizabeth**. Heb. "Pledged to God." The un-
likely pet name of Queen Elizabeth II of England.
   Lillibet, Lilybet
Lilith Arab. "Ghost, night demon." One Old Testament
translation refers to her as "the night hag." She was sup-
posed to descend on sleepers and suck their blood. Con-
notations of the name are so fearsome that it is rarely
used.
   Lillis
Lillian Lat. Very common variation of the flower name,

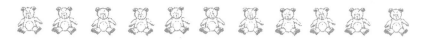

flourishing at the turn of the 20th century. Actress Lillian Gish and First Mother Lillian Carter were born during the name's peak of fashion, which faded after the 1930s. Writer Lillian Hellman.

Lila, Lili, Lilia, Lilian, Liliana, Liliane, Lilias, Lilli, Lillia, Lillianne, Lillie, Lilly, Lillyan, Lillyanne, Lily, Lilyan, Lilyann

Lily Lat. Flower name. Possibly because the lily plays such a large part in Christian iconography, this has been one of the most popular of the flower names and has produced many variants. The "-y" ending, usually thought of as feminine, has probably also boosted its use, though it has not been popular since 1900. Ripe for a revival among parents with a taste for nostalgia. Actress Lillie Langtry.

Lil, Lila, Lilas, Lili, Lilia, Lilian, Liliana, Liliane, Lilias, Lilie, Lilla, Lilley, Lilli, Lillia, Lillianne, Lillie, Lilly, Lily, Lilyan, Lilyanne

Lina Diminutive of names ending with "-line," like Caroline, Helena, Marlene. Var. **Lena**. Given as an independent name from the 1850s.

Linda Sp. "Pretty." Though the name existed as a particle of other English names (Belinda, Melinda) by the time of its great vogue in the 20th century (late 1930s to 1960s), it was probably interpreted as "pretty." Rather neglected now. President's daughter Lynda Bird Johnson; actresses Linda Evans, Linda Hunt; singer Linda Ronstadt; journalist Linda Ellerbee.

Lin, Lindee, Lindey, Lindi, Lindie, Lindy, Linn, Lynda, Lynde, Lyndy, Lyn, Lynn, Lynne, Lynnda, Lynndie

Lindsay OE. Place name: "Island of linden trees." Originally a surname, used for boys until the middle of this century, but now quite popular as a girl's name. Actress Lindsay Wagner.

Lind, Lindsea, Lindsee, Lindsey, Lindsy, Linzee, Linzy, Lyndsay, Lyndsey, Lyndsie, Lynnsey, Lynndsie, Lynnzey, Lynsey

Linette Welsh. "idol"; OF. "linnet" (a small bird). In historical terms, probably a variant of Lynette, which is not, surprisingly enough, a form of Lynn. These names and

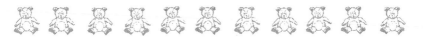

their variations were most popular from the 1940s into the 1960s.

Lanette, Linet, Linnet, Linnetta, Lynette, Lynnet, Lynnette

Linnea Scan. "lime or linden tree" is the meaning given by most sources, but an informal network of people named Linnea trace the name to a mountain flower growing in northern climates that botanist Carl Linnaeus named for himself.

Linea, Linnaea, Lynea, Lynnea

Lisa Dim. **Elizabeth**. Heb. "pledged to God." Used in numbers only since the 1950s, and quite a favorite in the last decade. Actress Lisa Bonet.

Leesa, Leeza, Liesa, Liesebet, Lise, Liseta, Lisetta, Lisette, Liszka

Lissa Dim. **Melissa**. Gk. "bee." May also be considered a variation of **Lisa**. Unusual.

Livia Dim. **Olivia**. Lat. "Olive." Though the historical connotations of Olivia should concern peace and harmony, in the modern era it is hard not to think of the little green morsel at the bottom of a martini glass. Joyce fans, on a higher plane, may use the name to pay homage to the character Anna Livia Plurabelle from *Finnegan's Wake*.

Liza Diminutive of **Elizabeth** and more particularly of **Eliza**. The vogue for Lisa has given Liza some reflected popularity. Entertainer Liza Minnelli.

Lizette, Lizzie, Lyza

Loelia Var. **Leila**. Arab. "Night." Unusual form used occasionally at the turn of the 20th century.

Lois Var. **Louise**. OG. "Renowned in battle." Also, surprisingly enough, a biblical name. Use peaked early in the 20th century. Superman's consort Lois Lane.

Lola Dim. **Dolores**. Sp. "Sorrows." The most famous Lola has been the 19th-century courtesan Lola Montez, which has given the name a slightly racy aura. It is fairly well used regardless.

Lolita Dim. **Lola**. Sp. "Sorrows." Made famous by Vladimir Nabokov's 1958 novel about the 12-year-old nymphet and her older admirer, Humbert Humbert.

Lona Var. **Leona**. Lat. "Lion." Uncommon.

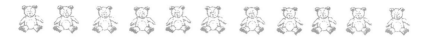

Lonee, Lonie, Lonna, Lonnie

Lora Var. **Laura**. Lat. "Laurel." Not, as it might seem, a modern phonetic variant, but a throwback to the 14th century, when this was the usual spelling of the name.
Loree, Lorey, Lori, Lorra, Lorree, Lorrie, Lory

Lorelei Ger. Place name. Derives from the name of a dangerous rock jutting into the Rhine. Though popularly supposed to be an old myth, the tale of a siren perched on the rock to lure ships to destruction actually dates from a novel of 1801. The name, however, carries connotations of risky allure.
Loralee, Loralie, Loralyn, Lorilee, Lorilyn, Lura, Lurette, Lurleen, Lurlene, Lurline

Lorelle Dim. **Laura** or **Laurel**. Lat. "Laurel tree."

Lorenza (fem. **Lorenzo**) Lat. "From Laurentium." Very unusual in English-speaking countries, being primarily an Italian name.

Loretta Dim. **Laura**. Lat. "Laurel." A name that cropped up with the 19th-century taste for elaboration, and became famous with actress Loretta Young. Country singer Loretta Lynn; actress Loretta Swit.
Larretta, Lauretta, Laurette, Lorretta

Lori Dim. **Laura**. Lat. "Laurel." Unlike Lora, this is a modern spelling and was very popular in the 1960s. The rage for the "-i" ending on names has diminished considerably since then.

Lorna Scot. Place name converted into a female name for the 19th-century romantic novel *Lorna Doone*. Used occasionally, but to most North Americans, is probably the name of a cookie. Entertainer Lorna Luft.
Lorrna

Lorraine Fr. "From Lorraine." Lorraine is an area in eastern France, but this is not just your average place name: It was often used for Joan of Arc (who was from Lorraine). It can also be considered an elaboration of **Lora**. Was well used from the 1930s, and in the U.S. its vogue peaked in the 1940s. Rare now. Actress Laraine Newman.
Laraine, Laurraine, Lorain, Loraine, Lori, Lorine, Lorrayne

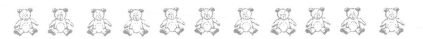

Lottie Dim. **Charlotte**. Fr. "Little, womanly." Mostly 19th-century use. Singer Lotte Lenya.
Lotta, Lotte, Lotie, Lotti, Lotty

Lotus Gk. "Lotus flower." The name signifies different plants in several different cultures: The Egyptians consider it a kind of water lily, while to the Greeks it is a shrub. It also has great significance in the Indian religions and in Homeric legend, where eating the lotus causes people to forget their homes and families and long for a life of idleness.

Lou Dim. **Louise**. Used mostly in America, and in combined forms such as Louann, Louella, etc.
Lu, Loulou

Louise (fem. **Louis**) OG. "Renowned in battle." Actually a French (and more euphonious) version of Ludwig. Louisa was the preferred form in the 18th and 19th centuries, eclipsed by Louise at the turn of the century. Currently experiencing a revival in Britain, but rare in the U.S. Author Louisa May Alcott, actresses Louise Brooks, Louise Lasser.
Aloisa, Aloise, Aloysia, Eloisa, Eloise, Heloisa, Heloise, Lois, Loise, Lola, Lolita, Lou, Louisa, Louisetta, Louisette, Louisina, Louisiana, Louisiane, Louisine, Louiza, Lovisa, Lowise, Loyise, Lu, Ludovica, Ludovika, Ludwiga, Luisa, Luise, Lujza, Lujzika, Lula, Lulita, Lulu

Love OE. "Love." Unromantically enough, probably not the name of the emotion but a transferred surname.
Loveday, Lovey

Luana OG. Com. form **Louise** and **Anne**. One of many possible phonetic versions of the name.
Lewanna, Louanna, Louanne, Luane, Luann, Luannie, Luwana

Lucerne Lat. "Lamp." Also the name of a city in Switzerland; parents have occasionally named children for the cities where they were born—or, in the modern era of frankness, conceived.
Lucerna

Lucetta Dim. **Lucy**. Lat. "Light." Mostly 19th century, now very unusual.
Lucette

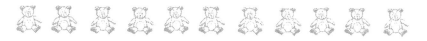

Lucia It. Var. **Lucy**. Lat. "Light." Uncommon form in English-speaking countries. Ballet patron Lucia Chase.

Lucille Fr. Var. **Lucy**. Lat. "Light." As Lucilla, used by the Romans and revived in the 19th century. Lucille came into use at the turn of the 20th century, and its considerable popularity (roughly 1940–1960) seems to have been inspired by comedienne Lucille Ball.
Lucila, Lucile, Lucilla

Lucinda var. **Lucy** (Lat. "light") Popular along with the other "-inda" names of the 18th century (Clarinda, Belinda), and boosted by the fondness for Lucille.
Cindy

Lucita Sp. Dim. **Lucy**. (Lat. "light") Also an allusion to the Virgin Mary as Santa Maria de Luz.

Lucretia Lat. Clan name of uncertain meaning, though some sources suggest "wealth." The famous story of the rape of Lucretia concerns a Roman matron who, having been raped, stabbed herself rather than live with the shame.
Lucrece, Lucrecia, Lucreecia, Lucrezia

Lucy Lat. "Light." The vernacular form of Lucia, and more widely used in modern times, peaking in the U.S. at the turn of the century. The 4th-century martyr Saint Lucy, patroness of sight, is often depicted with a pair of eyes in a dish, though her martyrdom did not involve being blinded. The Lucy in Charles Schulz's much-loved *Peanuts* comic strip is the prototypical bossy little girl. A few parents (especially in Britain) use the name regardless.
Lou, Loulou, Lu, Luce, Lucetta, Lucette, Luci, Lucia, Luciana, Lucida, Lucie, Lucienne, Lucile, Lucilia, Lucilla, Lucille, Lucina, Lucinda, Lucine, Lucita, Lucyna, Lucza, Luz

Ludmilla Slavic. "Beloved of the people."
Ludmila, Lyuba, Lyudmila

Luella OE. Com. form **Louise** OG. "renowned in battle," and **Ella**. OG. "all." Can also be said to come from Lucy; it's often not possible to trace a name's roots accurately. Columnist Louella Parsons.
Loella, Lou, Louella, Lu, Luelle, Lula, Lulu

Lulu Dim. **Louise**. OG. "Renowned in battle."
Luna Lat. "Moon."
Lunetta, Lunette, Lunneta
Lupe Sp. Allusion to the Virgin Mary as she miraculously appeared to a peasant boy in Guadalupe, Mexico.
Lurleen Modern variant of **Lorelei**. Ger. place name.
Lura, Lurette, Lurlene, Lurline
Luz Sp. "Light." Another name for the Virgin Mary: Santa Maria de Luz.
Lydia Gk. "From Lydia." Lydia was an area of Asia famous for its two rich kings, Midas and Croesus. The name (biblical in origin) was used heavily in the 18th and 19th centuries, less so in the 20th.
Lidia, Lidija, Lydie
Lynette Welsh. "Idol." Though it looks like a modern elaboration of Lynn, this is actually a French version of the Welsh Eiluned, and was popularized by the English poet Tennyson. However, its use (middling, since the 1940s) has certainly depended on the appeal of Lynn.
Lynn Dim. **Linda**. Sp. "Pretty." This is one of those names that, along with its variations, is so popular as to virtually swamp its source. Most used in the 20th century. Actress Lynn Redgrave.
Lin, Linell, Linn, Linnell, Lyn, Lyndel, Lyndell, Lynelle, Lynette, Lynna, Lynne, Lynell, Lynnelle, Lynnett, Lynette

Mab Ir. Gael. "joy, hilarity." Welsh. "baby." In old English, Welsh, and Irish stories, Queen Mab is monarch of the fairies.
Mave, Mavis, Meave
Mabel Dim. **Amabel**. Lat. "Lovable." Very popular at the turn of the 20th century, but uncommon now, perhaps because it has the air of being a period artifact. Singer Mabel Mercer.
Amabel, Amable, Amaybel, Amaybelle, Amayble, Mab, Mabelle, Mable, Maible, Maybel, Maybelle, Mayble

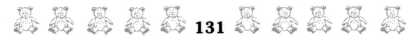

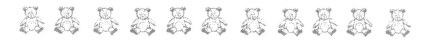

Madeline Gk. Place name: Magdala was a town on the Sea of Galilee, the home of Saint Mary Magdalen, whom Jesus healed and who was present at his crucifixion. Magdalen was the common form in the Middle Ages, but the *g* was dropped, leaving Madeline as the standard form. The French version, Madeleine, became more popular in the 1930s, but the name, pretty as it is, has never been a standard. Many people may be familiar with this name from Ludwig Bemelman's French school girl Madeline in her wide-brimmed hat, from the children's books. Actress Madeline Kahn.

Dalanna, Dalenna, Lena, Lina, Lynn, Mada, Madalaina, Madaleine, Madalena, Madalyn, Maddalena, Maddie, Maddy, Madel, Madelaine, Madelayne, Madeleine, Madelena, Madelene, Madelina, Madella, Madelle, Madelon, Madge, Madlen, Madlin, Madlyn, Mady, Magda, Magdala, Magdalen, Magdalena, Magdalene, Magdolna, Maidel, Maighdlin, Mala, Malena, Malina, Marleah, Marleen, Marlena, Marlene, Marline, Marlyne, Maud, Maude

Madge Dim. **Madeline, Margaret**. Gk. "Pearl."

Madonna Lat. "My lady." Used mostly by devout Catholic families, like the parents of rock star Madonna Louise Ciccone.

Madra Sp. "Mother."

Maeve Ir. Gael. Possibly "delicate, fragile." Name of a 1st-century queen of Ireland, and used mostly in that country.

Magda Ger. Var. **Madeline** Gk. "from Magdala" or **Maida** (OE. "maiden").

Maggie Dim. **Margaret**. Gk. "pearl." Used as an independent name in the late 19th century. Although babies are more likely to be given the full name these days, Maggie is precisely the kind of nostalgic-sounding nickname that is expected to be popular in the 1990s.

Maggey, Maggi, Maggy

Magnilda OG. "Strong in warfare."

Magnhilde

Magnolia Lat. Flower name. The tree was named after 17th-century French botanist Pierre Magnol. Because of

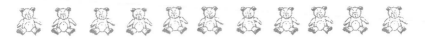

the tree's popularity on old southern plantations, the name is redolent of Dixie.

Maggie, Maggy, Nola

Mahala Heb. "Tender affection." Old Testament name that was well used in the 19th century. Singer Mahalia Jackson is keeping it alive today.

Mahalah, Mahalia, Mahaliah, Mahalla, Mahelia, Mehalia

Maia Gk. "Mother." In Greek myth, a nymph who became mother of Hermes; also the Roman goddess of the springtime, for whom the month of May is named. Writer Maya Angelou.

Maaja, Maiah, Maj, Maja, May, Maya, Mya

Maida OE. "Maiden." Used with some frequency in the 19th century, often in the diminutive form Maidie.

Maddie, Maddy, Mady, Magda, Maidel, Maidie, Mayda, Maydena, Maydey

Maisie Dim. Margaret. Gk. "Pearl." Originally a Scottish variation by way of Margery, it became more widespread early in the 20th century. Literary parents may be reminded of Henry James's novel *What Maisie Knew*.

Maisey, Maisy, Maizie, Mazie

Majesta Lat. "Majesty."

Majidah Arab. "Splendid."

Majida

Malka Heb. "Queen."

Malcah, Malkah, Malkie, Milcah

Mallory OF. "Unhappy, unlucky." Literally, *malheureux*. Originally a nickname, transferred to a last name and thus to a first name. Used for boys as well, but feminine use probably has the edge.

Malloreigh, Mallorey, Mallorie, Malorey, Malorie, Malory

Malva Gk. "Slender, delicate." Also a flower name.

Melva, Melvina

Malvina Literary name invented by a romantic poet of the 18th century: It may come from the Gaelic words for "smooth brow." Sculptor Malvina Hoffman.

Mal, Malva, Malvie, Mel, Melva, Melvie, Melvina, Melvine

Mamie Dim. Margaret. Gk. "pearl" or **Mary**. Heb. "bitter." First Lady Mamie Eisenhower.

Mame

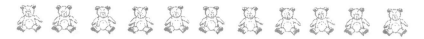

Manda Dim. **Amanda**. Lat. "Much-loved."
Mandee, Mandie, Mandy

Mandisa South African. "Sweet."

Mandy Dim. **Amanda**. Lat. "much-loved." Popular in Great Britain a generation ago.
Mandee, Mandie

Mansi Hopi. "Plucked flower."

Manuela (fem. **Emmanuel**) Sp. from Heb. "the Lord is among us."
Manuelita

Mara Heb. "Bitter." In the Old Testament, Naomi says, "Call me Mara, for the Almighty has dealt very bitterly with me." This is widely considered to be the root of that all-time favorite, **Mary**.
Mahra, Marah, Maralina, Maraline, Mari, Marra

Marcella (fem. **Marcellus**) Lat. "Warlike." First cropped up at the turn of the 20th century. Very unusual.
Marcela, Marcele, Marcelle, Marcellina, Marcelline, Marchella, Marchelle, Marcie, Marcile, Marcille, Marcy, Marquita, Marsella, Marselle, Marshella, Marsiella

Marcene (fem. **Mark**) Lat. "Warlike." An American variant that occurred in the 1940s and 1950s, following on the popularity of Marcia.
Marceen, Marcena, Marcenia, Marceyne, Marcina

Marcia (fem. **Mark**) Lat. "Warlike." Used in Imperial Rome and not revived until the late 19th century. It gradually became a great favorite in the middle of the 20th century, but was passé by the 1970s. Actress Marsha Mason.
Marcelia, Marcene, Marchita, Marci, Marciane, Marcie, Marcile, Marcille, Marcilyn, Marcilynn, Marcina, Marcita, Marcy, Marquita, Marsha, Martia

Marcy Dim. **Marcella**. Lat. "warlike." This is the most common form of Marcella's diminutives.
Marcee, Marcey, Marci, Marcie

Mare Ir. Var. **Mary**.
Maire

Marelda OG. "Renowned battle maid."
Marilda

Margaret Gk. "Pearl." One of the standard female names of the Western world. In the Middle Ages the virgin

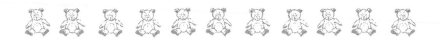

martyr Saint Margaret (swallowed by a dragon) was hugely popular, keeping the name current. An 11th-century queen of Scotland was also a saint, and the name is especially common in Scotland. It has been neck and neck with Mary from the 17th century until the 1970s, when more novel names have moved to the forefront. Britain's Princess Margaret and Prime Minister Margaret Thatcher; actress Margaret Sullavan; anthropologist Margaret Mead; writer Margaret Mitchell.

Greta, Gretal, Gretchen, Gretel, Grethel, Gretta, Grette, Gretl, Madge, Mag, Maggi, Maggie, Maggy, Maiga, Maighread, Mairead, Maisie, Maisy, Malgorzata, Marga, Margalit, Margalo, Margareta, Margarete, Margaretha, Margarethe, Margaretta, Margarette, Margarida, Margarit, Margarita, Margarite, Marge, Margeret, Margeretta, Margerie, Margerita, Margery, Marget, Margette, Margey, Margharita, Margherita, Margie, Margies, Margisia, Margit, Margo, Margot, Margret, Margreth, Margrett, Marguarette, Marguarita, Marguerita, Marguerite, Marguita, Margy, Marjery, Marjey, Marji, Marjie, Marjorey, Marjorie, Marjory, Marketa, Markita, Meg, Megan, Meggi, Meggie, Meggy, Meghan, Meta, Metta, Mette, Meyta, Peg, Pegeen, Peggie, Peggy, Rita

Margery Fr. dim. **Margaret**. Imported to England in the 12th century and steadily used there until a late–19th-century revival that lasted into the 1930s, usually as Marjorie. Because it is unusual but not outlandish, a good candidate for a 1990s revival. Novelists Margery Allingham, Margery Sharp.

Marge, Margeree, Margerey, Margerie, Margey, Margi, Margie, Margy, Marje, Marjerie, Marjery, Marjie, Marjorey, Marjori, Marjorie, Marjory, Marjy

Margo Fr. Dim. **Margaret**. Another import that never matched the popularity of Margery. Actress Margaux Hemingway changed the spelling of her name to match that of a famous Bordeaux wine, Chateau Margaux. Ballet star Dame Margot Fonteyn.

Margaux, Margot

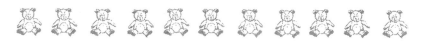

Marguerite Fr. Var. **Margaret**. Also botanical, the French name for Daisy, and popular at the same time (late 19th century to mid–20th) as that flower name.
Margarite, Margherita, Margherite, Marguerita, Margurite

Maria Lat. Var. **Mary**. Launched in English-speaking countries in the 18th century as a welcome alternative to the all-too-common Mary. Faded after some 200 years, but revived in the middle of the 20th century, particularly after the popularity of *West Side Story*, with its famous ballad "Maria." Singer Maria Muldaur, TV journalist Maria Shriver.
Mariah, Marie, Marja, Marya

Marian Fr. com. form **Mary** Heb. "Bitter" and **Ann** Heb. "Grace." Var. **Mary**. Actually an anglicization of Marion. Common in the Middle Ages, and after a period of neglect, revived in the early Victorian era when medieval history was very popular. Singer Marian Anderson; Robin Hood's love interest Maid Marian.
Mariam, Mariana, Mariane, Marion, Maryann, Maryanne

Marianne Fr. Com. form **Marie** Heb. "bitter" and **Anne** Heb. "grace." Like Annemarie, combines the names of the Virgin Mary and her mother, thus appealing powerfully to Catholic families. In English-speaking countries Mary Ann is the standard form, though Marianne has had moments of fashion, in the early 19th and mid–20th centuries. Marianne is the name of the official symbol who personifies the spirit of France.
Mariana, Mariane, Mariann, Marianna, Maryann, Maryanna

Maribel Com. form **Mary** Heb. "bitter" and **Belle** Fr. "beautiful." This is a modern name.
Maribelle, Marybelle

Marie Fr. Var. **Mary**. Also the earliest English spelling of the name, revived in the 19th century, and in the 1970s nearly as popular as Mary. Now much less in vogue. Scientist Madam Marie Curie; singer Marie Osmond.
Maree

Mariel Dutch. Var. of **Mary**. Actress Mariel Hemingway.
Marella, Marelle, Marial, Marieke, Mariela, Mariele, Mariella, Marielle, Mariet, Marijke, Marilla

Marietta Fr. Dim. **Mary**, via **Marie**. Current since the mid–19th century. Philanthropist Marietta Tree.
Maretta

Marigold Flower name. The golden yellow flower, whose name is a combination of Mary and gold. It cropped up in the 20th century, a bit later than the 19th-century craze for flower names.

Marika Dutch. Var. **Mary**.
Marieke, Marijke, Marike, Mariska, Mariske, Maryk

Marilyn Dim. **Mary**. Possibly also a combination of **Mary** and **Ellen**. In any case, a modern name promoted by show business, not in the person of Marilyn Monroe (whose career in the 1950s paralleled the name's decline), but by an earlier star, Marilyn Miller. As is often the case with modern names, there are numerous phonetic variations.
Maralin, Maralynn, Marelyn, Marilee, Marilin, Marillyn, Marilynne, Marralynn, Marrilin, Marrilyn, Marylin, Marylyn

Marina Lat. "From the sea." Also possibly, in the distant mists of time, related to the Latin god of war, Mars.
Marena, Marine, Marinna, Marna, Marne, Marni, Marnie

Marion Fr. Dim. **Mary**. Though it was turned into Marian when it arrived in Britain in the Middle Ages, this form was revived as well in the 19th century and is now just as common. It is occasionally used for boys as well.
Marian, Maryon, Maryonn

Maris Lat. "Of the sea." Comes from the phrase *stella maris*, or "star of the sea," which refers to the Virgin Mary.
Marisa, Marise, Marissa, Marisse, Marris, Marys, Maryse, Meris

Marisol Com. form **Mary** Heb. "Bitter" and *sol* (Sp. "sun"). A modern name particularly favored in Puerto Rico.

Marissa Var. **Maris**. Lat. "Of the sea."
Maressa, Marisa, Marisse, Marrissa, Merissa, Morissa

Marjolaine Fr. "Marjoram." Unusual botanical name.

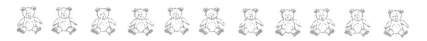

Marjorie Var. **Margery,** dim. **Margaret.** Imported to England in the 12th century as Margery, and steadily used there until a late–19th-century revival that lasted into the 1930s. This is currently the most common form, though the name is infrequently given.
Marge, Margeree, Margerey, Margerie, Margery, Margey, Margi, Margie, Margy, Marje, Marjerie, Marjery, Marjie, Marjorey, Marjori, Marjory, Marjy

Marla Var. **Marlene.** Appeared in the 1940s, but hard to find since the 1970s. Actress Marla Gibbs.

Marlene Com. form **Mary** Heb. "bitter" and **Magdalene** Gk. "from Magdala." Marlene Dietrich introduced the name in the 1920s, and it was widespread by the 1940s, but is now rare. Actress Marlee Matlin.
Marla, Marlaina, Marlane, Marlayne, Marlea, Marlee, Marleen, Marlena, Marley, Marlie, Marline, Marlyn, Marlynne, Marna

Marlo Modern name, possibly a variation of the last name **Marlow,** or a diminutive of **Marlene.** Briefly popular in the 1970s, perhaps following the TV career of comedienne Marlo Thomas.
Marlon, Marlow, Marlowe

Marmara Gk. "Sparkling, shining."
Marmee

Marna Origin disputed. May be a diminutive of **Marina** or of **Marlene.**
Marne, Marney, Marni, Marnia, Marnie, Marnja, Marnya

Marsha Var. **Marcia.** The more common form in America.

Martha Aramaic. "Lady." In the New Testament, Martha is the woman who bustles around resentfully getting dinner ready while her sister Mary listens to Jesus. She is patron saint of the helping professions. The name has been very widely used since the Puritans revived it, though it is less common in the last 40 years. First Lady Martha Washington; dancer Martha Graham; Martha "Calamity" Jane Burke.
Mariet, Marit, Mart, Marta, Martella, Martelle, Marth, Marthe, Marthena, Marti, Martie, Martina, Martita, Marty, Martynne, Martyne, Matti, Mattie, Pat, Pattie

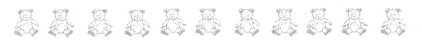

Martina (fem. **Martin**) Lat. "Warlike." Tennis star Martina Navratilova.
> **Marta, Martie, Martine, Marty, Tina, Tine**

Marvel OF. "Something to marvel at."
> **Marva, Marvela, Marvele, Marvella, Marvelle**

Mary Heb. Though "bitter, bitterness" is the most commonly accepted meaning, the *Facts on File Dictionary of First Names* disputes this. "Rebellious" is also sometimes suggested. Mary is the Greek version of Miriam. Although until the Middle Ages it was thought of as too sacred to use, it gradually became the most common female name. The numerous variants, both English and foreign, cropped up as a result of the name's great popularity. In the modern era it is frequently combined with other names (Mary Jo, Mary Lou, Mary Beth). Ironically, the name once thought of as completely commonplace is now very rare among young children. Actresses Mary Pickford and Mary Martin; Queens Marie Antoinette and Mary of Scots; artist Mary Cassatt; writer Mary Shelley.
> **Mair, Marie, Mal, Malia, Mallie, Mame, Mamie, Manette, Manon, Manya, Mara, Marabel, Marabelle, Mare, Maree, Marella, Marelle, Maren, Maretta, Marette, Maria, Mariam, Marian, Mariann, Marianna, Marianne, Marice, Maridel, Marie, Mariel, Mariella, Marielle, Marietta, Mariette, Marilee, Marilin, Marilla, Marilyn, Marin, Marion, Mariquilla, Mariquita, Mariska, Marita, Maritsa, Maritza, Marja, Marje, Marla, Marlo, Marya, Maryann, Maryanne, Marylin, Marysa, Maryse, Marysia, Masha, Maura, Maure, Maureen, Maurene, Maurine, Maurise, Maurita, Maurizia, Mavra, May, Mayme, Maymie, Meridel, Meriel, Mimi, Minette, Minnie, Minny, Miriam, Mitzi, Moira, Moire, Moll, Mollie, Molly, Morag, Moya, Muire, Murial, Muriel, Murielle, Poll, Polly**

Matilda OG. "Battle-mighty." William the Conqueror's wife took the name to Britain in the 11th century, when it was pronounced Maud. It was revived in the 18th century, but faded again in the 19th, and was never a real favorite in the U.S. Most parents know it only from the famous Australian song "Waltzing Matilda."

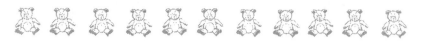

Maitilde, Mat, Matelda, Mathilda, Mathilde, Matilde, Matti, Mattie, Matty, Maud, Maude, Maudie, Tilda, Tilde, Tildie, Tildy, Tilli, Tillie, Tilly

Mattea (fem. **Matthew**) Heb. "Gift of God."
Mathea, Mathia, Matthea, Matthia, Mattia

Maud Var. of **Matilda**. OG. "Battle-mighty." Although a common enough name after the Middle Ages, its period of real popularity was 1840–1910, especially in Britain. Now rare. Actress Maude Adams.
Maude, Maudie

Maura Ir. Var. **Mary**.
Moira, Mora

Maureen Ir. Var. **Mary**. Popular in the baby boom era, but not among baby boomers who are now parents. Actresses Maureen O'Sullivan, Maureen O'Hara.
Maura, Maurene, Maurine, Maurise, Maurita, Maurizia, Mavra, Moira, Mora, Moreen, Morena, Morene, Moria, Morine

Mauve Fr. "Mallow plant." The petals of the mallow are purple, hence the use of this word for a color.
Malva

Mavis Fr. "Thrush." Popular mostly in Britain from the turn of the 20th century into the thirties.

Maxine Lat. "Greatest." A modern name that had its moment from the fifties through the seventies.
Massima, Max, Maxeen, Maxena, Maxene, Maxie, Maxime, Maxina, Maxy

May Several possible sources: a medieval form of **Matthew** (Mayhew), a nickname form of **Mary**, or an anglicization of **Maia**. It was very fashionable in the U.S. in the 1870s, some 50 years before month names (April and June) became current. Actress Mae West; writer Maya Angelou; poet May Sarton.
Mae, Maia, Maj, Mala, Maya, Maye, Mei

Mead OE. Place name: "Meadow." This is more common as a last name.
Meade

Meara Ir. Gael. "Jollity."

Medea Gk. "Ruling." Since the Medea of Greek myth was a witch who left a trail of dead bodies behind her (in-

cluding those of her two children), the name has grue-some connotations and is rarely used.

Madora, Medeia, Media, Medora, Medorah

Meg Dim. **Margaret**. Rarely given as an independent name. Actresses Meg Tilly, Meg Ryan.

Megan Welsh. Dim. **Margaret**. Fairly widespread in the 20th century, especially in the U.S.

Maegan, Meagan, Meaghan, Meg, Megen, Meggi,
Meggie, Meggy, Meghan, Meghann, Meghanne

Mehitabel Heb. "Benefited by God." Old Testament name rarely used, except by writer Don Marquis in his tales of the great friends *archy and mehitabel,* a cockroach and a cat.

Mehetabel, Mehitabelle, Hetty, Hitty

Meira Heb. "Light."

Melanie Gk. "Black, dark-skinned." Uncommon until the publication of *Gone With the Wind,* whose Melanie Wilkes launched it into fashion. Scarlett, though the more memorable character, did not inspire parents in the same way. Actresses Melanie Mayron, Melanie Griffith.

Malanie, Mel, Mela, Melaney, Melani, Melania, Melanney,
Melannie, Melantha, Melany, Mella, Mellanie, Melli,
Mellie, Melloney, Melly, Meloni, Melonie, Melonnie,
Melony, Milena

Melantha Gk. "Dark flower."

Melba Name coined in honor of the Australian operatic soprano Nellie Melba (the dessert peach Melba was also named after her). She, in turn, took her name from her hometown, Melbourne. Actress Melba Moore.

Malva, Melva

Melina Gk. "Honey." Use was mostly 19th century. Actress Melina Mercouri.

Meleana

Melinda Lat. "Honey." Names ending in "-inda" (Belinda, Clarinda) were very fashionable in the 18th century, when this name was coined. It became more widespread in the 19th century, but is still far from common.

Linda, Lindy, Linnie, Lynda, Maillie, Malina, Malinda,

Malinde, Mallie, Mally, Malynda, Mandy, Melina, Melinde, Meline, Mellinda, Melynda

Meliora Lat. "Better." Unusual Roman name used by the Puritans, but now rare.

Melisande Fr. Var. Melissa.
Lisandra, Malisande, Malissande, Malyssandre, Melesande, Melisandra, Melisandre, Melissande, Melissandre, Mellisande, Melysande, Melyssandre

Melissa Gk. "Bee." A name that existed in ancient Greece and occurred steadily through the 19th century, but had no real vogue in English-speaking countries until the 1970s. Now somewhat neglected. Singer Melissa Manchester; actress Melissa Gilbert.
Lissa, Malissa, Mallissa, Mel, Melesa, Melessa, Melicent, Melisa, Melisande, Melise, Melisenda, Melisent, Melisse, Melita, Melitta, Mellicent, Mellie, Mellisa, Melly, Melosa, Milli, Millicent, Millie, Millisent, Millissent, Milly, Misha, Missie, Missy

Melita Gk. "honey."

Melody Gk. "Song." Though it occurred as early as the 13th century, common usage didn't develop until the 1940s, and didn't endure.
Melodey, Melodia, Melodie

Melvina Celt. "Chieftain." A variation of Malvina, itself a literary name coined in the 18th century. Melva is the most common variant, but all forms are rare.
Malvina, Melva, Melvena

Mercedes Sp. "Mercies." Refers to Santa Maria de las Mercedes, or Our Lady of the Mercies. Mostly Catholic use. Actresses Mercedes McCambridge, Mercedes Ruehl.
Merced, Mercede

Mercia OE. Place name: Refers to the English Kingdom of Mercia, which comprised much of central England in the 6th through 9th centuries. The name has been used mostly in the 20th century.

Mercy Middle English. "Mercy." One of the names of virtues that were so popular among the Puritans (who, since they were very pious but couldn't use saints' names, were often hard put to find appropriate names for their children).
Merci, Mercie, Mersey

Meredith Old Welsh. "Great ruler." Occasionally used for boys, especially in Wales. Elsewhere a girl's name, used with some frequency. Actress Meredith Baxter.
Meredithe, Meridith, Merridie, Merry

Meriel Var. **Muriel**. Ir. Gael. "Sea-bright."
Merial, Meriol, Merrill, Meryl

Merle Fr. "Blackbird." Use probably inspired by actress Merle Oberon, whose middle name it was. Little used recently.
Merl, Merla, Merlina, Merline, Merola, Meryl, Myrle, Myrleen, Myrlene, Myrline

Merry OE. "Lighthearted, happy." Also dim. **Meredith, Mercy**. May also be considered a variant of its homonym Mary.
Marrilee, Marylea, Marylee, Merree, Merri, Merrie, Merrielle, Merrile, Merrilee, Merrili, Merrily

Meryl Var. **Muriel** via Meriel. Strictly a 20th-century name, which in the U.S. is strongly associated with actress Meryl Streep.
Meral, Merel, Merrall, Merrell, Merril, Merrill, Merryl, Meryle, Meryll

Messina Lat. "Middle." Also a place name: Messina is a town in Sicily.

Meta Ger. Dim. **Margaret**. Use is mostly German.

Mia It. "Mine." Probably owes much of its use to the career of actress Mia Farrow.

Michaela (fem. **Michael**) Heb. "Who is like the Lord?" The most common feminine form of Michael is the French Michelle, but Michaela is gaining ground in Britain. Actress Michael Learned.
Micaela, Michal, Michael, Michaelina, Michaeline, Michaila, Michalin, Michele, Michelina, Micheline, Michelle, Mickee, Mickie, Miguela, Miguelina, Miguelita, Mikaela, Mikhaila, Mikhayla

Michelle (fem. **Michael**) Fr. var. Heb. "Who is like the Lord?" Spelled with one or two *l*s, fashionable right from its 1940s appearance in English-speaking countries. The Beatles' famous song "Michelle" gave the name

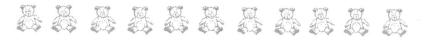

even more of a boost, putting it on some top-ten lists in the 1970s. Now past its prime. Actress Michelle Pfeiffer.

Mechelle, Mia, Micaela, Michaela, Michaelina, Michaeline, Michaella, Michal, Michele, Michelina, Micheline, Michell, Micki, Mickie, Midge, Miguela, Miguelita, Mikaela, Miquela, Misha, Mishelle

Michiko Jap. "The righteous way." The name of the first commoner ever to become empress of Japan.

Michee, Michi

Mignon Fr. "Cute." First used as a name by the German poet Goethe, and has spread from literary to real-life use, but not with great frequency.

Mignonette, Minyonne, Minyonette

Milada Czech. "My love."

Milagros Sp. "Miracles."

Mila, Milagritos, Miligrosa

Mildred OE. "Gentle strength." An Anglo-Saxon name that was revived in the 17th century, but its real popularity came in the U.S. 1900–1930. By the time of the 1945 film *Mildred Pierce,* it was already slightly dated.

Mildrid, Millie, Milly

Millicent OG. "Highborn power." Norman name that has been used mostly in Britain, at its most fashionable around 1900, but never a standard. U.S. Congresswoman Millicent Fenwick.

Lissa, Mel, Melicent, Melisande, Melisenda, Mellicent, Mellie, Mellisent, Melly, Milicent, Milissent, Millie, Millisent, Milly, Missie

Mimi Dim. **Mary, Miriam,** etc. First used by parents after the appearance of Puccini's famous opera *La Bohème,* whose tragic heroine is named Mimi.

Mindy Dim. **Melinda.**

Mindee, Mindie

Minerva The name of the Roman goddess of wisdom. Those great revivalists the Victorians brought it back for their daughters, but by the Jazz Age it was obsolete.

Min, Minette, Minnie, Myna

Minna Dim. **Wilhelmina.** Most common at the turn of the 20th century.

Min, Mina, Minetta, Minette, Minne, Minnie, Minny

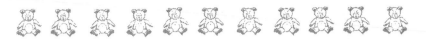

Minnie Dim. **Mary, Wilhelmina**. Enjoyed a great vogue as an independent name around the 1870s for no very clear reason. Most parents now will associate it with Mickey Mouse's girlfriend.

Minta Dim. **Araminta**. An 18th-century literary name.
Minty

Mira Lat. "Admirable." Dim. **Miranda** or var. **Myra**, although it is usually pronounced with a short *i*. In Spanish *mira* spelled this way means, "Look!" The name was most used in the 19th century.
Mireille, Mirella, Mirelle, Mireya, Mirielle, Mirilla, Mirra, Myra, Myrella, Myrène, Myrilla

Mirabel Lat. "Wonderful." In this case the "-bel" ending does not mean "beautiful," though the variations often spell it "-belle." In fact, it was at one period a man's name. Very rare.
Mira, Mirabella, Mirabelle

Miranda Lat. "Admirable." Another name contributed to us by Shakespeare, this time directly from the Latin: He used it for the heroine of *The Tempest*. Use has been steady but never widespread. Actress Miranda Richardson.
Mira, Miran, Myra, Myranda, Randa, Randi, Randie, Randy

Miriam Heb. Possibly "bitter" or "rebellious." This is the source of Mary, which is its Latin form, and its translation is not quite clear, though "bitter" is very widely accepted. Overlooked by the Puritan fervor for Old Testament names, but revived in the 18th century and quite common for some 250 years, peaking around 1900 in the U.S. Now unusual.
Mariam, Mimi, Mirham, Mirjam, Mirriam, Miryam, Mitzi, Mitzie

Missy Dim. **Melissa** or **Millicent**.

Misty OE. "Mist." Briefly popular in the U.S. in the middle of the 20th century.

Mitzi Ger. Var. **Mary**. Actress Mitzi Gaynor.
Mitzee, Mitzie

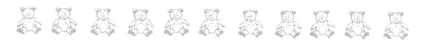

Modesty Lat. "Modesty." As Modesta, used by the Romans, but very rare ever since, even during the Puritan craze for virtue names.
Modesta, Modestia, Modestina, Modestine

Moira Ir. Var. **Mary**. Found mostly in Scotland. Dancer Moira Shearer.
Moyra

Mollie Dim. **Mary**. Not Irish, in spite of the famous song "Cockles and Mussels" about Dublin's "sweet Molly Malone." Since a "moll" has meant, at various times, a prostitute or a gangster's girlfriend, the name has had long periods of disuse, but now that these slang terms are obsolete, it may be ready for a revival. Actress Molly Ringwald.
Moll, Mollee, Molley, Molly

Mona Ir. Gael. "Aristocratic." Spread from Ireland in the mid–19th century. Never widespread, but common enough not to be outlandish.
Moina, Monah, Moyna

Monica Possibly Lat. "adviser" or "nun." Established by Saint Monica, the mother of Saint Augustine, and favored by Catholic families.
Mona, Monca, Monicka, Monika, Monike, Monique, Monnica

Morela Pol. "Apricot."

Morgana Different sources give different meanings, including Welsh "great and bright" and OE. "bright or white sea dweller." Morgan is most common in Wales as both a first and a last name, for both sexes. The current trend toward unisex names suggests that the feminizations are in for a spell of disuse. Actress Morgan Fairchild.
Morgan, Morgance, Morganica, Morganne, Morgen

Moriah Heb. "The Lord is my teacher."

Moselle (fem. **Moses**) Heb. Possibly "savior." Also a variety of delicately sweet white wine.

Mouna Arab. "Wish, desire."
Mounia, Muna

Muriel Ir. Gael. "Sea-bright." Some names, like this one, seem rooted in a certain period (in this case the first half of the 20th century), but Muriel actually dates back to

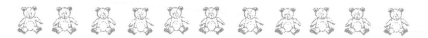

the Middle Ages. Perhaps the children of the 1990s will find it nostalgic enough to use for their children. Novelist Muriel Spark.
Meriel, Murial, Murielle

Musetta Middle French. "Little bagpipe." Musette came to be the term for a dance tune that employed the musette, an instrument fashionable in the 18th century.
Musette

Musidora Gk. "Gift of the Muses."

Myra (fem. **Myron**) Lat. "Scented oil." Literary name coined in the early 17th century, but real-life use dates from the 19th century. Harpsichordist Dame Myra Hess.

Myrna Ir. Gael. "Tender, beloved." Popularity, in the 1930s and 1940s, spans the career of actress Myrna Loy.
Merna, Mirna, Moina, Morna, Moyna, Muirna

Myrtle Botanical name. The myrtle is a dark green shrub with pink or white blossoms. The name first appeared in the 1850s, before the true vogue for flower names, but it became more popular along with those other names in the 1880s. Now dated.
Mertis, Mertle, Mirtle, Myrta, Myrtia, Myrtice, Myrtie, Myrtis

N

Naavah Heb. "Lovely."

Nabila Arab. "Highborn."
Nabeela

Nadette OG. "Bear/courageous." Dim. **Bernadette**.

Nadia Rus. "Hope." Nada appeared in English-speaking countries at the turn of the 20th century, but Nadia had taken root by the 1960s. Though not outlandish, it has a pleasantly foreign sound. Gymnast Nadia Comaneci; poet Nadezhda Mandelstam.
Nada, Nadege, Nadezhda, Nadiya, Nadja, Nady, Nadya, Nadyenka, Nadzia, Nata, Natka

Nadine Fr. Var. **Nadia**. Author Nadine Gordimer.

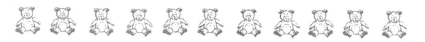

Nadeen, Nadena, Nadene, Nadina, Nadyna, Nadyne, Naydeen

Naida Gk. "Water nymph."

Naiad, Nayad, Nyad

Nan Var. **Ann.** Heb. "Grace." At its most common in the 18th century, but now occurs most often as a nickname for Ann. Its diminutives (Nana, Nanny) have come to mean grandmother or person who looks after children.

Nana, Nance, Nanci, Nancie, Nancy, Nanette, Nanine, Nanna, Nannie, Nanny, Nanon, Nettie

Nancy Var. **Ann.** Heb. "Grace." Also originally a nickname whose use as a given name began at roughly the same time as Nan, in the 18th century. Nancy, however, took root more firmly (perhaps because it had not acquired any other meanings) and was very popular in the U.S. in the middle of the 20th century. First Lady Nancy Reagan.

Nainsi, Nance, Nancee, Nanci, Nancie, Nancsi, Nanice, Nanncey, Nanncy, Nannie, Nanny, Nansee, Nansey

Nanette Fr. Dim. **Nan.**

Nannette, Nettie, Netty

Naomi Heb: "Pleasant." Old Testament name; the mother-in-law of Ruth, who, after her sons died, said, "Do not call me Naomi, call me Mara, for the Almighty has dealt very bitterly with me." Naomi came into English-speaking use not with the Puritan revival of biblical names, but in the 18th century.

Naoma, Naomia, Naomie, Navit, Noami, Noemi, Noemie

Narcissa Gk. "Daffodil." Not actually a flower name, but the unusual feminine version of the masculine (and equally unusual) Narcisse, which comes from the legend of the beautiful Greek youth who became enamored of his own reflection—hence "narcissism."

Narcisa, Narcisse, Narcyssa, Narkissa

Narda Lat. "Scented ointment."

Nastasia Gk. "Resurrection." Dim. **Anastasia**. Actress Nastassja Kinski.

Nastassia, Nastassja, Nastassiya, Nastassya

Nasya Heb. "The Lord's miracle."

Natalie Lat. "Birth day." More specifically, the Lord's birthday, or Christmas. This is probably the most common of all the Christmas names, and certainly the only one that is used for babies born at other times of the year (unlike Noel). Though there was a 4th-century Saint Natalia, this Frenchified form did not crop up until the late 19th century. Actress Natalie Wood.
Nat, Nata, Natala, Natalee, Natalene, Natalia, Natalja, Nataline, Natalya, Natasha, Natelie, Nathalia, Nathalie, Natilie, Natividad, Nattilie, Nattie, Nettie, Tasha

Natasha Rus. Var. Natalie.
Nastaliya, Nastalya, Natacha, Natascha, Natashenka

Nathania (fem. **Nathan**) Heb. "A gift or given of God."

Natividad Sp. "Christmas." See **Natalie**.

Neala (fem. **Neal**) Gael. "Champion." Unusual feminization of the male name that was quite popular in the middle of the 20th century.
Neila, Neile, Neilla, Neille

Neda (fem. **Edward**) OE. "wealthy defender" via the nickname Ned, or Rus. "born on Sunday." In any case, very unusual.
Nedda, Neddie, Nedi

Nelia Dim. **Cornelia**. Lat. "Horn."
Neelia, Neelie, Neelya, Nela, Nila

Nell Dim. **Eleanor**. Gk. "Light." Used sparingly as an independent name, though some of its variants like Nellie have had periods of popularity. Charles II's mistress Nell Gwynn; opera star Nellie Melba.
Nel, Nella, Nellie, Nelly

Neola Gk. "Young one." Comes from the same root as the widely used prefix "neo-."

Nerine Gk. "Sea nymph."
Nerice, Nerida, Nerina, Nerissa, Neryssa

Nessie Dim. **Agnes**. Gk. "Lamb." Also the name of the Loch Ness Monster, which might limit its appeal.
Nesha, Nessa, Nesta, Neta, Netia

Nettie Diminutive of "-ette" names like **Henrietta or Nanette**. Use as an independent name mostly around the turn of the 20th century.
Netta, Netty

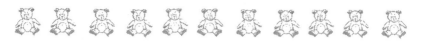

Neva Sp. "Snowy." Nevada, which means "covered with snow," is one of the American state names (like Florida) that adapts nicely to use as a girl's name.
Nevada

Nicole (fem. **Nicholas**) Gk. "Victory of the people." Nicola, the Italian form, is more common in Britain (though its vogue peaked in the 1970s). This French version has been more popular in other English-speaking countries, especially around the 1960s. Singer Nicolette Larson.
Colette, Cosetta, Cosette, Nichelle, Nichola, Nichole, Nicholette, Nicholle, Nicia, Nicki, Nickola, Nickole, Nicky, Nicola, Nicolea, Nicolene, Nicoleen, Nicolette, Nicolie, Nicolina, Nicoline, Nicolla, Nicolle, Niki, Nikki, Nikky, Nikola, Nikoleta, Nikoletta, Nikolia

Nike Gk. "Victory." Also, and more commonly to most Americans, the name of a very popular athletic shoe.
Nika

Nikki Var. **Nicole**. Used mostly in the 1960s.
Nickie, Nicky, Nikkey, Nikky

Nina Sp. "Girl." Dim. **Ann** (Heb. "grace") History buffs will remember that Nina was the name of one of Christopher Columbus's three ships. The name is rather uncommon. Ballerina Dame Ninette de Valois.
Neena, Ninacska, Nineta, Ninete, Ninetta, Ninette, Ninnette, Ninon, Ninochka, Ninotchka

Niobe Gk. "Fern." In myth, Niobe was a boastful queen of Thebes whose children were all killed as a reprimand for her arrogance. In her resulting misery she asked Zeus to turn her to stone. In art she is usually depicted weeping.

Nita Sp. Dim. **Juanita, Anita**, etc. Unusual.

Nixie OG. "Water sprite." Usually beautiful and antagonistic to men, unlike pixies, which, though mischievous, are content to share the world with humans.

Noel Fr. "Christmas." Though used since the Middle Ages for both boys and girls, it is more common for the latter.
Noela, Noeleen, Noelene, Noeline, Noella, Noelle, Noelleen, Noelynn, Nowel, Noweleen, Nowell

Nola Dim. **Finola**. Gael. "White shoulder." Related to Nuala but not, as many parents think, to Nolan.

Noleta Lat. "Unwilling."
Nolita

Nona Lat. "Ninth." Although it was originally used for a family's ninth baby, it would hardly have survived to this day if parents had not been willing to overlook its meaning.
Nonah, Noni, Nonie, Nonna, Nonnah

Nora Dim. **Eleanor, Honora.** Gk. "Light." Used independently, especially for the half century around 1900. Well-read parents will remember Nora as the heroine of Ibsen's *A Doll's House*; she sets a discouraging precedent, however. Writer Nora Ephron.
Norah

Norberta (fem. **Norbert**) OG. "Renowned northerner."

Noreen Ir. Dim. **Nora.** Originated in Ireland.
Norene, Norina, Norine

Norma Lat. "Pattern." From the same root that gave us "normal" or "the norm." Launched by Bellini's 1831 opera of the same name, and boosted in the 1920s by popular actress Norma Shearer. Out of fashion for the last couple of generations. Fashion designer Norma Kamali.
Norm, Normie

Novia Lat. "new"; Sp. "girlfriend."
Nova

Nuala Dim. **Fionnula** Ir. Gael. "White shoulder."
Nola, Nula

Nunzia It. "Messenger." See **Annunciata**.

Nur Arab. "Light." The Arabic name adopted by the current queen of Jordan, an American woman known formerly as Lisa Halaby.
Noor

Nydia Lat. "Nest."

Nyx Gk. "Night."

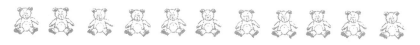

Octavia Lat. "Eighth." Used most often in the Victorian era of large families.
Octavie, Ottavia, Tavia, Tavie, Tavy

Odele Derivation disputed. Some sources relate it to either German "rich" or Greek "song," but *The Facts on File Dictionary of First Names* claims that it derives from an Old English place name: "woad hill." Woad is a blue dye reputedly used by the ancient Druids in their religious rites.
Odela, Odelet, Odelette, Odell, Odella, Odelle

Odelia Heb. "I will praise the Lord." Possibly also related to Odele.
Oda, Odeelia, Odele, Odelinda, Odella, Odilia

Odessa Gk. "Long voyage." As in "odyssey," more specifically Homer's epic poem about the wandering Odysseus. The Russian port of Odessa was supposedly named to honor *The Odyssey*.

Odette Fr. from Ger. "Wealthy." In the famous ballet *Swan Lake*, the same ballerina usually dances as both Odette, the good swan, and Odile, the evil black swan. Folk singer Odetta.
Odetta

Odile Fr. from Ger. "Wealthy." Related to Odette and also to Odelia. For balletomanes, the malevolent alter ego of Odette.
Odila, Odilia

Olena Rus. Var. **Helen**. Gk. "light."
Alena, Elena, Lena, Lenya, Olenya

Olesia Gr. "Man's defender."
Ola

Olethea Var. of **Alethea**. Gk. "Truth."
Oleta

Olga Rus. "Holy." The Russian form of Helga, and perhaps more common than Helga in English-speaking countries. The Russian Saint Olga was a princess from Kiev and a 10th-century Christian convert; the name was favored in the ill-fated Russian imperial family. Gymnast Olga Korbut.
Elga, Helga, Ola, Olenka, Olia

Oliana Polynesian. "Oleander."

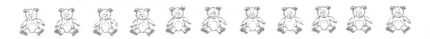

Olinda Lat. "Scented."

Olivia Lat. "Olive tree." The most common form of the name today, though Olive had a flurry of popularity with other nature names at the turn of the 20th century. It would be hard to use Olive today given the fame of Popeye's scrawny girlfriend, Olive Oyl. Actresses Olivia de Havilland, Olivia Hussey; singer Olivia Newton-John.
Liv, Liva, Livia, Livvie, Livvy, Olia, Oliva, Olive, Olivet, Olivette, Olivine, Ollie, Olva

Olwen Welsh. "White footprint." Along with Bronwen, one of the best-known Welsh-language first names. Nevertheless, it is very unusual outside Wales.
Olwenn, Olwin, Olwyn

Olympia Gk. "From Mount Olympus," the home of the gods. Slightly more common in Europe, where it may avoid the faintly commercial connotation of the Olympic Games. Actress Olympia Dukakis.
Olimpia, Olypme, Olympie

Oma Arab. "Leader." Infrequent use.

Omega Gk. "Last." It would seem to be tempting fate to use this name for a youngest child.

Ondine Lat. "Little wave." In myth, Undine is the spirit of the waters. Edith Wharton created a heroine in *The Custom of the Country* who was named Undine for the hair-curling tonic that had made her father rich.
Ondina, Ondyne, Undine

Oneida NAm. Ind. "Long-awaited." In the U.S. probably most familiar as a brand of silverware, which was originally manufactured by a utopian colony that was disbanded in the 19th century because its residents practiced polygamy.
Onida, Onyda

Onella Gk. "Light."

Onora Var. **Honoria.** Lat. "Honor."
Onoria, Onorine, Ornora

Oona Ir. Var. **Una.** Lat. "Unity."
Oonagh, Una

Opal Sanskrit. "Gem." One of the less common of the jewel names.
Opalina, Opaline

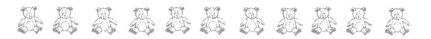

Ophelia Gk. "Help." Most famously, the young girl in *Hamlet* who goes mad. Mostly used in the late 19th century, but its connotations are far from happy.
Filia, Ofelia, Ofilia, Ophelie, Phelia

Ora Lat. "Prayer." Homonym for Aura, which means "gold" or "breeze."
Orabel, Orabelle, Orra

Oralee Heb. "My light."
Orali, Oralit, Orlee

Oralie Fr. Var. **Aurelia.** Lat. "Golden."
Aurelie, Oralee, Oralia, Orelie, Oriel, Orielda, Orielle, Orlena, Orlene

Orane Fr. "Rising." From the same Latin source as Oriana.
Orania, Oriane

Orela Lat. "Announcement from the gods." Related to "oracle."

Oriana Lat. "Dawning." From the same root as Aurora. Italian journalist Orianna Falacci.
Oria, Oriane, Orianna

Oriole Lat. "Golden." Most commonly the name of a bird with golden markings, or the name of the Baltimore baseball team.
Auriel, Oriel, Oriella, Oriola

Orpah Heb. "A fawn." Old Testament name rarely used. Talk-show star Oprah Winfrey's unusual name is the result of a misspelling of this name by her mother.

Orquidea Sp. "Orchid."

Orsa Var. **Ursula.** Lat. "Bear."
Orsaline, Orselina, Orseline, Ursa

Orszebet Hung. Var. **Elizabeth.** (Heb. "devoted to God").

Ortensia It. Var. **Hortense** Lat. clan name.

Otthild OG. "Prospers in battle."
Ottila, Ottilia, Ottilie, Ottiline, Ottoline, Otylia

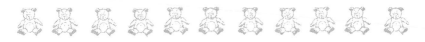

Page Fr. A young boy in training as a personal assistant to a knight. Usually a transferred surname, possibly indicating an ancestor who was a page. Use as a girl's name is quite recent.

Padget, Padgett, Paget, Pagett, Paige, Payge

Pallas Gk. "Wisdom." Another name for the Greek deity Athena, goddess of wisdom.

Palma Lat. "Palm tree." Also a place name used in several countries, no doubt to indicate locales where palm trees grew.

Pallma, Pallmirah, Pallmyra, Palmer, Palmira, Palmyra

Paloma Sp. "Dove." Little-known until the recent fame of designer Paloma Picasso, daughter of the artist.

Palloma, Palometa, Palomita, Peloma

Pamela Gk. "All-honey." Literary name coined at the end of the 16th century, growing gradually more common until a distinct vogue in the 1950s and 1960s. Likely to be neglected by the current generation of parents, precisely because it was popular among their parents. Actresses Pam Dawber, Pamela Reed; tennis star Pam Shriver.

Pam, Pamala, Pamalla, Pamelia, Pamelina, Pamella, Pamilla, Pammela, Pammie, Pammy

Pandora Gk. "All-gifted." In Greek myth Pandora was the first woman, endowed with gifts by all the gods. She is famous for the box that was her dowry; it contained all the world's evils, which flew out when the box was opened. One of the more common of the Greek names in English-speaking countries, but still highly unusual.

Panndora, Pandorra

Panphila Gk. "All-loving." A pleasant notion, though the name might require a lot of explanation.

Panfila, Panfyla, Panphyla

Pansy Flower name from the late 19th century: the name of the flower originally came from the French word for thought, *pensée*, possibly because the petals of the flower are thought to resemble wise little faces.

Pansey, Pansie

Panthea Gk. "All the gods." An early Middle Eastern

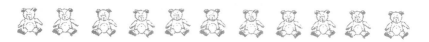

queen was named Panthea, but the name is more familiar from its close relative "pantheon," which means a temple to all gods.
Pantheia, Pantheya

Parthenia Gk. "Virginal." Used most often at the turn of the 20th century, when the attributes of the virgin were particularly highly valued.
Partheenia, Parthenie, Parthinia, Pathina

Pascale (fem. **Pascal**) Fr. "Easter." Despite some English-speaking use in the last 30 years, still primarily a French name.
Pascalette, Pascaline, Pascalle, Paschale

Paquita Sp. Dim. **Frances** (Lat. "from France") via **Paco**.

Pat Dim. **Patricia**. Used as an independent name, but neglected with the recent leaning toward the nostalgic and elaborate.

Patience Virtue name. One of the more popular of the 16th-century names, though eclipsed in the 20th century by **Hope**. Patience, after all, is not a very modern virtue.
Paciencia

Patricia (fem. **Patrick**) Lat. "Noble, patrician." Obscure until it was used for one of Queen Victoria's granddaughters, which launched its popularity for close to fifty years. It has now returned to neglect. Singers Patti LaBelle, Patsy Cline, Pat Benatar; choreographer Trisha Brown; actresses Patty Duke, Patricia Neal; First Lady Pat Nixon; Congresswoman Pat Schroeder.
Pat, Patreece, Patreice, Patrica, Patrice, Patricka,
Patrizia, Patsy, Patte, Pattee, Pattey, Patti, Pattie, Patty,
Tricia, Trish, Trisha

Paula (fem. **Paul**) Lat. "Small." Roman name that cropped up in English-speaking countries in this century and was rather well used in the Baby Boom era. Actress Paulette Godard; model Paulina Porizkova; singer Paula Abdul.
Paola, Paolina, Paule, Pauletta, Paulette, Paulie,
Paulina, Pauline, Paulita, Paulla, Paullette, Pauly, Pavia,
Pollie, Polly

Pauline (fem. **Paul**) Fr. from Lat. "Small." Popular earlier than Paula, having peaked at the turn of the 20th century in the U.S.
Pauleen, Polline, Paulyne

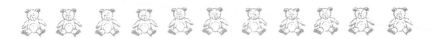

Paz Sp. "Peace."

Pazia Heb. "Golden."

Paza, Pazit

Peace Middle English. Word used as a name. Though not strictly a virtue name, this is the kind of abstract quality celebrated by the Puritans in their choice of names.

Pearl Lat. "Pearl." Probably the most common of the jewel names, though of course it is not a gemstone. The Greek form, Margaret, is far more widespread and has been used for centuries, while Pearl only appeared in the late Victorian era. Writer Pearl S. Buck; singer Pearl Bailey.

Pearla, Pearle, Pearleen, Pearlette, Pearline, Perl, Perla, Perle, Perlette, Perley, Perline, Perlline

Peggy Dim. **Margaret**. (Gk. "pearl.") Used as an independent name since the 18th century, and parents who choose it today probably do so without thinking of Margaret. Its greatest vogue came in the first third of the 20th century. Skater Peggy Fleming.

Peg, Pegeen, Pegg, Peggie

Pelagia Gk. "Ocean, sea."

Pelage, Pelageia, Pelagie, Pellagia

Penelope Gk. "Bobbin worker." The bobbin probably refers to part of the equipment for weaving, since the Penelope of Greek myth was the wife of Odysseus. To put off the many suitors who courted her when it seemed that the wandering Odysseus must be dead, she told them she couldn't marry until she finished the tapestry she was weaving. She would work all day and unravel her work at night, hoping that her husband would come home. The name was most popular in the middle of the 20th century, in Britain. Model Penelope Tree; parenting expert Penelope Leach.

Pen, Penelopa, Penina, Penna, Pennelope, Penney, Pennie, Penny

Peninah Heb. "Pearl."

Penny Dim. **Penelope**. Gk. "Bobbin worker." Given as an independent name mostly in the 20th century.

Penee, Pennee, Penney, Pennie

Peony Unusual flower name.

Pepita Sp. Dim. **Joseph** Heb. "Jehovah increases" via **Pepe**.
Pepa, Peta

Perdita Lat. "Lost." Coined by Shakespeare, and rarely used since his day.

Perfecta Sp. "Perfect, flawless." A daunting name to give any child.

Pernella (fem. **Peter**) Fr. from Gk. "rock."
Parnella, Pernelle

Perry Fr. "Pear tree." Dim. **Peregrine** (Lat. "voyager"). Originally a boy's name and common as a last name, but also used in America as a girl's name. The masculine names with "-y" or "-ie" endings (**Leslie**, for instance) seem more susceptible to feminine appropriation, which is irreversible. Author Perri Klass.
Perrey, Perri, Perrie

Persis Lat. "From Persia."
Perssis

Petra (fem. **Peter**) Gk. "Rock." The simplest feminization of a name that seems to resist being feminized.
Perrine, Pet, Peta, Peterina, Petrina, Petronela, Petronella, Petronelle, Petronia, Petronija, Petronilla, Petronille, Petrova, Petrovna, Pierette, Pierrette, Pietra

Petula Derivation unclear: may be a version of **Peter,** may come from a Latin word meaning "to seek." The name might even be an adaptation of the flower name Petunia. Its use is based entirely on the fame of singer Petula Clark.
Petulah

Petunia Flower name, for the rather humble trumpet-shaped flower with white or bright pink blossoms.

Phedra Gk. "Bright." In Greek myth, the daughter of King Minos, who was married to the hero Theseus and fell in love with her stepson Hippolytus. When he spurned her advances, she committed suicide. One of those pretty Greek names with a not-so-pretty history.
Faydra, Phaedra, Phaedre, Phaidra, Phedre

Pheodora (fem. **Theodore**) Rus. from Gk. "Gift of God."
Fedora, Feodora, Fyedora

Philana Gk. "Loving mankind."

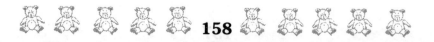

Filania, Filanna, Phila, Philene, Philina, Philine, Phillane

Philantha Gk. "Lover of flowers."

Philberta OE. "Very brilliant." Feminine of Filbert, which is the unusual modern form of Philibert, an Anglo-Saxon saint's name.

Filberta, Filiberta

Philippa (fem. **Philip**) Gk. "Horse lover." Another unusual feminization, though it was used somewhat in the 19th century. Something of a curiosity today.

Felipa, Filipa, Filippa, Phil, Philipa, Philippe, Philippine, Phillie, Phillipa, Phillipina, Philly, Pippa, Pippy

Philomena Gk. "Loved one." Name of a saint worshiped enthusiastically, especially in Italy, in the 19th and 20th centuries. However, her cult was based on nothing more than a set of bones discovered in Rome in 1802, which linked up very vaguely with a Roman inscription. It was assumed that she was a virgin martyr, and many miracles were attributed to Saint Philomena after a shrine was established to her. But in 1961, after archaeologists proved the bones in the shrine could not have been those of a young girl, her veneration was forbidden by Rome.

Philomène, Philomina, Filimena, Filomena

Phoebe Gk. "Shining, brilliant." One of the epithets of Apollo, the sun god, was Phoebus Apollo, referring to the fact that he brought light. A Phoebe appears in the New Testament, but the name didn't gain ground until the 18th century. Reached a peak in the last part of the 19th century, now pleasantly old-fashioned and ripe for revival. Singers Phoebe Legere, Phoebe Snow.

Pheabe, Phebe, Pheby, Phoebey

Phyllida Var. **Phyllis**. Gk. "Leafy bough." Rare name that appeared in the 16th century; mostly literary use.

Fillida, Phillida, Phillyda

Phyllis Gk. "Leafy bough." Name of a mythological woman, taken up by generations of poets to stand for the idealized country lass. Parents applied it to babies increasingly through the 19th century, but it died out after the 1930s. Poet Phyllis McGinley; comedienne Phyllis Diller.

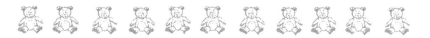

Fillys, Fyllis, Philis, Phillis, Philys, Phylis, Phyllida, Phylliss, Phyllys

Pia Lat. "Pious." More common in Europe than in English-speaking countries. Singer/actress Pia Zadora.

Piedad Sp. "Piety, devotion."

Pilar Sp. "Pillar." An allusion to the Virgin Mary, in her role as a "pillar" of the Church. Used mostly by Spanish-speaking parents.

Piper OE. Occupational name: "pipe player." Transferred to last name, and occasionally used as a first name, probably inspired, however indirectly, by actress Piper Laurie.

Pippa Dim. **Philippa**. Gk. "Lover of horses." Almost exclusively British use.

Placidia Lat. "Calm, tranquil." From the word that gives us "placid." It seems a bit dangerous, however, to make predictions about a baby's temperament at birth.
Placida, Plasida

Polly Var. **Molly**, Dim. **Mary**, Heb. "bitter." Independent name, used especially in the 19th century. Another old-fashioned choice that should be appealing to parents of the 1990s. Actress Polly Bergen.
Poll, Pollee, Polley, Polli, Pollie

Pomona Lat. "Apple." The Roman goddess of fruit trees.

Poppy Lat. Flower name that reached its peak in the 1920s.

Portia Lat. Clan name, obscure meaning. The heroine of Shakespeare's *Merchant of Venice*, an enterprising woman who disguises herself as a lawyer to save her husband's life. In spite of this worthy prototype, the name is uncommon.

Prima Lat. "First."
Primalia, Primetta, Primina, Priminia

Primavera It. "Spring." Pretty name for a spring baby.

Primrose Middle English. "First rose." The primrose does not actually belong to the rose family, but it is one of the flowers that blooms early in spring. 19th-century flower name.
Primula

Priscilla Lat. "Ancient." New Testament name and com-

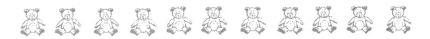

mon in the early Christian era, then revived strongly by the Puritans. After generations of neglect, it was taken up in the 19th century, but has been scarce in the last half of the 20th century, possibly because the most natural nickname is "Prissy." Actress Priscilla Presley.
Cilla, Pris, Prisca, Priscella, Prisilla, Prissie, Prissy, Prysilla

Prudence Lat. "Caution, discretion." Virtue name most common in the 19th century after its first popularity in the 16th and 17th centuries. Use now is mostly British.
Pru, Prudencia, Prudie, Prudy, Prue

Prunella Lat. "Small plum." Actress Prunella Scales.

Psyche Gk. "Breath" and, by extension, life or soul. In myth Psyche was a mortal girl whom Cupid loved. In post-Freudian times someone's psyche is his innermost soul or mind.

Purity Middle English. The word as name; a virtue name comparable to Chastity.
Pureza

Rabab Arab. "Pale cloud."
Rabiah

Rachel Heb. "Ewe, female sheep." In the Old Testament Rachel is the wife of the patriarch Jacob. Like many Old Testament names, this one was taken up by the Puritans in the 17th century and remained current but not fashionable until parents of the late sixties and seventies used it in great numbers. Actress Raquel Welch; author Rachel Carson.
Rachael, Racheal, Rachele, Rachelle, Rachil, Rae, Rahel, Rahil, Rakel, Raquel, Raquela, Raquella, Raquelle, Ray, Raychel, Raychelle, Rashell, Rashelle, Shell, Shelley, Shellie, Shelly

Radmilla Slavic. "Industrious for the people."
Radmila

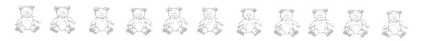

Rae Dim. **Rachel**. Heb. "Ewe." Used independently in modern times. Actress Rae Dawn Chong.
Raeann, Raelene, Ray, Raye, Rayette, Raylene
Rafa Arab. "Well-being, prosperity."
Rafah
Ragnild Teut. "All-knowing power."
Ragnhild, Ragnhilda, Ragnhilde, Ragnilda, Ranillda, Reinheld, Renilda, Renilde
Raina Var. **Regina** Lat. "queen" or fem. **Ray** OG. "wise guardian." Modern name of several possible origins. Like many names that have appeared in this century, it has numerous variations, none of which is clearly a favorite.
Raenah, Raene, Rainah, Raine, Raleine, Raya, Rayann, Rayette, Rayleine, Raylene, Rayline, Rayna, Rayne, Raynelle
Raja Arab. "Hope."
Ramona (fem. **Raymond**) Sp. "Wise guardian." A 19th-century historical novel of the same title was immensely successful, and brought the name to wide attention, but it is scarce now. Character in a very popular children's book of the same name by Beverly Cleary.
Mona, Ramonda, Ramonde, Ramonna, Romona, Romonda, Romonde
Randy Dim. **Miranda**. Lat. "admirable." Mostly U.S. use.
Randa, Randee, Randene, Randi, Randie
Rani Sanskrit. "Queen."
Raine, Rana, Ranee, Rania, Ranice, Ranique, Ranit, Rayna, Raynell
Ranita Heb. "Song."
Ranit, Ranite, Ranith, Ranitra, Ranitta
Raphaela (fem. **Raphael**) Heb. "God heals." The feminization is very unusual in English-speaking countries, though Italian parents use it with some frequency.
Rafa, Rafaela, Rafaelia, Rafaella, Raffaela, Raffaele, Rafella, Rafelle, Raphaelle
Rashida (fem. **Rashid**) Turkish. "Righteous, rightly advised."
Rasheda, Rasheeda, Rasheida, Rashidah

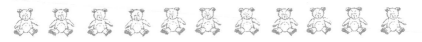

Raven Name of the large black bird that is closely related to the crow. A fanciful name for a black-haired baby.
Ravenne

Reba Dim. Rebecca. Singer Reba McEntire.
Reyba, Rheba

Rebecca Heb. "Joined." A prominent Old Testament name; Rebecca is the wife of Isaac and mother of Jacob and Esau. Predictably, the name was taken up by the Puritans and remained fairly common through the 19th century. Subsequent revivals (in the thirties in the U.S., in the late sixties in Britain) may have been prompted by literary and cinematic use of the name, especially in the novel and film *Rebecca*. Philanthropist Rebekah Harkness; author Rebecca West.
Becca, Becka, Beckie, Becky, Bekka, Reba, Rebeca, Rebecka, Rebeka, Rebekah, Rebekkah, Ree, Reeba, Rheba, Riva, Rivah, Rivalee, Rivi, Rivkah, Rivy

Regan Ir. Celt. "Son of the small ruler." Use for girls may hark back to Shakespeare's play *King Lear,* but the king's daughter of that name is so cruel that this seems unlikely.

Regina Lat. "Queen." Cropped up at the end of the Victorian era, possibly encouraged by the fact that Her Majesty was often known as Victoria Regina. It may also be an allusion to the Virgin Mary, Regina Coelis ("Queen of the Heavens"). Nightclub founder Regine.
Gina, Raina, Raine, Regan, Reggi, Reggie, Regine, Reina, Reine, Reyna, Rina

Remedios Sp. "Help, remedy." Currently popular in South America.

Remy Fr. "From Rheims." Champagne, and the fine brandies made from champagne, are the principal product of Rheims, a town in central France.
Remi, Remie

Rena Heb. "Melody."
Reena

Renata Lat. "Reborn." The Latin (and less popular) form of Renée. It was used in this guise by the Puritans. Author Renata Adler.
Renae, Renate, René, Renée, Renie, Rennie

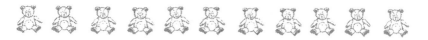

Rene Dim. **Irene**. Gk. "peace." Used on its own, primarily around the turn of the 20th century.
Renie, Rennie

Renée Fr. "Reborn." The French form of **Renata**, more common (though not really widespread) in modern times. Tennis star Renée Richards.
Renae, René, Renell, Renelle, Renie, Rennie, Renny

Renita Lat. "Resistant." Has come into use since the 1980s.
Reneeta

Reseda Latin term for a flower more commonly known as mignonette.

Reta Var. **Rita**, dim. **Margaret**, Gk. "pearl."
Reeta, Rheta, Rhetta

Rexana It is possible to translate this name by its parts, *rex* being Latin for "king," and *anna* a variant of the Hebrew word for "grace." Or it may be a feminization of Rex, or a variant of Roxane.
Rexanne, Rexanna

Rhea Gk. "Earth." In Greek myth, Rhea was an earth-mother who bore Zeus, Demeter, Hera, and Poseidon, among other gods. Actress Rhea Perlman.
Rea, Rhia, Ria

Rheta Gk. "A speaker, eloquent." From the same root as the word "rhetoric."

Rhiannon Welsh. "Witch, goddess."
Rhianna, Rhianon, Rianon, Riannon

Rhoda Gk. "Rose," Lat. "from Rhodes." Rhodes is a Greek island originally named for its roses. The name is found in the New Testament, and was used mostly in the 18th and 19th centuries.
Rhodia, Rhodie, Rhody, Roda, Rodi, Rodie, Rodina

Rhodanthe Gk. "Rose blossom."
Rhodante

Rhona ONorse. "Rough island." A form of Rona more common in Britain.
Rhona, Roana

Rhonda Welsh place name: The Rhondda Valley is a significant landmark in southern Wales, named for the river that runs through it. (In Welsh, the name means

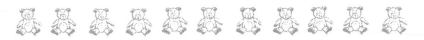

"noisy.") Today's parents will probably associate it with the Beach Boys' song, "Help Me, Rhonda!"

Rhonnda, Ronda

Ria Dim. **Victoria**. Lat. "Victor." Used occasionally as an independent name.

Rea

Riane (fem. **Ryan**) Ir. last name. Uncommon, but analogous to the more widely used **Briana**.

Rhiane, Rhianna, Riana, Rianne, Ryann, Ryanne

Rica Familiar form of **Erica**. Scan. "ruler forever"; **Frederica** (OG. "Peaceful ruler"), Sp. "Rich."

Ricca, Ricki, Rickie, Ricky, Rieca, Riecka, Rieka, Riki, Rikki, Riqua, Rycca

Ricarda (fem. **Richard**) OG. "Powerful ruler." One of many feminine forms of a very popular man's name, none of which has been adopted in large numbers.

Richarda, Richel, Richela, Richele, Richella, Richelle, Richenda, Richenza, Richia, Richilene, Richmal, Richmalle

Rickie Dim. **Frederica**. OG. "Peaceful ruler." Also possibly a feminine version of **Richard**, and certainly more popular than the longer forms. Occurred most often in the middle of the 20th century. Singer Rickie Lee Jones.

Rickie, Ricki, Ricky, Ricquie, Riki, Rikki, Rikky, Ryckie

Rilla Middle German. "Small brook."

Rilletta, Rillette

Rima Arab. "Antelope."

Risa Lat. "Laughter." A pretty name, but very unusual in English-speaking countries. Opera singer Rise Stevens.

Riesa, Rise, Rysa

Rita Dim. **Margaret**. (Gk. "pearl") Comes via the Spanish form, Margarita. First used on its own some hundred years ago, and quite popular for 50 years. Actresses Rita Hayworth, Rita Moreno.

Reeta, Reita, Rheeta, Riet, Rieta, Ritta

Ritsa Gk. Dim. **Alexander**. Gk. "Man's defender."

Riva Var. **Rebecca**. Heb. "Joined." Also possibly from the French for "shore," but the Jewish families who use it most often probably have the Old Testament associations in mind.

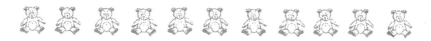

Ree, Reeva, Reevabel, Rivalee, Rivi, Rivka, Rivkah, Rivy

Roanna Var. **Rosanne.**

Ranna, Roanne, Ronni, Ronnie, Ronny

Roberta (fem. **Robert**) OE. "Bright fame." While Ricarda, another simple feminization of an Old German name, never caught on, Roberta was rather widespread between its introduction in the late 19th century and its fall from favor some eighty years later. Singers Roberta Peters, Roberta Flack.

Berta, Bertie, Berty, Bobbe, Bobbee, Bobbette, Bobbie, Bobby, Bobbye, Bobette, Bobi, Bobina, Bobine, Bobinette, Robbee, Robbey, Robbi, Robbie, Robby, Robeena, Robena, Robenia, Robertena, Robertene, Robertina, Robin, Robina, Robinett, Robinette, Robinia, Robyn, Robyna, Robynna, Ruperta, Rupetta

Robin dim. **Robert** OE "Bright fame." Originally a boy's nickname (as in Winnie the Pooh's friend Christopher Robin), but appropriated for girls in increasing numbers starting in the middle of the 20th century. Now out of fashion for both sexes. Actress Robin Givens.

Robee, Robbey, Robbi, Robbie, Robbin, Robby, Robbyn, Robena, Robene, Robenia, Robi, Robina, Robine, Robinet, Robinett, Robinette, Robinia, Robyn, Robyna, Robynette

Rochelle Fr. Place name: "Little rock." Enthusiastically used as a first name starting in the 1940s, but rare now.

Roch, Rochell, Rochella, Rochette, Roshelle, Shell, Shelley, Shelly

Roderica (fem. **Roderick**) OG. "Renowned ruler."

Rica, Roddie, Roderiqua, Roderique

Rohana Sanskrit. "Sandalwood."

Rohanna

Rolanda (fem. **Roland**) OG. "Famous land."

Orlanda, Orlande, Rolande, Rollande

Roline Dim. **Caroline.** (OG. "Man.") Unusual diminutive that appears from time to time in the South.

Roelene, Rolene

Roma It. Place name: the capital city, Rome. Rather widely used since it first appeared in the late 19th century,

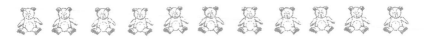

though of course, it never approached the popularity of Florence.

Romelle, Romilda, Romina, Romma

Romaine (fem. **Romain**) Fr. "From Rome." A pretty name that might be associated with a common variety of lettuce.

Romayne, Romeine, Romene

Romola Lat. "Roman woman."

Romella, Romelle, Rommola, Romolla, Romula

Rona ONorse. "Rough island." In Britain, used interchangeably with Rhona. Both versions cropped up at the turn of the century and have occurred steadily without ever being fashionable. Gossip columnist Rona Barrett.

Rhona, Ronella, Ronelle, Ronna

Ronni (fem. **Ronald**) OE. "Strong counsel" or Dim. **Veronica** Lat. "image."

Ronee, Ronette, Roni, Ronna, Ronnee, Ronney, Ronnie, Ronny

Rosabel Com. form **Rose** and **Belle**. A combination that appeared in the mid–19th century. Its meaning ("beautiful rose") probably appealed as much to parents of the era as the name itself, which lost favor in the unsentimental 20th century.

Rosabella, Rosabelle

Rosalba Lat. "White rose." Artist Rosalba Carriera.

Rosalie Fr. Var. It. **Rosalia**. Possibly "rose garden." Mostly 19th-century use.

Rosalee, Rosaleen, Rosaley, Rosalia, Rosalina, Rosaline, Rosalyne, Rosella, Rozalia, Rozalie, Rozele, Rozelie, Rozely, Rozella, Rozelle, Rozellia

Rosalind Sp. "Pretty rose" is the most common interpretation, though the name was actually coined in 16th-century Britain. A German form also existed, formed of words that meant "horse" or "renown" and "shield" or "snake." It has been used since the mid–19th century, with a surge in the middle of the 20th century. Actress Rosalind Russell.

Ros, Rosalen, Rosalin, Rosalina, Rosalinda, Rosalinde, Rosaline, Rosalinn, Rosalyn, Rosalynd, Rosalynda, Roselin, Roselina, Roselind, Roselinda, Roselinde,

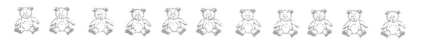

Roseline, Roselinn, Roselyn, Roselynda, Roselynde, Rosina, Roslyn, Roslynn, Roslynne, Roz, Rozali, Rozalia, Rozalin, Rozalind, Rozalinda, Rozalynn, Rozalynne, Rozelin, Rozelind, Rozelinda, Rozelyn, Rozelynda

Rosalyn Com. form. **Rose** and **Lynn** (Sp. "pretty"). The most common of the modern variants of **Rosalind**. First Lady Rosalynn Carter.

Rosalin, Rosalynn, Roselynn, Roslyn, Rozlynn

Rosamond OG. "Renowned protector." Also translatable (from the Latin) as "rose of the world." More popular in the 19th century than it is today. Author Rosamond Bernier.

Ros, Rosamonde, Rosamund, Rosamunda, Rosemond, Rosemonda, Rosmund, Rosmunda, Roz, Rozamond

Rose Lat. Flower name. Scholars actually trace the name (which the Normans imported to Britain in the 11th century) to an Old German name meaning something like "renown," but the flower meaning has had much more currency, particularly given the Christian symbolic meaning of the rose. (The "rosa mystica" is the Virgin Mary.) It reached its peak use at the turn of the 20th century, along with other flower names.

Rasia, Rasine, Rasja, Rasya, Rhoda, Rhodea, Rhodia, Rhody, Rosa, Rosaleen, Rosalia, Rosalie, Rosalin, Rosalina, Rosalind, Rosaline, Rosalinn, Rosalynn, Roselia, Roselina, Roseline, Rosella, Roselle, Rosena, Rosenah, Rosene, Rosetta, Rosette, Rosie, Rosina, Rosita, Roslyn, Rosy, Roza, Rozalie, Rozaline, Rozalyne, Roze, Rozele, Rozella, Rozina, Rozsa, Rozsi, Rozsika, Zita

Roseanne Com. form. **Rose** and **Anne**. The pairing of the two names appeared in the 18th century, and various forms have drifted in and out of popularity. Actresses Roseanne Barr, Rosanna Arquette.

Ranna, Roanna, Roanne, Rosanagh, Rosanna, Rosannah, Rosanne, Roseann, Roseanna, Rosehannah, Rozanna, Rozanne, Rozeanna

Rosemary Lat. "Dew of the sea" is the correct meaning, though the name gained great currency with the flower name fad of the late 19th century. The fact that most

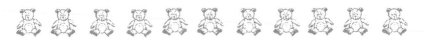

parents read it as a combination of Rose and Mary (both already popular, and with strong religious resonance for Catholics) can't have hurt. Singer Rosemary Clooney.

Rosemaree, Rosemarey, Rosemaria, Rosemarie, Rosmarie, Rozmary, Romy

Rowena Welsh. "Slender and fair." This meaning is an approximation. The name was actually brought to public notice by novelist Sir Walter Scott with his immensely popular *Ivanhoe*, in the early 19th century.

Roweena, Roweina, Rowina

Roxanne Per. "Dawn." In history, the wife of Alexander the Great was named Roxane, but 20th-century parents may be more familiar with the Roxane who is the heroine of Rostand's play *Cyrano de Bergerac*. Favored in the U.S.

Roksanne, Roxana, Roxane, Roxann, Roxanna, Roxene, Roxey, Roxie, Roxine, Roxy

Royale OF. "Regal one." Something of a curiosity in the democratic United States.

Royalene, Royall, Royalle, Royalyn

Ruby Jewel name. Launched in the 1870s with other jewel names, but passé by the mid–20th century. Dancer Ruby Keeler.

Rubee, Rubetta, Rubey, Rubi, Rubia, Rubie, Rubinia, Rubyna

Rudelle OG. "Renowned." From the same root that produces the male name Rudolph.

Rudella

Rufina Lat. "Red-haired." Can be considered a feminine version of Rufus, which is given to boys regardless of their hair color.

Rufeena, Rufeine, Ruffina, Ruphyna

Ruth Heb. "Friend, companion." The Old Testament Book of Ruth is about the widowed Moabite woman who refuses to leave her Hebrew mother-in-law, Naomi, and says, "Whither thou goest, I will go." Her sentiments appealed greatly to Victorian poets. The name has been consistently used ever since the 17th century, peaking at the turn of the century. Actresses Ruth Gordon, Ruth Buzzi; author Ruth Rendell.

Ruthe, Ruthelle, Ruthetta, Ruthi, Ruthie, Ruthina, Ruthine

Ruthann Com. form. **Ruth** and **Ann**.
Ruthanna, Ruthanne

S **Saba** Gk. "from Sheba"; Arab. "morning." The queen of Sheba is mentioned in the Old Testament as having been hugely rich and very ostentatious.
Sabah, Sheba, Shebah

Sabina Lat. "Sabine." The Sabines were a tribe living in central Italy around the time Romulus and Remus established the city of Rome. In an effort to provide wives for the citizens of Rome, Romulus arranged the mass kidnapping of the Sabine women, which came to be known (and frequently portrayed in art and literature) as the "Rape of the Sabines." The name was used among the ancient Romans and in English-speaking countries after the 17th century, but has been very rare lately.
Bina, Byna, Sabine, Sabinna, Sabiny, Sabyna, Savina, Savine, Sebina, Sebinah

Sabra Origin disputed: may be Heb. "to rest." Is now used as a term for a native-born Israeli.
Sabrah

Sabrina Lat. Place name: the Latin term for the Severn River in England. Though Milton (among others) writes about a Sabrina, she appeared most vividly in modern culture as *Sabrina Fair* in the play and movie. The name was used in the 19th century and cropped up again in the last part of the 20th century.
Brina, Sabreena, Sabrinna, Sabryna

Sachi Jap. "child of joy."
Sachiko

Sadie Dim. **Sarah**. Heb. "Princess." Use as an independent name occurred mostly at the turn of the 20th century. Actress Sada Thompson.

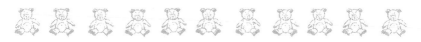

Sada, Sadah, Sadelle, Saidee, Saydie, Sydell, Sydella, Sydelle

Sadira Per. "Lotus tree." The lotus has great significance in several of the Eastern religions.

Saffron Flower name: Saffron refers to a substance (the dried stamens of saffron crocuses) used as a spice in Mediterranean and other Southern cuisines. It produces a bright orange-yellow color, and is sometimes used as a dye. Monks of some Eastern religions wear saffron robes, which may explain why the name was used occasionally in the 1960s, an era when saffron robes and Eastern religions went mainstream.

Saffren, Saffronia, Saphron

Sage Lat. "Wise, healthy." More likely to be a boy's name, perhaps via associations with sagebrush, cowboys, and the Wild West.

Saige, Sayge

Salena Var. **Selina**. Gk. "Moon goddess."

Salina

Salimah Arab. "Healthy, sound." Currently popular in Arabic countries.

Salima

Sally Dim. **Sarah**. Heb. "Princess." A popular independent name in the 18th, and again in the 20th, centuries. Talk-show host Sally Jessy Raphael; actress Sally Field; astronaut Sally K. Ride.

Sal, Saletta, Sallee, Salletta, Sallette, Salley, Sallianne, Sallie, Sallyann

Salome Heb. "Peace." Possibly from the same root that gives us the greeting "Shalom." The most famous biblical Salome is the woman who danced for King Herod and demanded, as her reward, the head of John the Baptist on a platter. In spite of this unsavory antecedent, the name was used somewhat in the 19th century, but its connotations make it an unlikely choice.

Saloma, Salomey, Salomi

Salvadora Sp. "Savior." Referring, of course, to Jesus Christ.

Salvia Lat. "Whole, healthy." The Latin name for the herb

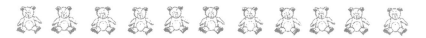

known as Sage, which has mild healing powers as well as being an aromatic used in cooking.
Sallvia, Salvina

Samala Heb. "Requested of God."
Samale, Sammala

Samantha (fem. **Samuel**) Heb. "Told by God." Occasionally used in the 17th–19th centuries, but truly popular in the 1960s and 1970s, possibly triggered by the TV series "Bewitched." Having a resurgence of popularity in the 1990s. Actress Samantha Eggar.
Sam, Samentha, Sammantha, Sammee, Sammey, Sammie, Semantha, Semanntha, Simantha, Symantha

Samara Heb. "Under God's rule."
Samaria, Sammara

Samuela (fem. **Samuel**) Heb. "Told by God." Very scarce, particularly compared with Samantha.
Samella, Samelle, Samuella, Samuelle

Sancia Lat. "Sacred."
Sancha, Sanchia, Santsia, Sanzia

Sandra Dim. **Alexandra** Gk. "Defender of mankind." Via It. **Alessandra**. Popular in the middle of the 20th century, but today's parents are more inclined to prefer the full four syllables of the original name. Comedienne Sandra Bernhard; actresses Sandrine Bonnaire, Sondra Locke, Sandra Dee; Supreme Court Justice Sandra Day O'Connor.
Sahndra, Sandee, Sandie, Sandreea, Sandria, Sandrina, Sandrine, Sandy, Sanndra, Sanndria, Saundra, Sohndra, Sondra, Sonndra, Zandra

Sandy Dim. **Sandra**. Mostly used post–1950.
Sandee, Sandi, Sandie, Sanndi

Sapphire Heb. Jewel name. Unusual biblical name, and the birthstone for September. One of the least used of the jewel names.
Safira, Saphira, Sapphira, Sephira

Sarah Heb. "Princess." In the Old Testament, the wife of the patriarch Abraham. Came into vogue with other biblical names in the 16th century and was enough of a staple for 400 years to have spawned a variety of nicknames (though not as many as the multisyllabic Eliza-

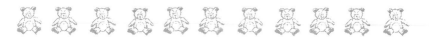

beth, for instance). Actresses Sarah Bernhardt, Sarah Siddons; singer Sarah Vaughan; poet Sara Teasdale; Sarah Ferguson, Duchess of York.

Sadee, Sadella, Sadelle, Sadellia, Sadie, Sadye, Saidee, Sal, Sallee, Salley, Sallie, Sally, Sara, Sareen, Sarena, Sarette, Sari, Sarika, Sarine, Sarita, Sarra, Sarrah, Sasa, Serita, Shara, Sorcha, Sydel, Sydelle, Zahra, Zara, Zarah, Zaria, Zarita

Sasha (fem. and dim. **Alexander**) Rus. The "-a" ending is not necessarily feminine in Russia, and Sasha is more commonly a male nickname.

Sacha, Sascha, Saschenka

Saskia Dutch name of unknown meaning. It would probably have been forgotten, but it was the name of Rembrandt's wife, who is depicted in some of his finest canvases.

Savanna Sp. "Treeless." Most familiar as a place name, as in the city in Georgia. A savannah is a wide, treeless plain, characteristic of the South.

Savana, Savannah, Sevanna

Scarlett Middle English. "Scarlet." Given its fame by the inimitable Scarlett O'Hara, heroine of *Gone With the Wind*. Not hugely popular, possibly because the young lady in the novel is so headstrong. It is nevertheless the middle name of one of Mick Jagger's children by Jerry Hall.

Scarlette

Season Lat. "Time of sowing." The word used as a name. Cropped up in the 1970s (along with Spring and Summer), when children were given counterculture names, but seems unlikely to endure. Actress Season Hubley.

Seema Heb. "Precious thing, treasure."

Cima, Cyma, Seemah, Sima, Simah, Sina

Sebastiane (fem. **Sebastian**) Lat. "From Sebastia." Unusual feminization of a name that is very infrequent in America.

Sebastiana, Sebastienne

Secunda Lat. "Second."

Selena Gk. "Moon goddess." Most popular in the 19th century.

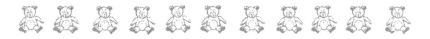

Celene, Celie, Celina, Celinda, Celine, Cellina, Celyna, Saleena, Salena, Salina, Sela, Selene, Selia, Selie, Selina, Selinda, Seline, Sena

Selima Heb. "Tranquil."

Selimah

Selma (fem. **Anselm** by way of **Anselma**) OG. "godly helmet." Selma is the more common form, though it is far from an everyday choice.

Anselma, Sellma, Selmah, Zelma

Semiramis Heb. "Highest heaven." Semiramis was an Assyrian queen who, myth has it, built Babylon and turned into a dove after death. Her legend inspired both Voltaire and Rossini.

Semira

Senalda Sp. "A sign."

Senga Var. **Agnes**. Gk. "Pure." A rare Scottish name; it is **Agnes** spelled backward.

September Month name. Much less common than April, May, or June.

Septima Lat. "Seventh." If one has a seventh child, why not celebrate with her name?

Seraphina Heb. "Ardent." The seraphim are the highest-ranking angels in Heaven (above angels, archangels, cherubim, etc.). They have six wings and are noted for their zealous love.

Sarafina, Serafina, Serafine, Seraphe, Seraphine

Serena Lat. "Tranquil, serene." Used by Roman Christians, and periodically popular since, though never in a big way.

Reena, Sarina, Saryna, Serene, Serina, Seryna

Serilda OG. "Armed warrior woman."

Sarilda, Serhilda, Serhilde, Serrilda

Shaina Heb. "Beautiful."

Shaine, Shanie, Shayna, Shayne

Shaka Modern name: "Sha-," like "La-," is a very fashionable prefix, attached to any number of other particles to form names that have no specific meaning but sound attractive.

Shakeela, Shakeita, Shakeera, Shakette, Shakila, Shakina, Shakira, Shakitra, Shaquina, Shaquita

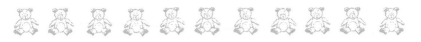

Shana Dim. **Shannon**. Uncommon, but kept in the public eye by journalist and biographer Shana Alexander.
Shanna

Shaneika Modern U.S. Another elaboration of the popular "Sha-" prefix. Some of the more common of these names are the ones that sound like *"Ashanti,"* which is an important name in Western Africa, where many American slaves originally came from. Other "Sha-" names, like the "La-" names, are limited in form only by parental imagination.
Shandee, Shandeigh, Shandey, Shanecka, Shaneese, Shaneikah, Shanequa, Shaneyka, Shaniece, Shanika, Shanique, Shanisse, Shanneice, Shanta, Shantee, Shanteigh, Shantella, Shantelle, Shantey, Sheniece, Shenika, Sheniqua, Shonyce

Shanelle Modern U.S. name which is a phonetic spelling of "Chanel," the name of the great French couturier. It has double-barreled appeal, since it combines the "Sha-" prefix with an evocation of great feminine elegance.
Shanel, Shanella, Shannel, Shanisse, Shanita, Shenelle, Shonelle, Shynelle

Shannon Ir. Gael. "Old, ancient." The name of an important river, county, and airport in Ireland, used as a first name in this century. Most popular among families with Irish roots, but little found in Ireland.
Channa, Shana, Shandy, Shane, Shani, Shanon, Shanna, Shannen

Shantal Var. **Chantal**. Fr. place name. Its popularity may be associated with both Shanelle and the other "Sha-" names, rather than with the rather obscure French first name.
Shanta, Shantay, Shantalle, Shante, Shantella, Shantelle, Shontal, Shontalle, Shontelle

Sharlene (fem and dim. **Charles**) OG. "Man." Var. **Caroline**. One of the numerous variations that were popular in the 1950s and 1960s.
Sharleen, Sharleyne, Sharlina, Sharline, Sharlyne

Sharon Heb. Place name: "A plain." In the Old Testament, refers to flat land at the foot of Mount Carmel. Not picked up by the 16th-century Puritans, probably

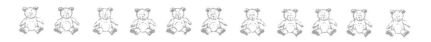

since it wasn't a personal name, but by mid–20th century it was quite popular in America. Now much less common.

Charin, Cheron, Shara, Sharan, Sharen, Shari, Sharie, Sharla, Sharolyn, Sharona, Sharonda, Sharren, Sharrin, Sharronne, Sheran, Sheron, Sherri, Sherry

Shavonne Phonetic var. **Siobhan** (Ir. Gael. var. **Joan**, fem. **John**). Heb. "The Lord is gracious."

Shevon, Shevonne, Shivonne, Shyvon, Shyvonne

Shawn (fem. var. **Sean**, Ir. var. **John**) Heb. "The Lord is gracious." Use of Sean and its variants, feminine and masculine, is on the wane since the late 1970s. Actress Sean Young.

Sean, Seana, Shana, Shanna, Shaun, Shauna, Shawna, Shawnee, Shawneen, Shawnette, Sianna

Sheba Heb. "From Sheba." Also a short version of **Bathsheba**. Heb. "Daughter of the oath." The queen of Sheba is mentioned in the Old Testament as having been hugely rich and very ostentatious.

Saba, Sabah, Shebah

Shea Ir. Gael. "From the fairy fort." More commonly an Irish last name.

Shae, Shayla, Shaylyn

Sheena Ir. Var. **Jane**. Heb. "The Lord is gracious." Many of the "Sh" names are Gaelic versions of Jane, Jean, and Joan, which are in turn variations on that old staple, John. Rock star Sheena Easton.

Sheenagh, Sheenah, Sheina, Shena, Shiona

Sheila Ir. Var. **Cecilia**. Lat. "Blind." Popular mid–20th century in Britain and the Commonwealth; in Australian slang, a "sheila" is a woman.

Seila, Selia, Shayla, Shaylah, Sheela, Sheelagh, Sheelah, Sheilagh, Sheilah, Shela, Shelagh, Shelia, Shiela

Shelby OE. Place name: "Estate on the ledge." More commonly a man's name.

Shelbee, Shelbey, Shellby

Shelley OE. Place name: "Meadow on the ledge." Last name made famous by the poet Percy Bysshe Shelley. Use as a feminine first name seems to have been related

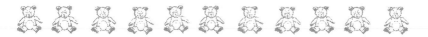

to Shirley. Actresses Shelley Winters, Shelley Duvall, Shelley Long.
Shellee, Shellie, Shelly

Sherry Var. **Cher** (Fr. "dear"), **Sharon** (Heb. "the plain"), or **Cheryl** (var. **Charlotte**, OG. "man"). In the 1950s and 1960s these three names and their variants were all popular, giving rise to a parade of further forms, spellings, and elaborations. Tracing the exact origin of any of them is difficult.
Sharee, Shari, Sharie, Sheree, Sherey, Sheri, Shericia, Sherie, Sherina, Sherita, Sherree, Sherrey, Sherri, Sherryn, Sherye

Sheryl Var. **Cheryl** (var. **Charlotte**, OG. "man"). Actress Sherilyn Fenn.
Sheralyn, Sheralin, Sherileen, Sherill, Sherilyn, Sherryl, Sheryll

Shifra Heb. "Lovely."
Schifra, Shifrah

Shiri Heb. "My song."
Shira, Shirah, Shirit

Shirley OE. Place name: "Bright meadow." Originally a last name, brought to immense fame and popularity as a girl's name with the career of child star Shirley Temple. Now widely neglected. Actress Shirley MacLaine; politician Shirley Chisholm.
Sherlee, Sherlie, Sheryl, Shirl, Shirlee, Shirleen, Shirlene, Shirline, Shirlley, Shirly, Shurlee

Shona Ir. Gael. Var. **John**. Closely related to Sinead, but spelled phonetically, which is a help to non-Gaelic-speaking parents.

Shoshana Heb. "Lily." The more common form is the anglicized Susan.
Shosha, Shoshanah

Shulamith Heb. "Peace." Composer Shulamit Ran; writer Shulamith Firestone.
Shula, Shulamit, Sula, Sulamith

Sibyl Gk. "Seer, oracle." In ancient myth, sibyls interpreted the messages from oracles devoted to particular Gods, but their legend was also taken up and Christianized, and the name was common in the Middle Ages.

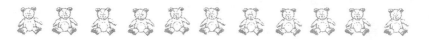

Use dropped off and was revived at the turn of the 20th century, but the name (more commonly spelled Sybil) now has a slightly dated aura. Actress Cybill Shepherd.
Cybele, Cybil, Cybill, Cybilla, Sabilla, Sabylla, Sib, Sibbell, Sibel, Sibell, Sibella, Sibelle, Sibilla, Sibyll, Sibylla, Sybel, Sybella, Sybelle, Sybill, Sybilla, Sybille

Sidonie Lat. "From Sidonia." Sidon was an area in the Middle East.
Sidaine, Sidonia, Sidony, Sydonia, Syndonia

Sidra Lat. "Of the stars."

Sigfreda OG. "Peaceful victory."
Sigfreida, Sigfrida, Sigfrieda, Sigfryda

Sigismonda It. From OG. "Victorious shield."
Sigismunda, Sigmonda, Sigmunda

Signa Unknown Scandinavian meaning: "Victory" is a possibility. The name is very unusual.
Signe, Signild, Signilda, Signilde

Silvia Var. **Sylvia**. Lat. "From the woods." This was the original form of the name, eclipsed by the "-y" spelling in the 19th century.
Silvie, Sylvia, Sylvie

Simcha Heb. "Joy."

Simone (fem. **Simon**) Heb. "listening intently." Used outside of France from the middle of the 20th century. Actress Simone Signoret.
Simona, Simonetta, Simonette, Simonia, Simonina, Symona, Symone

Sinead Ir. Var. **Janet** (fem. **John**, Heb. "the Lord is gracious"). This name and Siobhan are a little more common than most Gaelic names, possibly influenced by actresses Sinead Cusack and Siobhan McKenna. Sheena is a short version of Sinead. Singer Sinead O'Connor.
Seonaid, Sine

Siobhan Ir. Var. **Joan** (fem. **John**, Heb. "the Lord is gracious"). Many of the phonetic forms of this name are probably intended as a combination of the "Sha-" prefix and Yvonne. Actress Siobhan McKenna.
Chavonne, Chevonne, Chivon, Shavaun, Shavon, Shevonne, Shivahn, Shivaun, Shovonne, Shyvonne, Siobahn

Sirena Gk. "Entangler." In Greek myth, sirens were creatures that were half-woman, half-bird, and sang so sweetly that men dropped everything to listen, and starved to death. Odysseus encountered them in his travels.
Sireena, Sirene, Syrena

Sissy Dim. **Cecilia**. Lat. "blind." Also a common nickname for a sister, since this is the way a younger sibling may say that word. Actress Sissy Spacek.
Sissee, Sissey, Sissie

Skye Scot. Place name: the name of a spectacular island off the west coast of Scotland.

Skyler Dutch. "Giving shelter." Most probably an adaptation of the Dutch last name of Schuyler, which was brought to New York by 17th-century settlers.
Schyler, Schuyler, Skyla, Skylar, Skyllar

Socorro Sp. "Aid, help." Currently popular in Spain. Most likely refers to the aid or help provided by the Almighty.

Solange Fr. "With dignity."
Souline, Zeline

Soledad Sp. "Solitude."

Solveig Scan. "Woman of the house."
Solvag

Sondra Var. **Sandra** (dim. **Alexandra**, Gk. "defender of mankind"). Actress Sondra Locke.
Saundra, Sohndra, Zohndra, Zondra

Sonia Var. **Sophia**. Gk. "Wisdom." Used since early in the 20th century. Skater/actress Sonja Henie; painter Sonia Delaunay.
Sonja, Sonnja, Sonya

Sophia Gk. "Wisdom." Used in English-speaking countries since the 17th century, though the French form, Sophie, has given it much competition in Britain. The famous Istanbul mosque Hagia Sofia was once a Christian church, but it was dedicated, not to Saint Sophia (an obscure and possibly nonexistent martyr), but to the Holy Wisdom, i.e., the Word of God. The name is not particularly common, but ripe for revival. Actress Sophia Loren.

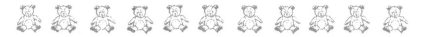

Saffi, Sofia, Sofie, Sofy, Sonia, Sonja, Sonnie, Sonya, Sophey, Sophie, Sophy, Zofia, Zofi

Sophronia Gk. "Sensible, prudent."
Sofronia

Sorcha Ir. Gael. "Bright, shining." Used almost exclusively in Ireland. Actress Sorcha Cusack.

Sorrel Botanical name. Sorrel is a wild herb. Much less common, however, than Laurel or Rosemary.
Sorrell, Sorrelle

Speranza It. "Hope."
Esperance, Speranca

Spring OE. "Springtime." Use as a given name dates from (and is almost exclusive to) the 1970s.

Stacy Gk. "Resurrection." Dim. **Anastasia**. Most popular since the 1970s, and has long since outstripped its source.
Stace, Stacee, Stacey, Staci, Stacia, Stacie, Stasee, Stasey, Stasia, Stasie, Stasey, Stasy

Star Word as name. Translations, such as Stella (Greek) and Esther (Persian), are far more common.
Starla, Starlene, Starr

Stella Lat. "Star." Use was mostly literary until the 19th century, when the name became fashionable. For this generation of parents brought up on classic movies, it is hard to dissociate from Marlon Brando bellowing "Stella!" in *A Streetcar Named Desire*.
Estelle, Estella, Estrella, Stelle

Stephanie (fem. **Stephen**) Gk. "Crowned." Cropped up in the 1920s and current since then, if never a real mainstay for parents. Tennis star Steffi Graff; actresses Stefanie Powers, Stephanie Zimbalist; poet Stevie Smith.
Stefa, Stefanie, Stefenney, Steffaney, Steffanie, Steffie, Stefinney, Stepfanie, Stepha, Stephana, Stephania, Stephannie, Stepheney, Stephine, Stevana, Stevena, Stevie, Stevey

Stina Dim. **Christina**. Gk. "Anointed, Christian."
Stine

Storm OE. Use of the word as a name: may be a last name transferred.
Stormie, Stormy

Sukey Dim. **Susan**. Heb. "lily." Appeared in the 18th cen-

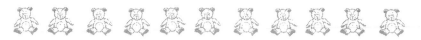

tury and revived in the 20th, following the popularity of Susan itself.

Sukee, Sukie, Suky

Summer OE. Name of the season. Like Spring and Season, a phenomenon of the 1970s.

Sunny Eng. Word as name: most likely to be a nickname characterizing a child's temperament.

Sunshine

Susan Heb. "Lily." After 18th-century use, neglected until a huge surge of popularity made it a top choice in the middle years of the 20th century. Parents who had three Susans in their first grade class are likely to pass over the name for their own children. Suffragette Susan B. Anthony; author Susan Cheever; actresses Susan Hampshire, Susan Dey, Susan Sarandon.

Shoshana, Shoshanah, Shoshanna, Shushana, Sioux, Siouxsie, Soosan, Soosanna, Sosanna, Sue, Suesann, Suezanne, Sukee, Sukey, Sukie, Susana, Susanetta, Susann, Susanna, Susannagh, Susannah, Susanne, Susette, Susi, Susie, Susy, Suzan, Suzane, Suzanna, Suzanne, Suze, Suzee, Suzette, Suzie, Suzy, Suzzanne

Susannah Heb. "Lily." The original version of the name, and ripe for revival, combining as it does the nostalgic and the unusual (like Molly and Emma).

Suesanna, Susana, Susanna, Susannagh, Suzanna

Suzanne Fr. Var. **Susan**. It has more or less followed **Susan** into and out of fashion. Ballerina Suzanne Farrell; actresses Suzanne Pleshette, Suzanne Sommers.

Suesana, Susanna, Susanne, Suzane, Suzannah, Suzette, Suzzanne

Sybil Var. **Sibyl**. The most common spelling of the name, though it only became prevalent in the last century.

Cybele, Cybill, Sibilla, Sibyl, Sibylla, Sybel, Sybella, Sybelle, Sybill, Sybilla

Sydney OF. Place name: "Saint Denis." Originally Saint Denis would have been the name of a village, and the name Sidney would have indicated a resident there. The name is almost exclusively male, but was given prominence as a woman's name in the 1980s by madam/celebrity Sydney Biddle Barrows.

Sydel, Sydelle, Sydnie

Sylvia Lat. "From the forest." The Latin form, Silvia, predominated for centuries, but when the name was at its most popular (from the 19th century into the 1940s), Sylvia was the spelling of choice. Poet Sylvia Plath; actress Silvana Mangano.

Silva, Silvaine, Silvana, Silvanna, Silvia, Silviana, Silvianne, Silvie, Sylva, Sylvana, Sylvanna, Sylvee, Sylvette, Sylviana, Sylvianne, Sylvie, Sylvine, Sylwia, Zilvia, Zylvia

Tabina Arab. "Muhammad's follower."

Tabitha Aramaic. "Gazelle." New Testament name reintroduced in the 17th century passion for biblical names. Neglected in this century until a minor revival in the 1960s.

Tabatha, Tabbee, Tabbey, Tabbi, Tabbie, Tabbitha, Tabby, Tabetha, Tabotha, Tabytha

Tacita Lat. "Silence." Never a standard, but somewhat more common in eras when a woman's role was to be quiet.

Tacey

Taffy Welsh. "Loved one."

Tahira Arab. "Virginal, pure."

Talia Heb. "Heaven's dew." May also be a variant of Thalia, or a derivative of Natalie. A pretty name, but infrequently used. Actress Talia Shire.

Talley, Tallia, Tallie, Tally, Tallya, Talya

Talitha Aramaic. "Young girl." Actress Talitha Soto.

Taleetha, Taletha, Talita

Tallulah Choctaw Indian. "leaping water." Not, as one might expect, an invented name, nor even one assumed by its most famous bearer, actress Tallulah Bankhead. It was a Bankhead family name, and is also a place name in Georgia. Could not now be used without reference to the actress, however.

Talley, Tallie, Tally

Tamara Heb. "Palm tree." Old Testament name with a hint of the picturesque. Tamar was the more common version until this century, when Tamara, the Russian form, overtook it. Quite fashionable in the 1970s. Skiing champion Tamara McKinney; author Tama Janowitz.
Tama, Tamar, Tamarah, Tamarra, Tamary, Tamera, Tamma, Tammara, Tammi, Tammy, Thamar, Thamara, Thamarra

Tamika Modern U.S. name of unknown origin. Some sources suggest a Japanese root meaning "people," but this seems farfetched since the name is not used in the Japanese community. More likely to be a variant of the popular Tanisha.
Tameeka, Tamiecka, Tamieka, Tamike, Tamiko, Tamiqua, Timeeka, Tomika, Tonica, Tonique, Tymmeeka, Tymmiecka

Tammy Dim. **Tamara** (or other "Tam-" names). A nickname that took on a life of its own in the 1950s and 1960s, and was probably used without much interest in its source or meaning. Now out of fashion. Actress Tammy Grimes; singer Tammy Wynette; evangelist Tammy Faye Bakker.
Tami, Tammee, Tammey, Tammie

Tamsin Var. **Thomasina**. Very old name that was revived by British parents in the middle of the 20th century.
Tamasin, Tamasine, Tamzen

Tanisha Modern name of unclear meaning, though several sources propose an African origin. Its popularity may stem from a contemporary fondness for 3-syllable names ending in "-a." And while the "Ta-" prefix doesn't approach the popularity of "La-" or "Sha-," the similarity of sound may contribute to Tanisha's widespread use. This is probably a combination of "Ta-" and the much-favored **Aisha**.
Taneesha, Taniesha, Tanitia, Tannicia, Tanniece, Tannisha, Teneesha, Tinecia, Tiniesha, Tynisha

Tansy Gk. "Everlasting life." Also the name of a common herb. Used mostly since the 1960s.
Tandie, Tansee, Tansey, Tanzey

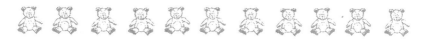

Tanya Dim. **Tatiana**, an ancient Italian name. This diminutive has been more popular than the full name, especially in the 1970s. Photographer Tana Hoban; skater Tonya Harding.
Tana, Tahnee, Tahnya, Taneea, Tania, Tanita, Tanja, Tawnya, Tonya, Tonyah

Tara Ir. Gael. "Rocky hill." Though Irish legends mention a place called Tara, its real prominence came in the 1940s when most Americans knew that Scarlett O'Hara's plantation home was called Tara. This seems to have launched the use of the name.
Tarah, Tarra, Tarrah

Taryn Var. **Tara**. Probably depends somewhat on the success of Karen, Sharon, and Darren in the 1950s and 1960s.
Taran, Tarin, Tarina, Tarren, Tarryn, Teryn

Tasha Dim. **Natasha**. Rus. "Christmas." Author Tasha Tudor.
Tahsha, Tasia, Tasya

Tatiana Rus. Var. of an ancient Italian name. Has penetrated the U.S. somewhat in recent years. Opera star Tatiana Troyannos.
Tania, Tanya, Tati, Tatie, Tatyana, Tatyanna, Tonya

Taylor Middle English. Occupational name: "Tailor." Probably considered a girl's name based on the fame of novelist Taylor Caldwell, whose middle name it is. But last names used as first names are increasingly popular for girls, and Taylor may become more fashionable.
Tailor, Tayler

Tecla Gk. "Fame of God." Traditionally Saint Thecla, converted by Saint Paul, was the first female Christian martyr, but her legend seems to be largely fantastic. The name has been most popular in Greece.
Tekli, Telca, Telka, Thecla, Thekla

Temira Heb. "Tall."
Temora, Timora

Tempest OF. "Storm." Rare usage is probably a matter of a family name transposed, since few parents wish for a child with a stormy temperament. Actress Tempest Bledsoe.

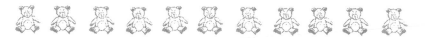

Terena (fem. **Terence**) Roman clan name. Used mostly in the middle of the 20th century.
Tereena, Terina, Terrena, Teryna

Terry Dim. **Theresa**. This and other nicknames for **Theresa** were at their most popular in the middle of the 20th century. Actress Teri Garr.
Terall, Teree, Terell, Terella, Teri, Terie, Terrey, Terri, Terrye

Tertia Lat. "Third." Unusual, as most of these number names (Prima, Secunda) are. Curiously, **Octavia** is the only one that has taken on a life of its own.

Tessa Dim. **Theresa**. Some sources also suggest Gk. "fourth child." Pretty, simple, and uncommon.
Tess, Tessie, Tessy

Thaddea (fem. **Thaddeus**) Gk., meaning unsure: "Brave" is one possibility.
Thada, Thadda

Thalassa Gk. "Sea, ocean."

Thalia Gk. "Blooming, in flower." In Greek legend Thalia is one of the Three Graces (along with Aglaia and Euphosyne); she is also one of the nine Muses, daughters of Zeus and Mnemosyne, each of whom represents an art or a science. Thalia represents Comedy.
Talia, Talie, Talley, Tally, Thalie, Thalya

Thana Arab. "Thanksgiving."

Thea Gk. "Goddess." Also dim. **Dorothea** (Gk. "gift of God").

Thelma Gk. "Will." Literary name coined in the late 19th century, at its peak in the first third of this century. It has the aura of a bygone era, but not so bygone that it is attractive to modern parents.

Theodora Gk. "Gift of God." Much less common than its synonym, Dorothy. At its peak in the middle third of the 20th century, but never a standard. Actress/vamp Theda Bara.
Dora, Fedora, Feodora, Fyodora, Teddey, Teddie, Tedra, Teodora, Teodory, Theadora, Theda, Theo, Theodosia

Theodosia Gk. "Gift of God." Little-used variant given some prominence by Anya Seton's 1941 historical novel *My Theodosia*, about Aaron Burr's daughter.
Feodosia, Theda, Teodosia

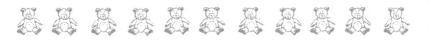

Theone Gk. "Name of God." Costume designer Theoni V. Aldredge.
Theoni

Theophania Gk. "God's appearance." Immensely popular in its contracted modern form, Tiffany.
Theophanie

Theophila Gk. "God-loving."
Theofila

Theresa Gk. "Harvest." May also stem from a Greek place name. The name owes its popularity to two important Catholic saints, the astringent, intellectual mystic Saint Teresa of Avila, and the humble young nun, St. Thérèse of Lisieux. It seems to have spread from Catholic families to wider acceptance, and was especially common in the 1960s. Actress Teresa Russell; Mother Teresa.
Taresa, Tera, Terasa, Teresa, Terese, Teresia, Teresina, Teresita, Teressa, Tereza, Terezinha, Terezsa, Teri, Terrasa, Terresa, Terresia, Terri, Terrosina, Terry, Terrya, Terza, Tess, Tessa, Tessey, Tessi, Tessie, Tessy, Thérèse, Theresina, Theresita, Tracey, Tracie, Tracy, Treesa, Tresa, Tressa, Trescha, Treza, Zita

Thomasina (fem. **Thomas**) Heb. "Twin." Thomasin was the earliest form, replaced by Thomasina in the Victorian era, and Tamsin a hundred years later. Now quite scarce.
Tammi, Tammie, Thomasa, Thomasin, Thomasine, Thomazine, Toma, Tomasina, Tomasine, Tommie, Tommy

Thora Scan. "Thor's struggle."
Thordia, Thordis, Thyra, Tyra

Thurayya Arab. "Star."
Thuraia

Tia Sp. "Aunt." Probably used as a first name with little reference to its actual meaning, but fondness for its sound.
Tiana, Tiara

Tiberia Lat. Place name: The river Tiber flows through Rome, and Tiberius was a Roman clan name.
Tibbie, Tibby

Tiffany Gk. "God's appearance." Literally, Theophania.

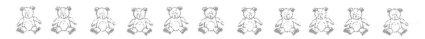

Traditionally used for babies born on Epiphany, the day when the Three Kings first saw the Christ Child. Now associated with Tiffany & Co., the New York City jeweler. The name has become shorthand for upper-class luxury, and was hugely popular in the 1980s.
Theophanie, Tifennie, Tiffaney, Tiffani, Tiffanie, Tiffenie, Tiffie, Tiffney, Tiphanie, Tyffany

Tilda Dim. **Matilda**. OG. "Battle-mighty."
Tildie, Tildy, Tilley, Tillie, Tilly

Timothea (fem. **Timothy**) Gk. "Honoring God." Uncommon feminization of a well-established boy's name.
Thea, Timmie

Tina Dim. **Christina**, etc. Used in the 20th century, but especially popular in the 1960s. Rock star Tina Turner; actress Tina Louise.
Teena, Teina, Tena, Tine

Tirza Heb. "Pleasantness." Although many versions of the name exist, it is rarely used in modern times. It is one of the few Old Testament female names that was not used widely in the Puritan era.
Thersa, Thirsa, Thirza, Thirzah, Thursa, Thurza, Tierza, Tirzah, Tyrzah

Tita Probably derived from Spanish diminutives like Martita; may be considered a feminization of Titus (or Tito).

Titania Gk. "Giant." The Titans in Greek myth were a race of giants. A more familiar use of the name, though, is the Queen of the Fairies in Shakespeare's *A Midsummer Night's Dream.*
Tania, Tita, Titanya, Tiziana

Toby Heb. "God is good." More commonly a boy's name, used from time to time for girls.
Tobe, Tobee, Tobey, Tobi, Tova, Tovah, Tove

Toni Dim. **Antoinette**. Lat. "Beyond price, invaluable."
Toinette, Tonee, Toney, Tonia, Tonie, Tony, Tonya, Twanette

Topaz Lat. Jewel name. Less common than Ruby and Pearl, but a good candidate for a November baby (it is that month's birthstone) or for a baby with topaz (golden) coloring.

Tory Dim. **Victoria**. Lat. "Victory."

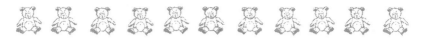

Torey, Tori, Toria, Torie, Torrey, Torrye

Toya Modern U.S. name, perhaps a diminutive of **Latoya**, one of the most popular "La-" names. It has no particular meaning.

Toia

Tracy Dim. **Theresa**. First used in numbers in the 1940s, probably in response to the film *The Philadelphia Story*. This touched off a long period of popularity that is now distinctly fading. Actress Tracey Ullman; tennis player Tracy Austin.

Tracee, Tracey, Traci, Tracie, Trasey

Traviata It. "One who goes astray." As in the great Verdi opera, *La Traviata.*

Tricia Dim. **Patricia**. Lat. "Aristocratic." Choreographer Trisha Brown.

Treasha, Trichia, Trish, Trisha

Trilby Literary name coined at the turn of the 20th century. Trilby, the central character of the eponymous novel and play, became a great singer. (The name may refer to vocal trills.) A trilby hat, worn by the character in the 1895 stage production, is a soft felt hat with a dented crown.

Trilbie, Trillby

Trina Dim. **Katrina**. Gk. "Pure."

Treena, Treina, Trine, Trinette

Trinity Lat. "Triad." Refers to the Holy Trinity, the three forms of God in the Christian faith. Used mostly among Spanish-speaking families. Actress Trini Alvarado.

Trini, Trinidad, Trinidade

Trista Lat. "Sad." An inauspicious name for a baby, however pretty it sounds.

Trixie Dim. **Beatrice**. Lat. "Bringer of gladness."

Trix, Trixy

Trudy Dim. **Gertrude**. OG. "Strength of a spear." Cropped up in the middle of the 20th century, but little heard now.

Truda, Trude, Trudey, Trudi, Trudie

Tsifira Heb. "Crown, diadem."

Tuesday OE. Day of the week. Given exposure by actress Tuesday Weld, but not in general use.

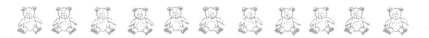

Twyla Modern name of uncertain meaning and derivation. Choreographer Twyla Tharp.
Twila
Tzigane Hung. "Gypsy."
Tsigana, Tsigane

Udele OE. "Wealthy."
Uda, Udella, Udelle, Yudella, Yudelle
Ula Celt. "Gem of the sea."
Eula, Ulla, Yulla
Ulima Arab. "Astute, wise."
Ulima, Ullima
Ulrica (fem. **Ulric**) OG. "Power of the wolf" or "power of the home." Very unusual outside of Germany.
Rieka, Rica, Ricka, Ulka, Ullrica, Ullricka, Ulrika, Ulrike
Ultima Lat. "End, farthest point." In English, hard to dissociate from "ultimate." There is a brand of cosmetics called Ultima.
Ulva OG. "Wolf."
Una Lat. "One." The origin of the name may be Irish, though its Celtic meaning is lost. Very unusual.
Oona, Oonagh
Undine Lat. "Little wave." In myth, Undine is the spirit of the waters. Edith Wharton created a character in *The Custom of the Country* who was named Undine for the hair-curling tonic that had made her father rich.
Ondina, Ondine, Undeen, Undene
Unity Middle English. "Oneness." Used by the Puritans and extremely uncommon. Most people have heard of it only in connection with Unity Mitford, one of the famous English Mitford sisters.
Unita
Urania Gk. "Heavenly." Urania was one of the Greek Muses, the nine daughters of Zeus and Mnemosyne identified with particular arts and sciences. Urania was in charge of astronomy.
Urainia, Uraniya, Uranya

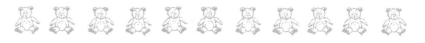

Urbana Lat. "Of the city." The male form, Urban, is a bit more familiar, having been used by eight popes. The female version is rare even in Europe.
Urbanna

Urit Heb. "Brightness."

Ursula Lat. "Little female bear." Saint Ursula was a much-venerated virgin martyr, allegedly executed by Attila the Hun, though her story has little basis in fact. The name was most popular in the 17th century. Fans of Disney cartoons will be bound to associate it with the overweight octopus sea-witch in *The Little Mermaid*. Author Ursula K. Le Guin; actress Ursula Andress.
Orsa, Orsala, Orsola, Orsolla, Seula, Sula, Ulla, Ursa, Ursala, Ursella, Ursie, Ursola, Ursule, Ursulina, Ursuline, Ursy, Urszuli

Uta Origin unclear: possibly dim. **Otthild**. OG. "Prospers in battle." Actress Uta Hagen.
Yuta

Val Dim. **Valentina, Valerie**. Occasionally an independent name.

Vala OG. "Singled out."
Valla

Valda (fem. **Waldemar**) OG. "Renowned ruler." Occurs in some Northern European countries, and from time to time in Britain, but very scarce in the U.S.
Vallda, Velda

Valentina Lat. "Strong." This name and Valerie come from the same Latin root. Valentia was the earliest form, but it entered the modern age as Valentina. Valentine is used for both boys and girls, and the early Christian martyr for whom the holiday is named was male. Cosmonaut Valentina Tereshkova.
Teena, Teina, Tena, Tina, Val, Vale, Valeda, Valena,

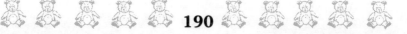

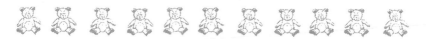

Valencia, Valentia, Valentijn, Valentine, Valenzia, Valera, Valida, Valina, Valli, Vallie, Vally, Velora

Valerie Lat. "Strong." The French form of an early Christian name (Valeria) that was revived at the turn of the 20th century. It was very popular in the middle of the 20th century, less so now. Actresses Valerie Harper, Valerie Bertinelli, Valerie Perrine.
Val, Valaree, Valarey, Valaria, Valarie, Vale, Valeree, Valeria, Valery, Valerye, Vallarie, Valleree, Vallerie, Vallery, Vallie, Valorie, Valry

Valeska (fem. **Vladislav**) Old Slavic. "splendid leader."
Valonia Lat. Place name. "Shallow valley."
Valora Lat. "Courageous."
Valoria, Valorie, Valory, Valorya

Vanda Var. **Wanda**. OG. tribal name. Mostly used at the turn of the century.
Vannda

Vanessa Literary name, invented by *Gulliver's Travels* author Jonathan Swift. Suddenly leapt into everyday use in the middle years of the 20th century, achieving some popularity in the 1970s. Actress Vanessa Redgrave; celebrity Vanna White; Singer Vanessa Williams.
Nessa, Nessie, Nessy, Van, Vanesa, Vanesse, Vanetta, Vannessa, Vannetta, Vania, Vanija, Vanna, Vannie, Vanya, Venesa, Venessa, Venetta

Vanora Old Welsh. "White wave."
Vannora

Varda Heb. "Rose."
Vardit

Varvara Var. **Barbara**. Gk. "Stranger." In Greek pronunciation the *v* and *b* sounds are quite close, hence the ties between these names.
Varenka, Varina, Varinka, Varya

Vashti Per. "Lovely." In the Old Testament, the wife of the proud King Ahasuerus of Persia. Passed over by the Puritans (perhaps because she became a divorcée), but revived very slightly in the 19th century.
Vashtee

Veda Sanskrit. "Knowledge, wisdom." The Vedas are the four sacred books of the Hindus.
Vedis, Veeda, Veida, Vida

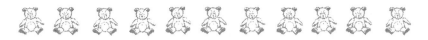

Vedette It. "Sentry, scout." By extension, because a sentry or a scout is often singled out or separated from the group, the French term *vedette* means something (like a headline) that is singled out graphically. And by further extension, in everyday usage, *vedette* is the French word for a movie star.

Vedetta

Vega Arab. "Falling." Vega is the name of one of the larger stars. It is also the name of a car manufactured by Chevrolet, and any parent who has ever driven one is unlikely to use that name for a daughter.

Velda Var. **Valda**.

Vellda

Velika Old Slavic. "Great, wondrous."

Velma Origin disputed. Possibly dim. **Wilhelmina** (OG. "will-helmet"), possibly a late–19th-century invention. In general use since the 1920s, but not fashionable.

Vellma

Venetia Place name. Never reached the stature of that other great Italian tourist mecca, Florence. Cropped up from the 17th century onward; use increased in the 19th century, but the name would still be considered a bit fanciful. The English form, Venice, is also used occasionally.

Vanecia, Vanetia, Venecia, Venezia, Venice, Venise, Venize, Venitia, Vonitia, Vonizia

Venus Name of the Roman goddess of love and beauty. Used in Britain in the 16th century through the 19th, but very scarce now. It creates a lot of expectations for a female baby.

Venusa, Venusina

Vera Slavic. "faith"; Lat. "truth." Use by two popular novelists in the late 19th century promoted the name to high fashion, but it is hardly found now. Actress Vera Miles.

Veradis, Veera, Veira, Vere, Verena, Verene, Verina, Verine, Verla, Verochka, Veroshka, Veruschka, Verushka

Verbena Lat. "Holy plants." Originally referred to olive,

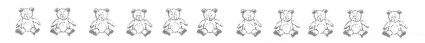

laurel, and myrtle, plants with spiritual significance to the Romans. In modern times, a class of plants with medicinal properties and, frequently, pleasant scents.

Verbeena, Verbina

Verdad Sp. "Truth."

Verena Lat. "True." Derives from the same root as **Vera**.

Vereena, Verina, Veruchka, Veruschka, Veryna

Verity Lat. "Truth." Puritan virtue name, much less common than Constance, Prudence, Hope, etc.

Verita, Veritie

Verna Lat. "Springtime." Use spans the late years of the 19th century to the middle of the 20th, but the name has a dated air and is rare today. Actress Virna Lisi.

Verda, Verne, Verneta, Vernetta, Vernette,
Vernice, Vernie, Vernis, Vernise, Vernisse,
Vernita, Virna

Verona Dim. **Veronica**. Also the name of a northern Italian city well-known to tourists, so it may be used by reminiscent parents.

Veron, Verone

Veronica Lat. "True image." Or var. **Bernice**, Gk. "she who brings victory." According to a legend that sprang up in the Middle Ages, a young girl wiped Jesus' sweating brow on his way to Calvary. The handkerchief she used later showed a perfect image of his face. (Three Italian churches now claim to own this holy relic.) The name first appeared in Britain in the 17th century, spread beyond Catholic families in the 19th century, and became popular in the 1950s. To baby boomers, reminiscent of the Archie and Veronica comic books. Actress Veronica Lake.

Rana, Ranna, Roni, Ronica, Ronna, Ronnee, Ronni,
Ronnica, Ronnie, Ronny, Veera, Veira, Vera, Veranica,
Veranique, Verohnica, Verohnicca, Veronice, Veronicka,
Veronika, Veronike, Veroniqua, Veronique, Vonnie

Vespera Lat. "Evening star."

Vesta Lat. The Roman household goddess. Her altar was tended by six virgins (the "vestal virgins"), who were kept under severe discipline. They were buried alive if

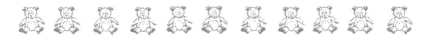

they lost their virginity. Most common late 19th to early 20th century.

Vicky Dim. **Victoria**. Author Vicki Baum; actress Vicki Lawrence.

Vicci, Vickee, Vickey, Vicki, Vicky, Vikkey, Vikki, Vikky

Victoria (fem. **Victor**) Lat. "Victory." Extremely common in Christian Rome, but curiously not fashionable during the reign (1837–1901) of the woman who gave her name to the Victorian age. Most recently popular in the 1950s and 1960s, but daughters in those days were probably called "Vicky." Parents who use it now are more likely to insist on the whole mouthful, or Tory in a pinch. Actress Victoria Principal.

Vic, Vicci, Vickee, Vickey, Vicki, Vickie, Vicky, Victorie, Victorina, Victorine, Vikkey, Vikki, Vikky, Viktoria, Viktorija, Viktorina, Viktorine, Vitoria, Vittoria

Vida Dim. **Davita**. Heb. "Loved one."

Veda, Veeda, Vidette, Vieda, Vita, Vitia

Vidonia Port. "Branch of a vine."

Veedonia, Vidonya

Vigilia Lat. "Wakefulness."

Vigdis Nor. "War goddess."

Vigdess

Vilhelmina Var. **Wilhelmina**. OG. "Will-helmet."

Vilhelmine, Villhelmina, Wilhelmina

Villette Fr. "Small town." The name of one of Charlotte Brontë's lesser-known novels.

Vilma Rus. Dim. **Vilhelmina**.

Wilma

Vina dim. **Davina,** etc. Sp. "vineyard" In either case, probably a name whose use was promoted by the feminine ending "-a."

Veena, Vena, Vinetta, Vinette, Vinita, Vyna, Vynetta, Vynette

Vincentia (fem. **Vincent**) Lat. "Conquering." An unusual feminization of a name that has not been very common in America.

Vincenta, Vincentena, Vincentina, Vincentine

Violet Lat. "Purple." A flower name in longer use than most. Occurred first in the 1830s and lasted nearly a hun-

dred years, but always more popular in Britain (whose cool, damp climate is more hospitable to the spring flowers). **Viola** has been a less-used choice. Ballerina Violette Verdy.

Eolande, Iolande, Iolanthe, Jolanda, Jolande, Jolanta, Jolantha, Jolanthe, Vi, Viola, Violaine, Violanta, Violante, Violanthe, Viole, Violeine, Violetta, Violette, Vyolet, Vyoletta, Vyolette, Yolanda, Yolande, Yolane, Yolantha, Yolanthe

Virginia Lat. "Virgin." The name probably derives from a Roman clan name, but the current meaning has been assumed for hundreds of years. A great favorite in the U.S. from the mid–19th century to the mid–20th; the first child born in the U.S. was Virginia Dare, in 1597. The state of Virginia was named in compliment to the Virgin Queen, Elizabeth I. A good candidate for 1990s revival. Author Virginia Woolf.

Geena, Geenia, Geenya, Gina, Ginella, Ginelle, Ginger, Gingia, Ginia, Ginnee, Ginni, Ginnie, Ginny, Ginya, Jenell, Jenella, Jenelle, Jinia, Jinjer, Jinnie, Jinny, Verginia, Verginya, Virge, Virgenya, Virgie, Virgine, Virginie, Virginnia

Viridis Lat. "Green."

Virdis, Viridia, Viridiana

Vita Lat. "Life."

Veeta, Vitel, Vitella, Vitka

Viveca Scan. "Alive." Var. **Viva**. Actress Viveca Lindfors.

Vivecka, Viveka

Viva Lat. "Alive." Most familiar from the expression meaning "Long live . . ." as in *"Viva l'España"* or *"Vive la France."* Actress Viva.

Veeva, Viveca, Vivva

Vivian Lat. "Full of life." Used for boys in Britain (although infrequently), generally for girls in the U.S. In spite of the early martyr Saint Vivian, the name has been current only since the 19th century, and has never been a real favorite. Actresses Vivien Leigh, Vivian Vance.

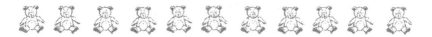

Bibi, Bibiana, Bibiane, Bibianna, Bibianne, Bibyana,
Vevay, Vi, Vibiana, Viv, Vivee, Vivi, Vivia, Viviana,
Viviane, Vivianna, Vivianne, Vivie, Vivien, Vivienne,
Vivyan, Vivyana, Vivyanne, Vyvyan, Vyvyana, Vyvyanne

Walburga OG. "Strong protection." Saint's name very rarely trotted out in modern times. Saint Walburga was an 8th-century missionary in Germany whose feast day was May 1, the traditional pagan festival day. *Walpurgisnacht* has come down in legend as the night of the witches' sabbath.

Walberga, Wallburga, Walpurgis

Walda (fem. **Waldo**) OG. "Ruler." Extremely unusual feminization of a name that is also unusual for boys.

Wallda, Welda, Wellda

Walker OE. Occupational name: "Cloth-walker." The era that saw the rise of last names was also the great English era of the wool trade, giving us such cloth-manufacturing names as Fuller, Tailor, and Weaver. In that medieval era, workers trod on the wool to clean it. This name is very unusual for girls.

Wallker

Wallis Var. **Wallace**. OE. "From Wales." Famous as a feminine name because of Wallis Simpson, the woman who very badly wanted to be queen of England, but became Duchess of Windsor instead.

Wallie, Walliss, Wally, Wallys

Wanda Probably a Slavic tribal name, though some sources suggest OG. "wanderer." Use has been pretty well confined to the middle of the 20th century.

**Vanda, Wahnda, Wandah, Wandie, Wandis, Wandy,
Wannda, Wenda, Wendaline, Wendall, Wendeline,
Wendy, Wonda, Wonnda**

Wanetta OE. "pale-skinned." From the same root that gives us "wan," which is not exactly a complimentary term.

Wanette

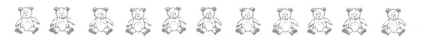

Warda (fem. **Ward**) OG. "Guardian."
Wardia, Wardine

Wendy Literary name: coined by James Barrie for the human heroine of *Peter Pan*. The parents who used it in great numbers in the middle of the 20th century may have been inspired by either the musical play or the animated movie. Some, wishing to call a daughter Wendy, no doubt named her Gwendolyn, but the names aren't actually related.
Wenda, Wendee, Wendeline, Wendey, Wendi, Wendie, Wendye, Windy

Whitney OE. Place name: "White island." Boy's name that became hugely popular for girls in the early 1980s, possibly because of its connotations of old wealth. Singer Whitney Houston.
Whitnee, Whitnie, Whitny

Wilda OE. "willow"; OG. "untamed."
Willda, Wylda

Wilhelmina OGer. "Will-helmet." Despite the number of variants spawned by the name, it hasn't been very popular in any form. Probably used more often to honor a beloved relative named William rather than on its own merits. Actress Billie Burke; author Willa Cather.
Billa, Billee, Billey, Billie, Billy, Ellma, Elma, Guglielma, Guillelmina, Guillelmine, Guillema, Guillemette, Guillemine, Helma, Helmina, Helmine, Helminette, Min, Mina, Minna, Minnie, Minny, Valma, Velma, Vilhelmina, Villhelmina, Villhelmine, Vilma, Wileen, Wilene, Wilhelmine, Willa, Willabella, Willabelle, Willamina, Willamine, Willeen, Willene, Willemina, Willetta, Willette, Williamina, Willie, Williebelle, Willmina, Willmine, Willy, Willybella, Wilma, Wilmette, Wilmina, Wilna, Wylma

Willow Tree name. A phenomenon of the 1970s. Fashion model Willow Bay.

Wilma Dim. **Wilhelmina**. Less of a mouthful than its source, but reminiscent of the dizzy Stone Age housewife Wilma Flintstone in the TV cartoon show "The Flintstones."
Valma, Vilma, Willma, Wilmina, Wylma

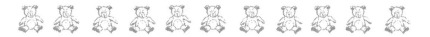

Wilona OE. "Longed-for."
Wilone

Winifred Welsh. "Holy peacemaking." Often explained as Old German "friend of peace." Popular in Britain for fifty years around the turn of the 20th century, but little used otherwise.
Fred, Freddie, Freddy, Fredi, Fredy, Wina, Winafred, Winefred, Winefride, Winefried, Winfreda, Winfrieda, Winifryd, Winne, Winnie, Winnifred, Wynafred, Wynifred, Wynn, Wynne, Wynnifred

Winola OG. "Charming friend."

Winona Sioux Indian. "Firstborn daughter." Actress Winona Ryder; country singer Winona Judd.
Wenona, Wenonah, Winnie, Winonah, Wynnona, Wynona, Wyomia

Winter OE. Season name. Like Summer, used mostly in the 1970s.

Wren OE. Bird name: A wren is a small brown songbird.

Wynne Welsh. "Fair, pure." Uncommon, but distinctive in a way that may appeal to parents of the 1990s.
Win, Winne, Winnie, Winny, Wyn, Wynn

Xanthe Gk. "Yellow." A description of someone's coloring. Almost unknown.
Xantha, Xanthia, Zanthe

Xaviera (fem. **Xavier**). Basque. "New house." Given some exposure by Xaviera Hollander, the author of a book that caused some stir in the early 1970s. It was called *The Happy Hooker*.
Xavyera, Zaviera

Xenia Gk. "Welcoming." Occasionally spelled with the X; occurs once in a while with a Z.
Xeenia, Xena, Zeena, Zena, Zenia, Zina, Zyna

Xylia Gk. "Wood-dweller." Related to the far more common Sylvia.
Xylina, Xylona

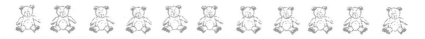

Yaffa Heb. "Lovely."
 Jaffa, Yaffah
Yalena Rus. Var. **Helen**. Gk. "Light."
 Yelena, Lenuschka, Lenushka, Lenya,
 Lenyushka
Yaminah Arab. "Suitable, proper."
Yamina, Yemina

Yasmin Arab. "Jasmine." A variation of a flower name that has been quite popular in the late eighties and early nineties. Princess Yasmin Aga Khan.
 Yasmeen, Yasmeena, Yasmena, Yasmene, Yasmina,
 Yasmine

Yehudit Heb. "Praise."
 Judit, Judith, Yudita, Yuta

Yetta OE. Dim. **Henrietta**. OG. "Ruler of the house." Used at the turn of the 20th century, but virtually unheard-of now.
 Yette

Ynez Sp. Var. **Agnes**. Gk. "Pure."
 Ines, Inez, Ynes

Yoko Jap. "Good, positive." Would probably be unknown outside Japanese families without the fame of Beatle wife Yoko Ono.

Yolanda Gk. "Violet flower." The Spanish version of Violet. Used in English-speaking countries in the 20th century, particularly during the 1960s.
 Eolande, Eolantha, Iola, Iolanda, Iolande, Iolantha,
 Iolanthe, Jolan, Jolanna, Jolanne, Jolanta, Jolantha,
 Jolanthe, Yalonda, Yola, Yoland, Yolande, Yollande,
 Yolantha, Yolanthe, Yulanda

Yonina Heb. "Dove."
 Jona, Jonati, Jonina, Yona, Yonah, Yoninah, Yonit,
 Yonita

Yosepha (fem. **Joseph**) Heb. "Jehovah increases." A possibility for parents who don't like Josephine.
 Josefa, Josepha, Yosefa, Yuseffa

Ysabel Var. **Elizabeth** Heb. "Pledged to God." Via **Isabel**.
 Ysabell, Ysabella, Ysabelle, Ysbel, Ysbella, Ysobel

Ysanne Modern name, combination of **Ysabel** and **Anne**. Found in Britain.

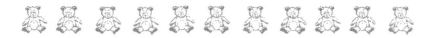

Ysande, Ysanna
Yuliya Rus. Var. **Julia**. Lat. "Youthful."
   Yulenka
Yvette Dim. **Yvonne**.
   Ivett, Ivetta, Ivette, Yevette, Yvetta
Yvonne (fem. **Ivo**) Fr. from OG. "yew wood." Since yew wood was used for bows, **Ivo** may have been an occupational name meaning "archer." The most common male form is probably Yves, but Yvonne is more widespread in English-speaking countries. It was particularly popular in Britain in the 1970s. Tennis star Evonne Goolagong; actress Yvonne DeCarlo.
   Eevonne, Evonne, Ivonne, Yevette, Yvetta, Yvette

    Zada Arab. "Fortunate, prosperous."
      Zaida, Zayeeda, Zayda
    Zahavah Heb. "Gilded."
      Zachava, Zachavah, Zahava, Zechava,
      Zehavah, Zehavit
    Zahira Arab. "Brilliant, shining."
   Zaheera, Zahirah
Zahra Arab. "White." Currently popular in Arabic-speaking countries.
   Zahrah
Zandra Var. **Sandra**, dim. **Alexandra**. Gk. "Defender of mankind." Fashion designer Zandra Rhodes.
   Zahndra, Zanndra, Zohndra, Zondra
Zanna Dim. **Susanna**. Heb. "Lily."
   Zana
Zara Heb. "Eastern brightness, dawn." May also be a form of **Sarah** (Heb. "princess"). Literary name used often over the centuries for exotic characters. Taken up in the 1960s in Britain (Princess Anne's daughter is named Zara), but unusual in the U.S.
   Zaira, Zarah, Zaria, Zayeera
Zelda Dim. **Griselda**. OG. "Gray fighting maid." The orig-

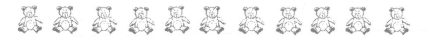

inal name has long been eclipsed by this nickname, which was made famous by F. Scott Fitzgerald's neurotic wife.

Selda, Zelde, Zellda

Zelia Origin unclear; perhaps Gk. "zeal" or Fr. "solemn," from a saint's name. Rare.

Zele, Zelene, Zelie, Zelina, Zeline

Zelma Dim. **Anselma.** OG. "God-helmet." A less common form than **Selma.**

Zena Var. **Xenia.** Gk. "Welcoming." This is the slightly more common form of the name. Tennis star Zina Garrison.

Zeena, Zeenia, Zeenya, Zenia, Zenya, Zina

Zenaïde Var. **Zenobia.**

Zenaida

Zenobia Gk. "Power of Zeus." A 3rd-century empress of Palmyra, whose name was revived in the 19th century but has a rather quaint sound today.

Cenobia, Cenobie, Zeba, Zeena, Zena, Zenaida, Zenaïde, Zenayda, Zenda, Zenina, Zenobie, Zenna

Zephyr Gk. "West wind."

Zefeera, Zefir, Zefiryn, Zephira, Zephyra

Zerlinda Heb./Sp. "Beautiful dawn."

Zerlina

Zetta Heb. "Olive."

Zeta, Zetana

Zia Lat. "Grain."

Zea

Zigana Hung. "Gypsy."

Tsigana, Tsigane, Tzigana, Tzigane

Zilla Heb. "Shadow." Old Testament name revived by the Puritans and again in the 19th century, when it was more popular than one might suppose, given its current obscurity.

Zillah, Zylla

Zinnia Lat. Flower name. In this case the flower itself was named for its classifier, 18th-century German botanist Johann Zinn.

Zinia, Zinnya, Zinya

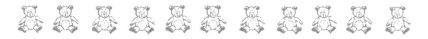

Zilpha Heb. Meaning unclear. Old Testament name revived in the 18th century and gradually fading ever since. Children's author Zilpha Keatley Snyder.
Zilpah, Zillpha, Zylpha

Zippora Heb. "Bird." Another Old Testament name; Zipporah was the wife of Moses. This biblical prominence has not translated into great popularity for the name, which sounds to some people like a way to do up a skirt.
Zipora, Ziporah, Zipporah

Zita Gk. "Seeker." Also dim. **Teresita, Rosita**, etc. The name of the last Hapsburg empress, who was given the name when it was at its most popular, at the turn of the century.
Zeeta, Zyta

Ziva Heb. "Brilliance, brightness."
Zeeva, Ziv

Zizi Hung. Dim. **Elizabeth**. Analogous to the Hungarian diminutive for Susan, Zsa Zsa. French singer Zizi Jeanmaire.
ZsiZsi

Zoe Gk. "Life." Currently popular in Greece, and catching on in English-speaking countries. Sufficiently unusual to appeal strongly to parents of the 1990s. Actress Zoe Caldwell.
Zoee, Zoelie, Zoeline, Zoelle, Zoey, Zoie, Zoya

Zola It. "Lump of earth." Like Zona, probably used more for its sound than for its meaning.
Zoela

Zona Lat. "Belt, girdle." The name given to the constellation in Orion's belt. Generally U.S. use.
Zonia

Zora Slavic. "Dawn's light." Author Zora Neale Hurston.
Zorah, Zorana, Zorina, Zorine, Zorra, Zorrah, Zorya

Zoya Rus. Var. **Zoe**.
Zoia, Zoyenka, Zoyya

Zsa Zsa Hung. Dim. **Susan**. Heb. "Lily." Made famous by actress and celebrity Zsa Zsa Gabor.
Zsuzsanna

Zsofia Hung. Var. **Sofia**. Gk. "Wisdom."

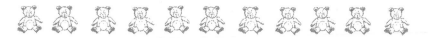

Zuleika Arab. "Brilliant and lovely." Inseparable from Max Beerbohm's comic heroine *Zuleika Dobson*, for the sake of whose love all the undergraduates of Oxford University drown themselves. Not, perhaps, an inspiring example for parents.

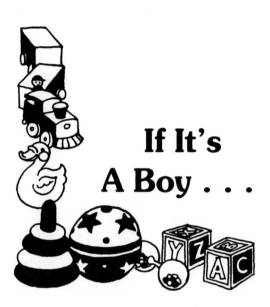

If It's
A Boy . . .

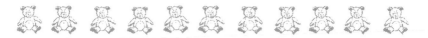

Aaron Heb. "Exalted, on high." In the Old Testament, Aaron was the brother of Moses. The name was unusual until the 17th century, when so many Old Testament names first came into prominence. It has been fashionable, especially in the U.S., since the 1970s. U.S. Vice President Aaron Burr; baseball star Hank Aaron; composer Aaron Copeland.

Aaran, Aaren, Aarron, Aeron, Aharon, Ari, Arin, Arnie, Arny, Aron, Arran, Arron, Erin, Haroun, Ron, Ronnie, Ronny

Abbey Dim. **Abbot, Abelard, Abner.** Political activist Abbie Hoffman.

Abbie, Abby

Abbott Heb. "Father." An abbot is the head of a monastic community, so the original bearers of this name (as a surname) may have worked for an abbot. Its use as a first name occurred mostly in the 19th century.

Ab, Abad, Abba, Abbe, Abe, Abbey, Abbie, Abbot, Abby, Abot, Abott

Abda Arab. "Servant."

Abdul Arab. "Servant of." Often used in combination with another name, as in "Abdullah," or "servant of Allah." Basketball star Kareem Abdul-Jabar.

Ab, Abdel, Abdullah, Del

Abe Dim. **Abraham.** Heb. "Father of many."

Abey, Abie

Abel Heb. "Breath." Abel was the younger son of Adam and Eve, who was slain by his older brother, Cain. Abel has survived with steady use ever since the 6th century, and surprisingly enough, Cain also occurs from time to time.

Abe, Abey, Abie, Able

Abelard OG. "Highborn and steadfast." Made famous by the 12th-century French philosopher Pierre Abelard, who fell in love with and seduced his student Heloise. Her uncle and guardian had him emasculated, even though he married Heloise. She became a nun, he became a monk.

Ab, Abbey, Abby, Abe, Abel

Abiah Heb. "My father is the Lord." Another Old Testament name, used for women as well as men in the Bible. Unusual in real life.
Abia, Abija, Abijah

Abida Heb. "God knows."

Abiel Heb. "My father is God." Old Testament name that the Puritans used in the U.S., but rare since.

Abimelech Heb. "My father is king." Occurred occasionally in the 19th century.

Abir Heb. "Strong."

Abisha Heb. "Gift of God."
Abijah, Abishai

Abner Heb. "My father is light." Old Testament name that came to some prominence in the late 16th century. Use fell off in this century, and the name is now mostly associated with Al Capp's comic strip *Li'l Abner*.
Ab, Abbey, Abbie, Abby, Abna, Abnar, Abnor, Avner, Eb, Ebbie, Ebby, Ebner

Abraham Heb. "Father of many." First of the Hebrew patriarchs. In the Bible, Abraham has a son named Isaac when he is 100 and his wife Sarah is 90. The name was popular while Abraham Lincoln was president (even more so after his assassination), but has faded from use since 1900.
Abarran, Abe, Abey, Abie, Abrahamo, Abrahan, Abram, Abrami, Abramo, Abran, Avram, Avrom, Bram, Ibrahim

Abram Heb. "He who is high is father." Var. **Abraham**.
Abe, Abey, Abie, Abramo, Avram, Avrom, Bram

Absalom Heb. "Father is peace." The handsome son of King David who connived to steal his father's throne. He died in battle, and his father lamented, "Would God I had died for thee, O Absalom, my son!" Also the title of a tragic novel by William Faulkner. Little used today.
Absolon

Ace Lat. "Unity." Connotations of superiority come from the fact that the ace is the playing card with highest face value.
Acer, Acey, Acie

Achilles Gk. Place name; also hero of the *Iliad*, as the greatest of the Greek heroes fighting the Trojans. He was

all but invulnerable, having been dipped in the River
Styx by his mother. She held him, however, by the heel,
which was thus his one weak point: hence "Achilles'
heel."

Achill, Achille, Achillea, Akil, Akilles

Achim Heb. "God will judge."

Acim

Ackerley OE. Place name: "Oak meadow." Surname
transferred to first name.

**Accerly, Acklea, Ackleigh, Ackley, Acklie, Ackerlea,
Ackerleigh, Ackerly**

Acton OE. Place name: "Oak tree settlement." Another
surname transferred to a first name: also the pseudonym
used by Charlotte Bronte's sister Anne, who wrote as
"Acton Bell." (The three sisters purposely chose mas-
culine-sounding pseudonyms.)

Adair Scot. Gael. Place name: "Oak tree ford." Recently
becoming more popular.

Adaire, Adare

Adalard OG. "Noble and courageous."

Adelard

Adalfieri It. from Ger. "Noble oath."

Adalric OG. "Highborn ruler."

Adelric

Adam Heb. "Son of the red earth." In the Bible, God created Adam—the first man—out of the "red earth" and
breathed life into him. An appropriate name for the first
boy in a family that has produced many girls. Congressman Adam Clayton Powell, Jr.

**Ad, Adamo, Adams, Adan, Adao, Addam, Addams,
Addie, Addis, Addison, Addy, Ade, Adhamh, Adnet,
Adnot**

Adamson OE. "Son of Adam."

Adamsson, Addamson

Adar Heb. "noble."

Addison OE. "Son of Adam." Transferred surname. The
English poet and essayist Joseph Addison was popular
and influential through the 18th century.

Ad, Addie, Addy, Adison, Adisson

Addy Teut. "Awe-inspiring; highborn." Also short for **Adam**, etc.
Addie, Ade, Ado

Adel OG. "Noble, highborn." More familiar as a particle of other names.
Adal

Adelar OG. "Noble eagle." Var. **Abelard**.
Adal, Adalar, Adalard, Adelard

Adelphe Fr. from Gk. "Brother."
Adelphus

Aden Possibly place name (for a region of South Yemen, formerly a British colony) or a variation on **Aidan**.
Aiden

Adham Arab. "Black."

Adlai Heb. "My ornament." Used in the Old Testament, and very rare, though brought to public notice by statesman Adlai Stevenson.
Ad, Addie, Addy, Adley

Adler OG. "Eagle." More common as a surname, especially in the U.S.
Ad, Addler, Adlar

Adnah Heb. "Ornamented."

Adney OE. Place name: "The noble's island."

Adolph OG. "Noble wolf." The Latinized form Adolphus arrived in Britain in mid–19th century, having been a German royal name. Almost unheard-of since the rise of Adolf Hitler and World War II. Filmmaker Adolph Zukor; French actor Adolphe Menjou.
Ad, Adolf, Adolfo, Adolfus, Adolphe, Adolpho, Adolphus, Dolf, Dolph, Dolphus

Adonis Gk. In Greek myth, Adonis was a young man so beautiful that Aphrodite, goddess of love, became enamored of him. The name has come to epitomize male beauty.

Adrian Lat. "From Adria"—a north Italian city. First popular in the 1950s in Britain, and used also as a woman's name. Hollywood costume designer Adrian; 12th-century pope Adrian IV (the only English pope in history).
Ade, Adiran, Adriano, Adrien, Adryan, Hadrian, Hadrien

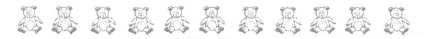

Aeneas Gk. "He who is praised." The Trojan hero of Virgil's Aeneid. Legend has it that he founded the Italian colony that was the origin of Rome.
Eneas, Enné

Afif Arab. "Chaste."

Afton OE. Place name. A surname that has come into use as a first name.
Affton

Agnolo It. "Angel."

Ahab Heb. "Father's brother." Pleasant way to honor an uncle, though literary types may be reminded of the mad sea captain in Herman Melville's novel *Moby Dick*.

Ahearn Celt. "Horse-lord."
Ahearne, Aherin, Ahern, Aherne, Hearn, Hearne, Herin, Hern

Ahmed Arab. "Greatly praised." Name often used for the prophet Muhammad, and favored by Muslims in the U.S.
Achmad, Achmed, Ahmad

Ahsan Arab. "Compassion."
Ehsan, Ihsan

Aidan Gaelic. "Fire." Saint Aidan was a 7th-century Irish monk. The name is also used for women. Actor Aidan Quinn.
Aiden, Edan, Eden

Aiken OE. "Made of oak." English writer Conrad Aiken.
Aicken, Aikin, Ayken, Aykin

Aimé Fr. "Much loved." More common as Aimée, a girl's name.

Aimery Teut. "Hardworking ruler."
Aimerey, Aimeric, Amerey, Aymeric, Aymery, Imre

Aimon Fr. from Teut. "House." Also possibly phonetic variant of the Irish Eamon, in turn a version of Edmund.
Aimond, Aymon, Haimon, Heman

Ainsley Scot. Gael. Place name: "His very own meadow." A last name converted to a first name, used by both sexes.
Ainsley, Ainsleigh, Ainslie, Ansley, Aynslee, Aynsley, Aynslie

Akbar Arab. "Great."

Akim Rus. Dim. **Joachim**. Heb. "God will judge."

Akmal Arab. "Perfect."

Alaire Fr. from Lat. "Joyful." Var. **Hilary**. The root is the same as "hilarious," though the meaning has shifted a bit.

Alair, Helier, Hilaire, Hilary, Larie, Lary

Alan Ir. Gael. Possible meanings are "rock" or "comely." Widely used in the Middle Ages, then again from the 19th century to the late 20th, with a boom around the 1950s influenced by the popularity of actor Alan Ladd. Now waning, like most fifties names. South African author Alan Paton; lyricist Alan Jay Lerner; astronaut Alan Shepard; actor Alan Alda; poet Allen Ginsberg.

Ailean, Ailin, Al, Alain, Alair, Aland, Alann, Alano, Alanson, Alen, Alin, Allan, Allayne, Allen, Alley, Alleyn, Alleyne, Allie, Allin, Allon, Allyn, Alon, Alun

Alard OG. "Noble and steadfast."

Adlar, Adlard, Al, Allard

Alaric OG. "Ruler of all" or "highborn ruler." Alaric I was the 5th-century king of the Visigoths who sacked Rome.

Al, Alarick, Alarico, Aleric, Alerick, Allaric, Allarick, Alleric, Allerick, Alric, Alrick, Ulrich, Ulrick

Alastair Gael. var. **Alexander** Gk. "man's defender." Generally a Scottish name, though it appears occasionally throughout the English-speaking world. Most of the variants are different phonetic spellings of the name. TV commentator Alistair Cooke.

Al, Alasdair, Alasteir, Alaster, Alastor, Alaisdair, Alaistair, Alaister, Aleister, Alester, Alistair, Alistar, Alister, Allaistar, Allaster, Allastir, Allistair, Allister, Allistir, Allysdair, Allysdare, Allystair, Allyster, Alysdair, Alysdare, Alystair, Alyster

Alban Lat. "From Alba," a city on a "white" hill, the oldest city in the ancient kingdom of Latium. The first Christian martyr on British soil was Saint Alban. Not to be confused with Albin, which has a different root.

Al, Albain, Alban, Albany, Albie, Albin, Albinet, Albion, Alby, Alvan, Alvin, Alvy, Auban, Auben, Aubin

Albern OG. "Noble courage."

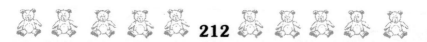

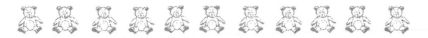

Albert OE. "Highborn, brilliant." Most widely used during the lifetime of Queen Victoria's German prince consort, Albert. Her many children and grandchildren carried the name to most of the royal families in Europe, but her eldest son's first move as king was to drop it. Out of style since the 1920s. Scientist Albert Einstein; Prince Albert of Monaco; actor Albert Finney; philosopher Albert Camus; artist Albrecht Dürer.

Adalbert, Adalbrecht, Adelbert, Adelbrecht, Ailbert, Al, Alberto, Albie, Albrecht, Albrekt, Aubert, Bert, Bertie, Berty, Elbert, Ulbricht

Albin Lat. "White, pale-skinned." From the root that gives us the word "albino." Common in Roman and medieval times, but not in the modern era.

Al, Albinson, Alpin, Aubin

Albion Celtic. "Mountain." Used in England until the 1930s; "Albion" is a poetic name for Britain.

Alcander Gk. "Strong."

Alcinder

Alcott OE. Place name: "The old cottage."

Alcot, Allcot, Allcott, Alkott

Alden OE. "Old friend." Surname transferred to first name, but unusual.

Al, Aldin, Aldwin, Aldwyn, Aldwynn, Elden, Eldin, Eldwin, Eldwyn, Eldwynn

Aldo OG. "Old." An Italian name that is occasionally used in the U.S.

Aldous OG. "Old." Medieval name that was brought back in the 19th century to slight popularity. Made most famous by writer Aldous Huxley.

Al, Aldis, Aldivin, Aldo, Aldon, Aldus, Eldin, Eldis, Eldon, Eldous

Aldred OE. "Old counsel."

Alldred, Eldred, Elldred

Aldrich OE. "Old leader."

Al, Aldric, Aldridge, Aldrige, Aldritch, Alldrich, Alldridge, Allric, Alrick, Audric, Eldrich, Eldridge, Eldritch, Elldrich, Rich, Richie, Richy, Ritch, Ritchey, Ritchie, Ritchy

Aldwin OE. "Old friend." See **Alden.**

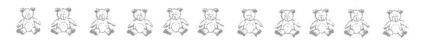

Aldwyn, Alswynn, Elden, Eldin, Eldwin, Eldwyn, Eldwynn

Alem Arab. "Wise man."

Alerio

Alex dim. Alexander

Alec, Aleck, Alick, Alik

Alexander Gk. "Man's defender." Given great prominence by Alexander the Great, and steadily used worldwide, as the numerous variants show. It was a royal
name in Scotland, where it is still highly popular. U.S.
statesman Alexander Hamilton; actors Sir Alec Guin-
ness, Alec Baldwin; U.S. Secretary of State Alexander
Haig; Soviet writer and dissident Aleksandr
Solzhenitsyn; writer Alexandre Dumas.

**Al, Alasdair, Alastair, Alaster, Alec, Alejandro, Alejo,
Alek, Aleksander, Aleksandr, Alessandre, Alessandri,
Alessandro, Alex, Alexandre, Alexandro, Alexandros,
Alexei, Alexi, Alexio, Alexis, Alic, Alick, Alik, Alisander,
Alissander, Alissandre, Alistair, Alister, Alistir, Alix,
Allistair, Allister, Allistir, Alsandair, Alsandare, Iskander,
Sacha, Sander, Sandero, Sandor, Sandro, Sandy,
Sascha, Sasha, Saunder, Saunders, Sikander**

Alexis Gk. "Helper." Usually thought of as a diminutive
of **Alexander**, though it has a different etymological root.
More commonly a girl's name.

Alejo, Alexei, Alexey, Alexi, Alexy

Alford OE. Place name: "The old river-ford."

Aldford

Alfred OE. "Counsel from the elves." After wide medieval
use, the name fell out of sight until a 19th-century revival; Queen Victoria even named her second son Alfred. Out of fashion since the 1920s. English King Alfred
the Great; poet Alfred Tennyson; movie director Alfred
Hitchcock.

**Ailfrid, Ailfryd, Al, Alf, Alfeo, Alfie, Alfredo, Alfy, Avery,
Fred, Freddie, Freddy, Fredo**

Alger OE. "Spear from the elves." Possibly a diminutive
of **Algernon**. Medieval name revived with the 19th-
century hunger for a picturesque past, but never common. State Department Official Alger Hiss.

Al, Algar, Allgar, Allger, Elgar, Elger, Ellgar, Ellger

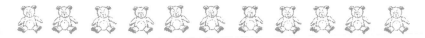

Algernon OF. "Wearing a mustache." A first name in several hugely powerful English aristocratic families, and given wider use in the latter half of the 19th century in Britain. Oscar Wilde used it for a brainless fop in *The Importance of Being Earnest*. All but unknown now. English poet Algernon Swinburne.
Al, Alger, Algey, Algie, Algy

Algis OG. "Spear."

Ali Arab. "The high, exalted one."
Aly

Alison OE. "Son of the highborn." More common as a girl's name.
Allison, Allisoun, Allson, Allyson

Allard OE. "Highborn and courageous."

Alonzo Var. **Alphonse**. OG. "Ready for battle."
Alonso, Lonnie, Lonny

Aloysius OG. "Famous fighter." Latinized version of Luigi or **Louis**, also related to **Clovis**. The 16th-century Italian Saint Aloysius is patron saint of students.
Alois, Aloisius, Aloisio, Aloys, Lewis, Louis, Ludwig

Alpheus Heb. "He who follows after." Biblical, used in the 19th century, now very unusual.
Alpheaus, Alphoeus

Alphonse OG. "Ready for battle." Alfonso is a royal name in Spain, thus very popular; Alphonse is probably the most common form in the U.S. French writer Alphonse Daudet.
Affonso, Al, Alfie, Alfo, Alfons, Alfonso, Alfonsus, Alfonzo, Alfonzus, Alford, Alfy, Alonso, Alonzo, Alphonso, Alphonsus, Alphonzo, Alphonzus, Fons, Fonsie, Fonz, Fonzie

Alpin Gael. "Fair one."
Alpine, Macalpin

Alston OE. Place name: "Noble one's settlement."
Allston

Altman OG. "Old man." Last name occasionally used as a first name.
Altmann

Alton OE. Place name: "Old town."
Allton, Alten

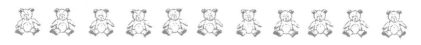

Alured Lat. Var. **Alfred**.

Alva Heb. Possibly "brilliance"; also related to Latin Albin. Old Testament name rarely used for men or women, in spite of Thomas Alva Edison's fame.
Alba, Alvah

Alvar OE. "Army of elves." Very rare. Architect Alvar Aalto.

Alvin OE. Several possible sources: the second element, "vin," means "friend," but Al could indicate "elf," "noble," or "old." Choreographer Alvin Ailey.
Ailwyn, Al, Aloin, Aluin, Aluino, Alva, Alvan, Alven, Alvie, Alvy, Alvyn, Alwin, Alwyn, Alwynn, Aylwin, Elvin, Elwin, Elwyn, Elwynn

Alvis Origin unclear. Possibly from an Old Norse legend involving the dwarf Alviss; possibly a modern blend. First appeared in the mid–20th century, but never widespread.

Amadeo Sp. from Lat. "Loved by God." The Latin version is Amadeus, given great prominence by the 1984 film about Mozart.
Amadée, Amadei, Amadeus, Amadi, Amadieu, Amadis, Amado, Amando, Amyas, Amyot

Amadour Fr. from Lat. "Lovable." A Saint Amadour, purportedly founder of a French shrine (Rocamadour), has been venerated by the Catholic church, but recent research indicates he probably never lived.

Amasa Heb. "Bearing a burden." Occasionally used in the 19th century, but little-known today.

Ambrose Gk. "Ever-living." Saint Ambrose was the 4th-century Bishop of Milan who baptized Saint Augustine. The name is more widely found on the Continent than in English-speaking countries. Writer Ambrose Bierce; Civil War General Ambrose E. Burnside.
Ambie, Ambrogio, Ambroise, Ambros, Ambrosi, Ambrosio, Ambrosius, Amby, Brose

Amerigo It. Var. **Emery** OG. "home ruler." Italian explorer Amerigo Vespucci.

Amiel Heb. "God of my people."

Amory OG. "Home ruler." Var. **Emery**.
Aimory, Amery, Amorey

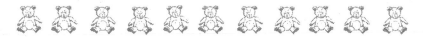

Amos Heb. "Borne, carried." A prophet of the Old Testament. The name has been little used in this century.

Amyas Lat. "Loved one." Possibly an anglicized version of Amadeus, though sometimes considered a masculine variant of Amy. Unusual.
Amias

Anastasius Gk. "Resurrection." Much more common in the feminine version, Anastasia.
Anastas, Anastase, Anastasio, Anastatius, Anastice, Anastius, Anasto, Anstas, Anstice, Stasio, Stasius

Anatole Gk. "From the east." Anatolia is a region of Turkey, which, of course, is east of Greece. French novelist Anatole France.
Anatol, Anatolio

Anders Scand. Var. **Andrew**.
Ander, Anderson, Andersson

André Fr. Var. **Andrew**. Pianist André Watts; actor André Gregory; composer/conductor André Previn.
Andras, Andres, Andris

Andrew Gk. "Masculine." In the Bible, Andrew was the first of the twelve apostles. Legend has it that after his crucifixion on an X-shaped cross, his bones were transported to Scotland, where he is patron saint. The "Saint Andrew's Cross," representing Scotland, appears on the flag of the United Kingdom. U.S. Presidents Andrew Jackson, Andrew Johnson; industrialist Andrew Carnegie; Prince Andrew, Duke of York; actors Andy Devine, Andy Griffith; artists Andrew Wyeth, Andy Warhol.
Aindrea, Aindreas, Anders, Andie, Andonis, André, Andrea, Andreas, Andrei, Andrej, Andres, Andresj, Andrezj, Andrey, Andro, Andy, Drew, Dru, Drud, Drugi

Aneurin Welsh. "Honor." Mostly limited to Wales.
Aneirin, Nye

Angel Gk. "Messenger." Angelo is most often used now, even in English-speaking countries, as Angel is usually considered a girl's name. Angel is popular in Spanish-speaking countries. Jockey Angel Cordero.
Ange, Angell, Angie, Angelo, Angy, Anjelo

Angus Scot. Gael. "Sole or only choice." In Celtic myth

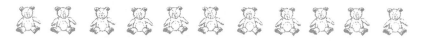

Angus Og is a god of such attractive traits as humor and wisdom.
Ennis, Gus

Annan Celt. "From the brook."

Anscom OE. Place name: "Valley of the awesome one." "Combe" is an Old English term for a deep, narrow valley.
Anscomb, Anscombe

Ansel OF. "Follower of a nobleman." Photographer Ansel Adams.
Ancell, Ansell

Anselm OG. "God-helmet." Saint Anselm was Archbishop of Canterbury in the 12th century, and one of the formative influences on medieval Christian thought.
Anse, Ansel, Anselme, Anselmi, Anselmo, Anshelm, Elmo

Ansley OE. Place name: "The awesome one's meadow."
Anslea, Ansleigh, Anslie, Ansly

Anson Unclear origin and meaning, perhaps OG. Possibly "son of Ann," though "son of the divine" seems more likely.
Annson, Ansson, Hanson

Anstice Var. Anastasius.
Anstiss

Anthony Lat. Clan name of the Romans, possibly meaning "beyond price, invaluable." The 3rd-century hermit Saint Anthony, who, according to legend, lived alone in the wilderness for over 80 of his hundred-some years, is patron saint of the poor. In England the name is usually spelled without the *h*. Actors Anthony Quinn, Anthony Hopkins, Anthony Perkins, Tony Curtis; photographer Antony Armstrong-Jones, Earl of Snowdon; Composer Anton Bruckner; playwright Anton Chekhov.
Anntoin, Antin, Antoine, Anton, Antone, Antonello, Antoney, Antoni, Antonin, Antonino, Antonio, Antonius, Antons, Antony, Toney, Toni, Tony

Antoine Fr. Var. Anthony. Popular in the U.S. in recent years.
Antione, Antjuan, Antuan, Antuwain, Antuwaine, Antuwayne, Antuwon, Antwahn, Antwain, Antwaine,

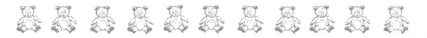

Antwan, Antwaun, Antwohn, Antwoin, Antwoine, Antwon, Antwone

Anwar   Arab. "Shafts of light." Made famous by Egyptian President Anwar Sadat.

Anwell   Welsh-Celt. "Loved one."
Anwel, Anwil, Anwill, Anwyl, Anwyll

Apollo   Gk. "Manly." In classical myth, Apollo is the god who drives the sun across the sky in a carriage, and also rules over healing and prophecy, speaking through the famous oracle at Delphi.
Apollon, Apollos

Aquila   Lat. "Eagle." Despite the feminine "a" ending, used in the 19th century as a revival of an ancient Roman name.
Acquila, Acquilla, Aquilla

Archard   Anglo-Ger. "Holy, powerful."
Archerd

Archelaus   Gk. "Ruler of the people." Not uncommon in the ancient world; Herod the Great had a son of that name who is mentioned in the Bible. Rare today.

Archer   OF. "Bowman." Originally surname indicating occupation (like Miller, Smith, or Baker), mildly popular in the 19th century. Philanthropist Archer Huntington.

Archibald   OG. "Noteworthy and valorous." Brought to Britain with the Norman Conquest, and popular largely in Scotland, where it was in the top 20 until the 1930s. Poet Archibald MacLeish.
Arch, Archaimbaud, Archambault, Archer, Archibaldo, Archibold, Archie, Archimbald, Archy

Arden   Lat. "Burning with enthusiasm." The Forest of Arden in Shakespeare's *As You Like It* is a magically beautiful place.
Ard, Ardie, Ardin, Ardy

Ardley   OE. Place name: "Home-lover's meadow."
Ardly, Ardsley, Ardsly

Ardmore   Lat. "More zealous."

Argus   Gk. "Vigilant guardian." In Greek myth, a creature with 100 eyes, later changed into a peacock with eyes on his tail-feathers.
Argos

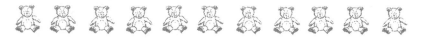

Argyle Scot. Place name. Also given to the indigenous knitting pattern of interlocking diamonds.
Argyll

Aric OG. "Ruler." Also an element of many other names, like Alaric and Frederick.
Arick, Arric, Arrick, Eric, Erick, Erric, Errick, Erik, Ric, Rickie, Ricky

Ariel Heb. "Lion of God." In Shakespeare's *The Tempest*, Ariel is a sprite who can disappear at will. The name has the connotation of something otherworldly, and though Shakespeare's Ariel is male, the name is used mostly for girls.
Aeriell, Airel, Airyel, Airyell, Arel, Arie, Ariell, Aryel, Aryell

Aries Lat. "A ram." Also the Greek God of war.
Ares, Arese, Ariese

Aristotle Gk. "Superior." Indelibly associated with the Greek philosopher Aristotle, though given prominence in recent years by the fame of Jacqueline Kennedy's second husband, shipping magnate Aristotle Onassis.
Ari, Arie, Arri, Ary

Arledge OE. Place name: "Lake with the hares."
Arlidge, Arlledge

Arlen Ir. Gael. "Pledge, Oath."
Arlan, Arles, Arlin, Arlyn, Arllen, Arrlen

Arley OE. Place name: "Hare-meadow."
Arlea, Arleigh, Arlie, Arly

Arlo Sp. "Barberry tree." Enjoyed a spurt of popularity in the early 1970s, possibly attendant on the fame of singer Arlo Guthrie.

Armand Fr. Var. **Herman**. OG. "Army man." Actor Armand Assante.
Arman, Armande, Armando, Armin, Armon, Armond, Armonde, Armondo, Ormond, Ormonde, Ormondo

Armstrong OE. "Strong arm."

Arnaud Fr. Var. **Arnold**.
Arnauld, Arnault

Arne OG. "Eagle." Var. **Arnold**.
Arney, Arni, Arnie

Arnett OF./Eng. "Little eagle."
Arnat, Arnet, Arnot, Arnott

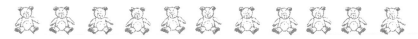

Arno OG. "Eagle-wolf."
Arnoe, Arnou, Arnoux

Arnold OG. "Strength of an eagle." Brought to Britain with the Norman invasion, faded out after the 13th century, and briefly revived in the late 19th century. Unusual today. English novelist Arnold Bennett; golfer Arnold Palmer; actor Arnold Schwarzenegger.
Arnaldo, Arnaud, Arnault, Arne, Arney, Arni, Arnie, Arnoldo, Arny

Arran Scot. Place name. The Isle of Arran is off the Atlantic coast. Also possibly a variant of **Aaron**.
Arren, Arrin, Arron

Arrio Sp. "Belligerent."
Ario, Arryo, Aryo

Artemus Gk. Probably "adherent of the goddess Artemis." New Testament name occasionally used in the 19th century.
Art, Artemas, Artemis, Artie, Artimas, Artimis, Artimus, Arty

Arthur Celt. Possibly "bear" or "rock." Linked with King Arthur, the legendary British hero of the Round Table, and often used in the Middle Ages, but unfashionable until the early 19th century, when Arthur Wellesley, the Duke of Wellington, vanquished Napoleon. Its popularity only began to wane in the 1920s. Columnist Art Buchwald; actor Art Carney; tennis star Arthur Ashe; writer Arthur C. Clarke.
Arrt, Art, Artair, Arte, Arther, Arthor, Arthuro, Artie, Artor, Artur, Arturo, Artus, Arty, Arthur

Arundel OE. Place name: "Eagle valley."

Arvad Heb. "Exile, voyager."
Arpad, Arv, Arvid, Arvie

Arvin OGer. "People's friend."
Arv, Arvie, Arvy, Arwin, Arwyn

Asa Heb. "Doctor." Another Old Testament name made popular by the Puritans in the 17th century. Now unusual.
Ase

Ascot OE. Place name: "Eastern cottage." More specifi-

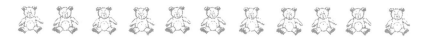

cally the name of England's famous racetrack near Windsor Castle, and also a style of tying a cravat.
Ascott

Ashby OE. Place name: "Ash tree farm."
Ash, Ashbie, Ashbey, Ashburn, Ashton

Asher Heb. "Felicitous." Old Testament name brought into English use by the Puritans.
Ash

Ashford OE. Place name: "Ford near ash trees."
Ash, Ashenford

Ashley OE. Place name: "Ash tree meadow." Originally a surname that migrated to first-name status, possibly helped along by Ashley Wilkes in Margaret Mitchell's *Gone With the Wind*. Though originally used for boys, it is now tremendously popular for girls.
Ash, Ashely, Asheley, Ashelie, Ashlan, Ashleigh, Ashlen, Ashlie, Ashlin, Ashling, Ashlinn, Ashly, Ashlyn, Ashlynn

Ashton OE. Place name: "Ash tree settlement." More popular in the 19th century than now, though this is the kind of name Anglophile parents of the 1990s may make more popular. Choreographer Sir Frederick Ashton.

Ashur Semitic. "Warlike one." A name used by various Assyrian kings, who lived up to its meaning.

Aston OE. Place name: "Eastern town." Famous for an English sports car, the Aston Martin.

Aswin OE. "Spear-friend."
Aswinn, Aswyn, Aswynn

Atherton OE. Place name: "Town by the spring."

Athelstan OE. "Highborn rock." Used by Anglo-Saxon royalty and revived slightly by Sir Walter Scott's use of it in *Ivanhoe*. Now extremely rare.

Athol Scot. Place name, meaning unclear.
Atholl

Atley OE. Place name: "The meadow." Indicates an ancestor who, once upon a time, lived in a house near (or "at") a meadow.
Atlea, Atlee, Atleigh, Attlee, Attleigh, Attley

Atwater OE. Place name: "The water."

Atwell OE. Place name: "The well."

Atwood OE. Place name: "The wood."

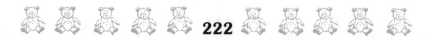

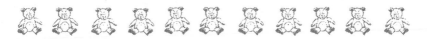

Atworth OE. Place name: "The farmstead."

Auberon OG. "Highborn and bearlike." Also possibly a form of Aubrey. Better-known, though no more common for it, as Oberon, King of the Fairies in Shakespeare's *Midsummer Night's Dream*. English writer Auberon Waugh.

Auberron, Oberon, Oberron, Oeberon

Aubrey OF. "Elf ruler." Originally a man's name that arrived in England with the Norman Conquest. Now used by girls as well, thus no doubt dooming its use as a boys' name. The 19th-century artist Aubrey Beardsley; biographer John Aubrey.

Alberic, Alberick, Alberik, Aube, Auberon, Aubry, Averey, Averie, Avery, Oberon

Audley OE. Place name of uncertain meaning.

Audric OG. "Noble ruler." Var. **Aldrich**.

August Lat. "Worthy of respect." The feminine version, Augusta, and the longer Latin version, Augustus, are more widely (though still infrequently) used in English-speaking countries. Sculptor Auguste Rodin, painter Auguste Renoir.

Agostino, Agosto, Aguistin, Agustin, Agustino, Augie, Auguste, Augustin, Augustine, Augustino, Augusto, Augustus, Augie, Augy, Austen, Austin, Gus, Guss

Augustine Lat. Dim. **August**. The 5th-century bishop Saint Augustine is famous for the frank *Confessions*, in which he says, "Oh God, make me chaste—but not yet."

Aguistin, Agustin, Augie, Augustin, Augy, Austen, Austin, Austyn

Augustus Lat. "Worthy of respect." Given historial glamor by Roman emperors and German princely families, who brought it to Britain in the 18th century, when it became very fashionable. Now little used. Sculptor Augustus Saint-Gaudens; painter Augustus John.

Augie, Augustin, Augy, Austen, Austin, Austyn

Aurelius Lat. "Golden."

Aurelio

Austin Oral form of **Augustine**, contracted by everyday speech. Now most often a family name transferred to a first name.

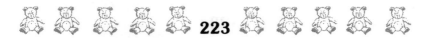

Austen, Austyn, Ostyn, Ostynn

Avenall OF. Place name: "Oat pasture."

Aveneil, Aveneill, Avenel, Avenell, Avenil, Avenill

Averill Most likely derivation is OE. "boar-warrior," though may also be related to French **Avril** or "April." Industrialist and statesman Averell Harriman.

Ave, Averel, Averell, Averil, Averyl, Averyll, Avrel, Avrell, Avrill, Avryll

Avery OE. "Elf-ruler." Var. **Alfred, Aubrey.** Philanthropist Avery Fisher.

Averey

Avram Heb. Var. **Abraham.**

Axel OGer. "Father of peace" and Scan. Var. **Absalom.**

Aksel, Ax, Axe, Axell, Axil, Axill

Aylmer OE. "Highborn and renowned." The homonym Elmer is the more common form of this very old English name.

Aillmer, Ailmer, Allmer, Ayllmer, Elmer, Eylmer

Aylward OE. "Awesome guardian" or "highborn guardian."

Azuriah Heb. "Aided by Jehovah." Although 28 different biblical characters are known by this name, it is all but obsolete today.

Azuria

B

Bailey OF. "Bailiff." Occupational name: in the Middle Ages a bailiff was a minor officer of the law.

Bail, Bailie, Baillie, Baily, Bayley, Bayly

Bainbridge Ir. Gael. "Pale bridge."

Bain, Baynbridge, Bayne, Baynebridge

Baird Gael. "One who sings ballads."

Bar, Bard, Barde, Barr, Bayerd, Bayrd

Baker OE. Occupational name transferred to surname and, in the 19th century, to a first name.

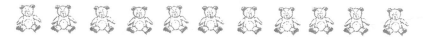

Balbo Lat. "Mutterer."
  Bailby, Balbi, Ballbo
Baldemar OG. "Bold and renowned."
  Baumar, Baumer
Balder OE. "Courageous army." In Norse myth the god Balder is called "the good," and reigns over summer, light, and innocence.
  Baldur, Baudier
Baldric OG. "Brave ruler."
  Baldrick, Baudric
Baldwin OG. "Brave friend." Unusual in English-speaking countries, though Baudoin is a royal name in Belgium. Author James Baldwin.
  Bald, Baldovino, Balduin, Baldwinn, Baldwyn,
  Baldwynn, Balldwin, Baudoin
Balfour Gael. "Grazing land." Also the name of a town in northern Scotland.
  Balfor, Balfore
Ballard OG. "Brave and strong."
Balthasar Gk. "God save the king." Along with Caspar and Melchior, one of the Three Kings who brought gifts to the baby Jesus, though they are not named in the Bible.
  Baldassare, Baltasar, Baltazar, Balthasaar, Balthazar,
  Belshazzar
Bancroft OE. Place name: "Field of beans." Many of the most common Anglo-Saxon place names that have become first names refer to simple, homely agricultural landmarks.
  Ban, Bancrofft, Bank, Binky
Banning Ir. Gael. "Small fair one" or "son of the fair one."
Barclay OE. Place name: "Where birches grow." This is the form most favored in Scotland; Berkeley is more common elsewhere.
  Bar, Barcley, Barklay, Barkley, Barklie, Barrclay, Berk,
  Berkeley, Berkie, Berkley, Berklie, Berky
Bard Ir. Var. Baird.
  Bar, Barde, Barr
Bardolf OE. "Axe-wolf." A drunken fool named Bardolph figures in four of Shakespeare's plays.
  Bardolph, Bardou, Bardoul, Bardulf, Bardulph

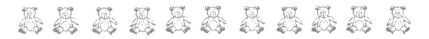

Bardrick Teut. "Axe-ruler." Just as many of the Anglo-Saxon names relate to farming, numerous Teutonic names relate to fighting.
Bardric

Barker OE. Possibly "shepherd." Used more often in the 19th century. In the U.S. a barker is also someone who delivers a glib sales talk to attract customers.

Barlow OE. Place name: "The bare hillside."
Barlowe, Barrlow

Barnabas Heb. "Son of comfort." In the New Testament, Barnabas is a companion of Paul's and uncle of the gospeler Mark. Barnaby is used more often now in Britain. One of Charles Dickens's lesser-known novels is entitled *Barnaby Rudge*.
Barna, Barnaba, Barnabé, Barnabee, Barnabey, Barnabie, Barnabus, Barnaby, Barnebas, Barnebus, Barney, Barnie, Barny, Burnaby

Barnes OE. Place name: "Near the barns."

Barnett OE. Place name: "From the land that was burned." Or possibly a contraction of the English aristocratic title "baronet." Duke, Earl, and Baron are used as first names from time to time.
Barnet, Barney, Barnie, Baronet, Baronett, Barrie, Barron, Barry

Barney Var. **Barnabas**.

Barnum OE. Possibly a contraction of "baron's home." In the U.S. inseparable from Phineas T. Barnum, founder of the circus, which is still going strong.
Barnham

Baron OE. The title of nobility used as a first name.
Barron

Barret OG. "Bear-strength." Used as a first name mostly in the 19th century, possibly because of the fame of English poet Elizabeth Barrett Browning.
Baret, Barrat, Barratt, Barrett, Barrey, Barrie, Barry

Barrington Eng. Place name now fairly common as a first name in Britain. Perhaps a bit of a mouthful for the more democratic U.S.

Barry Gael. "Sharp, pointed." Also a place name turned into a first name used by both sexes. Possibly influenced

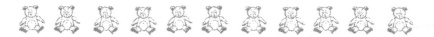

by the fame of Sir James Barrie, author of *Peter Pan*, since it cropped up as a first name during the height of his renown. Barry (with the *y*) was quite popular in the 1950s. Senator Barry M. Goldwater; singer Barry Manilow.

Bari, Barrie, Baris

Bart Dim. Bartholomew.

Bartholomew Heb. "Farmer's son." One of the twelve apostles. The name was common in the Middle Ages but was not revived in the 19th century, as so many medieval names were.

Bart, Bartel, Barth, Barthelemy, Bartho, Bartholomaus, Bartholome, Barthlomeo, Bartholomeus, Bartlet, Bartlett, Bartolome, Bartolomeo, Bartolommeo, Bartome, Bartt, Bat

Bartlet Dim. Bartholomew.

Bartlett

Barton OE. Place name: "Barley settlement."

Bart, Barrton

Bartram OE. "Bright raven." See **Bertram**.

Barthram

Baruch Heb. "Blessed."

Basil Gk. "Royal, kingly." Brought to England by the Crusaders, having been common in the eastern Mediterranean. Unusual in the U.S., but more often used in Britain. Also the name of a common herb. Actor Basil Rathbone.

Basile, Basilio, Basilius, Bazil, Bazyli, Vasilios, Vasilis, Vasilius, Vasilus, Vassilij, Vassily, Wassily

Bassett OE. "Little person." Descriptive surname transferred to first name. Also the name of a very short-legged hunting dog, the basset hound, possibly called that because its torso is so low (*bas* in French) to the ground.

Basset

Baxter OE. Occupational name: "Baker."

Bax

Bayard OE. "Russet-haired." A famous French knight of the 15th century, the Seigneur de Bayard, was known as "the irreproachable and fearless."

Baiardo, Bay

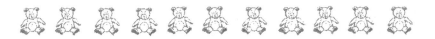

Beacher OE. Place name: "Near the beech trees." Generally a last name. The 19th-century preacher Henry Ward Beecher.
Beach, Beachy, Beech, Beecher, Beechy

Beagan Ir. Gael. "Small one."
Beagen, Beagin

Beal OF. "Handsome." Var. **Beau**.
Beale, Beall, Beals

Beaman OE. Occupational name: "Beekeeper."
Beamann, Beamen, Beeman

Beamer OE. "Trumpet player."

Beattie (masc. **Beatrice**) Ir. Gael. from Lat. "bringer of gladness."
Beatie, Beatty, Beaty

Beau Fr. "Handsome." Dim. **Beauregard**. Used somewhat in the U.S. in the last 30 years. English dandy Beau Brummel; actor Beau Bridges; sports star Bo Jackson.
Beal, Beale, Bo

Beaufort OF. Place name: "The beautiful fort."

Beaumont OF. Place name: "The beautiful mountain." More common in the 19th century than it is today.

Beauregard Fr. "Beautiful gaze." Could also be taken to mean, in modern parlance, "easy on the eye."
Beau

Beck OE. Place name: "Small stream." The term is still in use in rural Scotland.

Bede OE. "Prayer." Saint Bede was a 7th-century English church historian.

Belden OE./OF. Place name: "Pretty valley."
Beldon, Bellden, Belldon

Bellamy OF. "Handsome friend."
Belamy, Bell, Bellamey, Bellamie

Ben Heb. "Son." Also dim. **Benedict, Benjamin, Benson,** etc. Now given as an independent name. Playwright Ben Jonson; actor Ben Gazzara.
Benn, Benny

Benedict Lat. "Blessed." Saint Benedict, founder of a monastic order, brought the name to prominence. Bennett is the more common form, especially in the U.S., where every schoolchild learns the tale of Revolutionary War

traitor Benedict Arnold. Italian dictator Benito Mussolini.

Ben, Bendick, Bendict, Benedetto, Benedick, Benedicto, Benedictus, Benedikt, Bengt, Benito, Bennet, Bennett, Bennie, Bennt, Benoit, Bent

Benjamin Heb. "Son of the right hand." In the Old Testament, the younger son of Jacob and Rachel. Brought into use by the Puritan fondness for Old Testament names, and persistent until the end of the 19th century. After several decades of disuse, came back to great popularity by the 1970s, and is now quite common. Diplomat and inventor Benjamin Franklin; U.S. President Benjamin Harrison; jazz musician Benny Goodman; pediatrician and oracle Benjamin Spock; British Prime Minister Benjamin Disraeli.

Ben, Benejamen, Beniamino, Benjaman, Benjamen, Benjamino, Benjamon, Benji, Benjie, Benjiman, Benjimen, Benjy, Bennie, Benyamin, Benyamino

Bennett Fr. Var. **Benedict.** Choreographer Michael Bennett; humorist Bennett Cerf.

Benet, Benett, Bennet

Benoni Heb. "Son of my sorrow." In the Old Testament, Rachel, mother of Benjamin, knew she was dying after his birth and called him Benoni, but Jacob, his father, changed the name to Benjamin.

Benson "Son of Ben." Originally a surname, transferred to a first name in the 19th century.

Bensen, Benssen, Bensson

Bentley OE. "Meadow with coarse grass." Place name become surname become first name, more common for boys but used occasionally for girls. Irresistibly linked in most minds with the luxurious English cars.

Ben, Bentlea, Bentlee, Bentley, Bentlie, Bently, Lee

Benton OE. Place name. As in Bentley, refers to a kind of "bent" or coarse grass. Artist Thomas Hart Benton, film director Robert Benton.

Beresford OE. Place name: "Ford where barley grows." Used as a first name principally at the turn of the century. Film director Bruce Beresford.

Berg Ger. "Mountain." Often found as a suffix in German surnames.

Bergh, Burg, Burgh

Bergen Scan. "Lives on the hill." Bergen is a major port city in Norway.

Bergin, Birgin

Berger Fr. Occupational name: "Shepherd."

Berkeley OE. Place name: "Where birches grow." In the U.S. probably most famous as the San Francisco suburb that is home to a branch of the University of California.

Bar, Barcley, Barklay, Barkley, Barklie, Barrclay, Berk, Berkeley, Berkie, Berkley, Berky

Bern OG. "Bear." Also possible nickname for Bernard.

Berne, Bernie, Berny, Bjorn

Bernal OG. "Strength of a bear." Occasionally used in English-speaking countries, but more common on the Continent.

Bernald, Bernhald, Bernhold, Bernold

Bernard OGer. "Bear/courageous." Brought to England with the Norman Conquest. Two famous medieval saints bore the name; one was a founder of a monastic order. The other, for whom the shaggy brown and white dogs are named, is patron saint of mountain climbers. A fairly common name until the 18th century and revived a bit around 1920, but now unusual. Playwright George Bernard Shaw; statesman Bernard M. Baruch; film director Bernardo Bertolucci.

Barnard, Barnardo, Barney, Barnhard, Barnhardo, Barnie, Barny, Bear, Bearnard, Bern, Bernardo, Bernarr, Bernhard, Bernhardo, Bernie, Burnard

Berry Botanical name used for both boys and girls, though the boy's name is more likely a derivative of Bernard or a transferred surname.

Bert OE. "Shining brightly." Dim. **Albert, Egbert, Robert,** etc. Used more often as a nickname. Its popularity among show-business types of a certain age (Miss America emcee Bert Parks, actors Burt Lancaster and Burt Reynolds) suggests a certain jaunty, masculine connotation.

Bertie, Berty, Burt, Burty, Butch

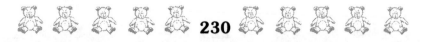

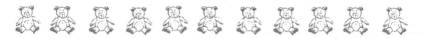

Berthold OG. "Bright strength." Unusual in English-speaking countries, but not unheard-of. Playwright Bertolt Brecht.
Bert, Berthoud, Bertold, Bertolde

Berton OE. Place name: "Bright settlement."
Bert, Bertie, Burt, Burton

Bertram OG. "Bright raven." Norman name revived in the Victorian era. Rare since the 1930s.
Bart, Bartram, Beltran, Beltrano, Berton, Bertrand, Bertrando, Bertranno

Bertrand OG. "Bright shield." Also possibly a variation on **Bertram**. Philosopher Bertrand Russell.

Berwyn OE. "Bear friend" or "bright friend."
Berwin, Berwynn, Berwynne

Bevan Welsh. "Son of Evan." Mostly 20th-century use.
Beavan, Beaven, Bev, Beven, Bevin, Bevon

Beverly OE. "Of the beaver-stream." Originally an English place name transferred to a surname, then a first name for both sexes. Probably still most famous as a place name, referring to Beverly Hills. The English spelling is usually Beverley.
Beverlea, Beverleigh, Beverley, Beverlie

Bevis OF. Place name: Beauvais is a town in France famous for the manufacture of tapestries. This anglicized version is very unusual.
Beauvais

Bickford OE. Place name: "Axe-man's ford."

Bill Dim. **William**. Used occasionally as an independent name. Before mid–19th century, Will was the more common nickname. Actors Bill Cosby, Bill Bixby; designer Bill Blass; singer Billy Joel; comedian/actor Billy Crystal.
Billie, Billy, Byll

Bing OG. Place name: "The hollow shaped like a pot." Another source claims that modern use of the name is inspired by singer Bing Crosby, who was given the nickname after a comic-strip character.

Birch OE. Place name: "Where birch trees grow." Not uncommon in the 19th century. Senator Birch Bayh.
Birk, Burch

Birkett Middle English. Place name: "Birch coastland."

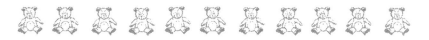

Birket, Birkit, Birkitt, Burket, Burkett, Burkitt

Birkey Middle English. Place name: "Island of birch trees."

Birkee, Birkie, Birky

Birley OE. Place name: "Meadow with the cow byre." Not related to the homonym Burleigh.

Birlie, Birly

Birney OE. Place name: "Island with the brook."

Birnie, Birny, Burney, Burnie

Birtle OE. Place name: "Hill of birds."

Bishop OE. "Bishop." Probably originally meant "one serving the bishop," or "bishop's man."

Bjorn Scan. Var. **Bernard**. The fame of tennis player Bjorn Borg is probably responsible for the use of this name in English-speaking countries.

Black OE. "Dark-skinned."

Blackburn OE. Place name: "Black brook." Used as a first name mostly in the 19th century. In Scotland, *burn* is still the term for a little brook.

Blagden OE. Place name: "Dark valley."

Blaine Ir. Gael. "Slender." Surname used since the 1930s as a first name, mostly for boys but occasionally for girls.

Blane, Blayne

Blair Scot. Gael. Place name: "Plain" or "flat area." Surname now used as first name, again more common for boys. Like many similarly transferred names, Blair was used for girls in greater numbers starting in the early 1980s.

Blaire, Blayr, Blayre

Blaise Lat./Fr. "One who stutters." Used for both sexes, though more common for men. The alternate spelling of Blaze probably refers to fire instead. French philosopher Blaise Pascal.

Blaize, Blase, Blayse, Blayze, Blaze

Blake OE. Paradoxically, could mean either "pale-skinned" or "dark." Surname used as a first name for either sex, most often in the U.S. Director Blake Edwards; "Dynasty" character Blake Carrington.

Blakely OE. Place name: "Dark meadow" or "pale meadow." See **Blake**.

Blakelee, Blakeleigh, Blakeley, Blakelie

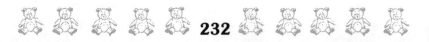

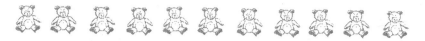

Blanco Sp. "Fair, white."

Blanford OE. Place name: "Gray man's ford."
  Blandford

Blaze Lat. "One who stutters." Anglicized form of **Blaise**.
  **Biaggio, Biagio, Blaise, Blaize, Blase, Blasien, Blasius,
  Blayse, Blayze**

Bliss OE. "Intense happiness."

Blythe OE. "Happy, carefree." Made famous by the opening lines of Shelley's poem "To a Skylark" (Hail to thee,
  blithe spirit!) and Noel Coward's play *Blithe Spirit*.
  Blithe

Bo Dim. **Robert, Beauregard**. Rare as a given name, more
  likely to be a nickname. Football coach Bo Schembechler;
  sports star Bo Jackson.

Boaz Heb. "Swiftness." Used for several Old Testament
  characters, and revived with the Puritan passion for Old
  Testament names. Now very rare.
  Boas, Boase

Bob Dim. **Robert**. OE. "Bright fame." Used independently
  from time to time. The usual habit for naming, however,
  is to give the full form of a name, even if the parents
  never intend to use anything but the nickname. Comedian Bob Hope; singer Bob Dylan; chess master Bobby
  Fischer.
  Bobbey, Bobbie, Bobby

Boden OF. "One who brings news."
  Bodin, Bowden, Bowdoin

Bogart OF. "Bow strength." In current use probably always refers to actor Humphrey Bogart.
  Bogey, Bogie, Bogy

Bonar OF. "Gentle, mannerly." From the French *débon-
  naire*. The famous line from the Sermon on the Mount,
  "Blessed are the meek," translates into French as *"Heu-
  reux sont les débonnaires."* In English, "debonair" now
  means something closer to "nonchalant" or "urbane," as
  personified by Fred Astaire.
  Bonnar, Bonner

Bond OE. Occupational name: "Man of the soil."

Boniface Lat. "Fortunate, of good fate." Also commonly,

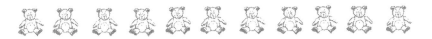

though erroneously, taken to mean "doing good." Name of a number of early popes.

Bonifacio, Bonifacius

Booker Uncertain origin; may allude to "the Book," i.e., the Bible. American reformer Booker T. Washington.

Boone OF. "Good." Backwoods connotations courtesy of 19th-century explorer Daniel Boone.

Booth OG. Place name: "Dwelling place." Surname whose 19th-century use as a first name was probably a tribute to Salvation Army founder William Booth. In the U.S. made famous also by Lincoln's assassin John Wilkes Booth. Author Booth Tarkington.

Boot, Boote, Boothe, Both

Borden OE. Place name: "Vale of the boar."

Boris Slavic. "Warrior." Russian playwright Pushkin and composer Mussorgsky both based works on the career of the bloodthirsty 16th-century czar Boris Godunov. Horror-movie actor Boris Karloff; author Boris Pasternak; tennis star Boris Becker, cartoon character Boris Badenov.

Boriss, Borris, Borys

Botolf OE. "Messenger wolf." An obscure 7th-century English saint who was very popular in the Middle Ages. He founded a monastery in England, which is thought to have been in the Lincolnshire town of Boston (Botolph's town).

Botolph, Botulf

Bourne OE. Place name: "The stream." A little stream is still called a *burn* in Scotland. Scottish poet Robert Burns.

Burn, Burne, Byrn

Bowen Welsh. "Son of the young one."

Bowie Scot. Gael. "Blond." Col. James Bowie, scout and originator of the knife that bears his name.

Bow, Bowen

Boyce OF. Place name: "Woods."

Boice, Boise

Boyd Scot. Gael. "Blond." Possibly also a place name, for the Scottish Isle of Bute.

Boid

Boyne Ir. Gael. "White cow."

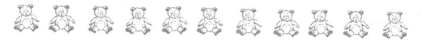

Brad OE. "Broad." Also diminutive for **Bradley** and other "Brad-" names.

Bradburn OE. Place name: "Wide stream."

Braden OE. Place name: "Wide valley."
Bradan, Bradin

Bradford OE. Place name: "Wide river-crossing." Name of the first governor of the Plymouth colony, William Bradford.
Braddford, Bradfurd

Bradley OE. Place name: "Wide meadow." Used since the mid–19th century, more in the U.S. than in other English-speaking countries.
Brad, Bradlea, Bradleigh, Bradlie, Bradly, Bradney, Lee

Bradshaw OE. Place name: "Broad forest."

Brady OE. Place name: "Wide island."

Brainard OE. "Courageous raven."
Brainerd

Bram Ir. Gael. "Raven." It is curious that so many names refer to the raven, a bird that historically has stood for death and destruction. *Dracula* author Bram Stoker.
Bramm, Bran, Brann

Bramwell OE. Place name: "Well where the broom grows." Author Bramwell Brontë.
Brammell, Bramwel, Bramwyll

Brand OE. "Firebrand." Also, diminutive of **Brandon**.
Brander, Brandt, Brant, Brantley, Brantlie

Brandon OE. Place name: "Broom-covered hill." Popular since around 1930, especially in the U.S. Also a variant of **Brendan**.
Band, Branden, Brandin, Brandyn, Brannon

Brant OE. "Proud."
Brannt

Brawley OE. Place name: "Meadow at the slope of the hill."

Brendan Ir. Gael. "Smelly hair." Very few names actually mean anything as negative as this. The Irish Saint Brendan, known as "the Voyager," is supposed to have sailed as far as the Canary Islands.
Brendon, Brennan, Brennen, Brennon

Brent OE. Place name: "Mount, hilltop." Use as a first

name dates back only 60 years or so, and has been particularly strong in Canada. Sportscaster Brent Musburger.

Brentan, Brenten, Brentin, Brenton, Brentyn

Brett Celt. "Man from Britain." Publicized by American writer Bret Harte. Quite popular in Australia.

Bret, Brette, Bretton, Brit, Britt

Brewster OE. Occupational name: "Brewer." Transferred to a surname, thence to a first name.

Brewer, Bruce

Brian Ir. Gael. Ancient name of obscure meaning, though many sources translate it as "strength." Ireland's most famous King, Brian Boru, liberated the country from the Danes in 1014, and the name has been much favored in Ireland. A spell of popularity lasted from the 1920s to the 1970s, but it is now out of fashion. Actor Brian Dennehy; film director Brian De Palma.

Briano, Briant, Brien, Brion, Bryan, Bryant, Bryen, Bryent, Bryon

Brice Var. Bryce. The *i* spelling was more common in the 19th century.

Bridgely OE. Place name: "Bridge meadow."

Bridgeley

Bridger OE. "Lives near the bridge."

Bridge

Brigham OE. Place name: "Little village near the bridge." Most uses of the name probably honor Mormon leader Brigham Young.

Brigg, Briggs

Brinley OE. Place name: "Burnt meadow." Used mostly in England and Wales.

Brindley, Brindly, Brinlee, Brinleigh, Brinly, Brynly

Brock OE. "Badger." Unusual transferred surname. Mostly American use.

Brockley OE. Place name: "Meadow of the badger."

Broderick ONorse. "Brother." Traveled from Ireland to Scotland as a surname. Actor Broderick Crawford.

Brod, Broddy, Broderic, Brodric, Brodrick, Ric, Rick, Rickey, Rickie, Ricky

Brody Ir. Gael. "Ditch."

Brodee, Brodey, Brodie, Broedy

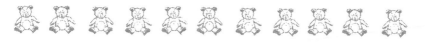

Bromley OE. Place name: "Meadow where broom grows."

Bronson OE. "Brown one's son." Actor Charles Bronson.
Bron, Bronnson, Bronsen, Bronsin, Bronsonn, Bronsson

Brook OE. Place name: "Near the stream or brook." Wide fame of actress Brooke Shields will probably go far to terminate use of this name for boys. Director Brooks Atkinson.
Brooke, Brookes, Brookie, Brooks

Broughton OE. Place name: "Settlement near the fortress."

Brown Middle English. "Russet-complected."

Bruce OF. "From the brushwood thicket." Norman place name brought to fame by the Scottish king Robert Bruce, who won Scotland's independence from England in 1327. Naturally popular as a first name in Scotland, and among Americans who cherish Scottish ancestry. Singer Bruce Springsteen; actor Bruce Willis.
Brucey, Brucie

Bruno OG. "Brown-skinned." Saint Bruno was the 11th-century founder of the Carthusian order of monks. Orchestral conductor Bruno Walter; actor Bruno Kirby.

Bryan Var. **Brian**. Actor Bryan Brown; singer Bryan Ferry.

Bryant Var. **Brian**. TV commentator Bryant Gumbel.

Bryce Unclear origin; may refer to followers of a 5th-century French bishop, Saint Brice.
Brice

Buck OE. "Buck deer." "Buck" was also a 19th-century term for a dandy, or a young man who cut a fine figure. It may have been used first as a nickname. Probably not related to the slang word for "dollar." Actor Buck Henry; baseball star Bucky Dent.
Buckey, Buckie, Bucky

Buckley OE. Place name: "Meadow of the deer." Author William F. Buckley.

Bud Modern slang, short for "buddy." Some sources think this is a child's pronunciation of "brother." Rarely given as a first name, but fairly common as a nickname in the middle years of the 20th century. Actor Buddy Ebsen; comedians Bud Abbott, Buddy Hackett.
Budd, Buddey, Buddie, Buddy

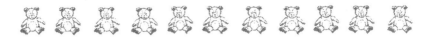

Burchard OE. "Castle strong."
  Burckhardt, Burgard, Burgaud, Burkhart
Burford OE. Place name: "Ford near the castle."
Burgess OE. "Citizen." Related to the French word *bourgeois*, which has come to mean something like "middle class." Actor Burgess Meredith; poet Gelett Burgess.
  Burges, Burgiss, Burr
Burke OF. "From the fortified settlement."
  Berk, Berke, Birk, Bourke, Burk
Burleigh OE. Place name: "Meadow with knotty-trunk trees."
  Burley, Burlie, Byrleigh, Byrley
Burnaby ONorse. "Fighter's estate."
Burne OE. Place name: "The brook." Related to **Bourne**.
  Beirne, Bourn, Bourne, Burn, Byrn, Byrne, Byrnes
Burnell OF. "Small brown one."
  Burnel
Burnet OE. Transferred surname of unclear origin, mostly used in the 19th century.
  Burnett
Burney OE. Place name: "Island of the brook."
Burton OE. Place name: "Fortified enclosure." Like many of the older place names, used as a first name in the 19th century. The exploits of explorer Sir Richard Burton may have influenced its use. Actors Richard Burton, Burt Lancaster.
  Bert, Burt, Burtt
Busby Scot./ONorse. Place name: "Village in the thicket." A busby is also a tall military hat made of fur, such as those worn by the British soldiers who guard Buckingham Palace. Choreographer Busby Berkeley.
Butcher OE. Occupational name: "Butcher." Nickname Butch is sometimes used to address a stranger in a slightly derogatory way: "Listen, Butch . . ."
Buster Nickname of unknown origin, made famous by silent film star Buster Keaton. A hugely popular comic strip character of the 1930s was called Buster Brown. His pageboy haircut, sailor hat, and round collar were all dubbed "Buster Brown" after him. The name continued

into the early 1960s as a brand of shoe with an advertising jingle that ended, ". . . with the boy and the dog and the foot inside." Swimmer/actor Buster Crabbe.

Byford OE. Place name: "By the ford."

Byram OE. Place name. Var. **Byron**.

Byrd OE. "Birdlike."
Bird, Byrdie

Byron OE. Place name: "Barn for cows." The term "byre" is still used. Use as a first name probably in tribute to the poet Lord Byron, since it dates from the 1850s.
Beyren, Beyron, Biren, Biron, Buiron, Byram, Byran, Byren, Byrom

Cadby OE. "Fighting man's settlement."

Caddock Welsh. "Eagerness for war."

Cadell Welsh. "Battle." Political consultant Patrick Cadell.
Caddell, Cadel

Cadman Anglo-Welsh. "Battle man."

Cadmus Gk. "From the east." In Greek myth, Cadmus is the founder of the city of Thebes, who ultimately turned into a serpent.

Caesar Lat. Clan name of obscure meaning, possibly "hairy, hirsute." The term "caesarean" for a surgical delivery of a baby came about because the famous Roman emperor Julius Caesar was born that way. It has become a generic term for emperor, translated into German (kaiser) and Russian (czar). Actor Cesar Romero.
Caezar, Casar, César, Cesare, Cesaro, Kaiser, Seasar, Sezar

Cain Heb. "Spear." Adam and Eve's elder son, who slew his brother Abel. Surprisingly enough, used with some frequency, at least in the 19th century. Homonym Kane has a different source.

Caius Lat. "Rejoice." Var. **Gaius**.
Cai, Caio

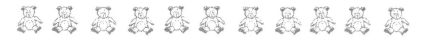

Cal Dim. **Calhoun, Calvin,** etc.

Calder OE. "Stream." Little rivulets are such important features in the English landscape that regional terms for them abound, and several (Brook, Burn) have traced the typical path from geographical feature to place name to surname to given name. Sculptor Alexander Calder.

Caldwell OE. Place name: "Cold well."

Caleb Heb. Either "dog" or "courageous." An Old Testament name brought to America with the Puritans, where it was fairly common until around 1920.
> **Cal, Cale, Kaleb**

Caley Ir. Gael. "Lean, slight."

Calhoun Ir. Gael. Place name: "The narrow woods."
> **Colhoun, Colquhoun**

Calvert OE. Occupational name: "Calf-herder." English surname. In the U.S. borne by George Calvert, founder of Maryland.
> **Calbert**

Calvin Lat. "Hairless." Roman clan name turned surname. Transferred to first name as a tribute to 16th-century Swiss religious reformer John Calvin. U.S. use also probably influenced by President Calvin Coolidge. Fashion designer Calvin Klein.
> **Cal, Calvino, Kalvin, Vinnie**

Camden Scot. Gael. Place name: "The twisting valley."

Cameron Scot. Gael. "Crooked nose." Clan name derived from the facial feature. Little used as a first name until the middle of this century.
> **Cam, Camron**

Campbell Scot. Gael. "Crooked mouth." Name of a very famous Scottish clan, again referring to a distinguishing feature. Use as a first name dates back only to the 1930s.

Canning Fr. Occupational name: "Official of the church." Var. **Cannon.**
> **Cannan**

Canute Scan. "Knot." Brought to Britain by the 11th-century King Canute of Denmark, who became King of England in 1016. Very rare, except in those of Scandinavian descent. Football coach Knute Rockne.
> **Knut, Knute**

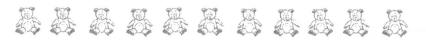

Cannon Fr. Occupational name: "Official of the church." Not, as might be expected by the spelling, related to fire-arms.
Canon

Carey Welsh. Place name: "Near the castle." Distinct from Cary, which has another source. By the 1950s, this form was usually a girl's name, often a nickname for Caroline.

Carl Var. **Charles**. OG. "Man." Use in America was fairly steady 1850–1950 (possibly as a result of intensive German and Scandinavian immigration), but dropped off in the 1960s. Poet Carl Sandburg; journalist Carl Bernstein; astronomer/author Carl Sagan.
Carel, Karl

Carleton OE. Place name: "Farmer's settlement." Only used as a first name since around 1880. In the U.S., usually spelled without the *e*.
Carl, Carlton, Charlton

Carlin Ir. Gael. "Little champion."
Carling, Carly

Carlisle OE. Place name: "The fortified tower." Also the name of a very old city in northwest England. Historian Thomas Carlyle.
Carley, Carly, Carlyle

Carlos Sp. Var. **Charles**. OG. "man." Film directors Carlos Saura, Carlo Ponti.
Carlo

Carmichael Scot. Gael. "Follower of Michael." Possibly referring to partisans of Saint Michael.

Carmine Lat. "Song." Though carmine also means "purplish red" (from an Aramaic word meaning "crimson"), the Latin source is more likely, since the name is almost exclusively used by families of Italian descent.

Carney Ir. Gael. "The winner."
Carny, Kearney

Carollan Ir. Gael. "Little champion." In the U.S., likely to be confused with a variant of **Caroline**.
Carlin, Carling, Carolan

Carr Scan. "From the Swampy place."
Kerr

Carroll Var. **Charles**. OG. "Man." The preferred mascu-

line spelling of the Latin form of Charles, but unusual, probably because it is so easily confused with the feminine Carol.

Carolus, Carrol, Cary, Caryl

Carson OE. "Son of the marsh-dwellers."

Carswell OE. Place name: "Well where the watercress grows."

Carter OE. Occupational name: "One who drives carts."

Carvell OF. "Swampy dwelling."
Carvel

Carver OE. Occupational name: "One who carves wood."

Cary OE. Place name: "Pretty brook." Distinct from Carey. Use in the 19th century as a first name was quite rare, but when actor Archibald Leach renamed himself Cary Grant, numerous families followed his lead.

Casey Ir. Gael. "Vigilant." Possibly also a short form of Casimir. Made famous by the song about the engineer of the Cannonball Express train, Casey Jones. Baseball personality Casey Stengel; radio disc jockey Casey Kasem.

Cacey, Cayce, Caycey, Kasey

Cash Dim. Cassius. Lat. "Vain."

Casimir Slavic. "Bringing peace." Associated with Poland for her famous 11th-century king, who brought peace to the nation.

Casimire, Kazimierz, Kazimir

Casper Origin unclear, though many sources suggest Per. "he who guards the treasure." Originally Jasper, Germanicized to Caspar. French is Gaspard. Traditionally one of the Three Kings (perhaps the one carrying the gold) was named Caspar. Americans who grew up in the 1960s will also be reminded of the cartoon character Casper the Friendly Ghost. Defense secretary Casper Weinberger.

Caspar, Cass, Gaspar, Gaspard, Gasparo, Gasper, Jasper, Kaspar

Cassidy Ir. Gael. "Ingenious, clever."
Cassady

Cassius Lat. "Vain." Historically, Cassius was a Roman

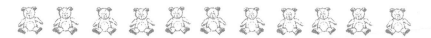

politician who was behind the plot to murder Julius Caesar. In Shakespeare's play, Caesar says, "Yon Cassius has a lean and hungry look; He thinks too much: Such men are dangerous."
Cash, Cass, Cassio

Castor Gk. "Beaver." In classical myth, along with Pollux, one of the heavenly twins immortalized in the constellation Gemini. They were considered the patron gods of seafarers, appearing to them in St. Elmo's fire.

Cato Lat. "All-knowing." Cato was a particularly high-minded Roman statesman of the time of Julius Caesar.

Cavan Ir. Gael. "Handsome."
Kavan

Cecil Lat. "Blind one," from a Roman clan name. Used in Roman times, then resurfaced in the Victorian era, possibly given a boost by the fame of industrialist (and founder of Rhodesia) Cecil Rhodes. Little used in this century. Film director Cecil B. De Mille; photographer Cecil Beaton.
Cecil, Cecilio, Cecilius, Celio

Cedric OE. "War leader." Used in two 19th-century literary landmarks (*Ivanhoe* and *Little Lord Fauntleroy*), which probably increased its popularity in Britain. Actor Sir Cedric Hardwicke.
Caddaric, Ced, Cedrick, Rick

Cephas Heb. "Rock." New Testament name; what Jesus called his apostle Simon. Peter is the Latin translation by which he is more commonly known. Cephas was in steady (if infrequent) use until the 20th century.

Chad Origin cloudy; possibly OE. "fierce." Saint Chad was a 7th-century English bishop. The name enjoyed an inexplicable burst of popularity in the late 1960s.
Chadd, Chaddie

Chadwick OE. Place name: "The fighter's settlement."

Chaim Heb. "Life." Male version of Eve. Hyman is more common in English-speaking countries. Author Chaim Potok.
Haim, Hayvim, Hayyim, Hy, Hyman, Hymen, Hymie, Manny

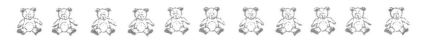

Chance Middle English. "Good fortune." Also var.
Chauncey.

Chancellor Middle English. Occupational name: "Chief
secretary, record keeper."
Chance, Chaunce

Chandler OF. Occupational name: "Candle merchant."

Chaney Fr. "Oak tree."
Cheney

Channing OF. Occupational name: "Official of the
church." Related to Cannon.
Canning, Cannon, Canon

Chapman OE. "Peddler."
Chap, Chappy, Manny

Charles OG. "Man." The English term "churl," meaning
"serf," comes from the same root. Has been a staple ever
since the era of the Emperor Charlemagne, and a royal
name in many European countries, including England,
where the next king will probably be Charles III. In
America, it was one of the top 5 names for the first three-
quarters of this century, but has since been displaced by
such exotics as Ryan, Zachary, and Justin. Naturalist
Charles Darwin; French president Charles de Gaulle; author Charles Dickens; actor Charlie Chaplin.
**Carel, Carl, Carlo, Carlos, Carrol, Carroll, Cary, Caryl,
Chad, Charley, Charlie, Charlot, Charlton, Chas, Chaz,
Chick, Chip, Chuck, Karel, Karl, Karoly**

Charlton OE. Place name: "Charles's dwelling." Also possibly a variation on Carlton. Used as a given name for
the last hundred years. Actor Charlton Heston.
Carleton, Carlton, Charleton

Chase OF. "Hunter." Painter William Merritt Chase.

Chauncey Middle English. Contraction of Chancellor.
Chance, Chancey

Chester Lat. "Soldier's camp." Place name from Roman
Britain, gradually evolved into a first name most com-
mon in the U.S. President Chester Arthur; newscaster
Chet Huntley.
Cheston, Chet

Chetwin OE. Place name: "Little house on the twisted
path."

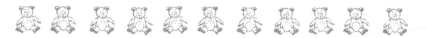

Chevalier Fr. "Knight." Comedian Chevy Chase.
  Chevy
Chick Dim. **Charles** OG. "Man."
Chico Sp. Dim. **Francis** (Lat. "Frenchman.") via Francisco.
Chilton OE. Place name: "Farm near the well."
Chris Dim. **Christian, Christopher.**
  Kris
Christian Gk. "Anointed, Christian." A girl's name that (contrary to the usual movement) became a male name, possibly after the huge success of John Bunyan's *Pilgrim's Progress* (1684), whose hero is called Christian. In Britain and Australia, especially popular in the 1970s. French fashion designers Christian Dior, Christian Lacroix; Dr. Christiaan Barnard.
  Chretien, Chris, Christiano, Christie, Cristian, Cristy, Kit, Kris, Kristian
Christmas Name of the holiday, used occasionally through the 19th century for Dec. 25 babies, but now usually replaced by the French, and somewhat subtler, form, Noel.
Christopher Gk. "Carrier of Christ." The much-loved story of Saint Christopher is that he lived alone by a river, carrying travelers across the ford on his back. A child whom he was carrying became almost too heavy to bear, and proved afterward to be the Christ child. Actually the tale has little basis in fact, and probably springs from the literal translation of the name, which originally meant carrying Christ in one's heart. Nevertheless, Christopher is still venerated as patron saint of travelers and drivers. In the modern era the name was little used until a revival in the 1940s, possibly influenced by the popularity of A. A. Milne's *Winnie the Pooh*, whose human hero is called Christopher Robin. Hugely popular right through the 1980s. Explorer Christopher Columbus; actor Christopher Plummer; architect Christopher Wren.
  Chris, Christie, Christof, Christoffer, Christoforo, Christoph, Christophe, Christophoros, Christos, Cris, Cristobal, Cristoforo, Kit, Kristo, Kristofer, Kristofor, Kristos

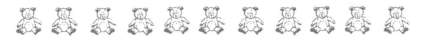

Chuck Dim. **Charles**. OG. "Man." Cartoon director Chuck Jones; musician Chuck Mangione; Colonel Chuck Yaeger.

Churchill OE. Place name: "Hill of the church." Use as a first name is probably homage to English statesman Sir Winston Churchill.

Cicero Lat. "Chickpea." Most famous for the Roman orator and statesman who lived in the 1st century B.C. Like Cato, probably came to the U.S. as a slave name.

Cid Sp. from Arab. "Lord." El Cid was a heroic Spanish knight of the 11th century whose story is told (and embroidered) in numerous medieval epics.
Cyd

Clancy Ir. Gael. "Red-haired fighter's child." An almost stereotypically Irish name.
Claney

Clare Dim. **Clarence**. Very unusual for boys.
Clair, Clarey

Clarence Lat. "Bright." An alternate source is the title Duke of Clarence, created for a 14th-century royal prince who married a girl from the Clare family. The bearers of the title have been ill fated: The third, for example, was said to have drowned in a barrel of wine. In the late 19th century Clarence was immensely popular, but gradually acquired the connotations of effete aristocracy and has been neglected recently. Lawyer Clarence Darrow.
Clair, Clarance, Clarrance, Clarrence, Klarance

Clark OF. Occupational name: "Cleric, scholar." Surname transferred to first name, heavily influenced by the fame of actor Clark Gable. Also made famous by "mild-mannered" Clark Kent, alter ego of Superman in the popular comic strip.
Clarke, Clerc, Clerk

Claude Lat. "Lame." Name of a Roman clan that produced the emperor immortalized in Robert Graves's novel (and subsequent TV dramatization) *I, Claudius*. Claud was used in the 19th century, but not in great

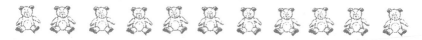

numbers. Painter Claude Monet; composer Claude Debussy; Congressman Claude Pepper; actor Claude Rains.
Claudan, Claudell, Claudianus, Claudien, Claudio, Claudius, Klaudio

Claus Dim. Nicholas. Gk. "People of victory."
Claes, Clause, Klaus

Clay OE. Occupational or place name involving clay. Most famous modern bearer was probably Cassius Clay, later Mohammad Ali, the boxing champion; he, in turn, had originally been named for a 19th-century abolitionist.

Clayborne OE. Place name: "Brook near a clay-bed."
Claiborn, Claiborne, Clay, Claybourne, Clayburn

Clayton OE. Place name: "Dwelling near the clay-bed." Given as a first name since the early 19th century.

Cleary Ir. Gael. "Learned one."

Clement Lat. "Mild, giving mercy." A name borne by six popes as well as the author (Clement Clark Moore) of "A Visit from St. Nicholas." Nevertheless, little used in English-speaking countries.
Clem, Clemens, Clemente, Clementius, Clemmie, Clemmy, Klemens, Klement, Kliment

Cleon Gk. "Renowned."
Kleon

Cleveland OE. Place name: "Hilly area." During the fame of U.S. President Grover Cleveland, several towns were named after him, and the surname became a first name, though only in the U.S. Writer Cleveland Amory.
Cleavon, Cleavland, Cleon, Cleve, Clevon

Cliff OE. "Steep slope." Or dim. **Clifford, Clifton.** Actor Cliff Robertson; singer Cliff Richard.
Clyff

Clifford OE. Place name: "Ford near the cliff." Surname transferred to first name, most popular in the late 19th century. Playwright Clifford Odets.
Cliff, Clyff, Clyfford

Clifton OE. Place name: "Town near the cliff." Another transferred surname, more common in the U.S. than in Britain.
Cliff, Clift, Clyfton

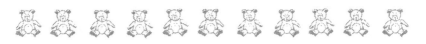

Clinton OE. Place name: "Settlement near the headland." An illustrious 18th-century governor of New York, De Witt Clinton, left his name on many locations. Actor Clint Eastwood.
Clint

Clive OE. Place name: "Cliff." Given some publicity by a famous English soldier, Robert Clive, for his exploits in India. Thackeray used it as a first name in an 1855 novel, but its real popularity in England didn't come for another hundred years. Never widely used in the U.S. Critic Clive Barnes.
Cleve, Clyve

Clovis OG. "Renowned fighter." Early form of the name that would eventually become Ludwig or Louis. King Clovis I was the first Christian king of the Franks, and later kings' use of the name Louis probably harks back to the dynasty he founded in the 5th century. The name is rare, however, in the 20th century.

Cluny Ir. Gael. "From the meadow."

Clyde Scot. place name: The River Clyde penetrates western Scotland as far as Glasgow.

Cody OE. "Pillow." Use as a first name was probably influenced by the fame of Buffalo Bill Cody, frontier scout and entrepreneur, who took his "Wild West Show" around the U.S. and Europe at the turn of the century.
Codey, Codie, Kody

Colbert OE. "Renowned mariner."
Cole, Colt, Colvert, Culbert

Colby OE. Place name: "The dark farmstead."
Collby

Cole Dim. **Nicholas** (Gk. "people of victory") and names beginning with Cole. Composer Cole Porter; outlaw Cole Younger.

Coleman OE. "Follower of Nicholas." Also contraction of the Latin word for "dove"; probably influenced by the Irish Saint Columba.
Colman

Colin Gael. "Young creature." Also dim. **Nicholas** (Gk. "people of victory"). Well-known in the Middle Ages,

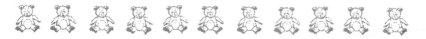

and popular in Britain in the middle of this century, but never spread in any numbers to the U.S.

Colan, Cole, Collin, Colyn

Colley OE. "Dark-haired." Use as a first name is rare.

Collis

Collier OE. Occupation name: "Coal miner."

Colier, Colis, Collayer, Collis, Collyer

Collins Ir. Gael. "Holly."

Colter OE. Occupational name: "Colt-herd."

Colton OE. Place name: "Dark settlement."

Collton, Colston

Colville OF. Place name of Norman origin and obscure meaning.

Colvile, Colvill

Colwyn Welsh. Place name, for a river in Wales.

Colwin, Colwynn

Conan Ir. Gael. "High, lifted up." Taken to Ireland some time after the Norman Conquest, but almost unknown until the fame of Sherlock Holmes's creator, Sir Arthur Conan Doyle. A more modern example is the movie character Conan the Barbarian, whose creators were probably unaware of the name's previous use or origin.

Con, Conant, Connie

Conlan Ir. Gael. "Hero."

Conlen, Conley, Conlin, Conlon, Connlyn

Connor Ir. Gael. "High longing."

Conor

Conrad OG. "Courageous advice." Despite occasional increases in its numbers, a name that has never been widely popular in English-speaking countries. Anthropologist Konrad Lorenz; hotelier Conrad Hilton; author Joseph Conrad.

Con, Connie, Conrade, Conrado, Cort, Curt, Konrad, Kort, Kurt

Conroy Ir. Gael. "Wise man."

Constantine Lat. "Steadfast." The form Constant was popular among the Puritans (as a virtue name) and was revived in the 19th century to occasional modern use. Constantine, the Latin form, was the name of the first

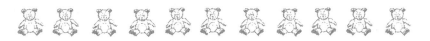

Roman emperor, and a royal name in Greece. Steady 19th-century use has now dwindled to neglect.
Constant, Constantin, Constantino, Costa, Konstantin, Konstantio, Konstanz

Conway Welsh. "Holy river." Rare.
Conwy

Cook Lat. "Cook." Occupational name, one of the 50 most common surnames in England, but an unusual first name in the 20th century.
Cooke

Cooper OE. Occupational name: "Barrel maker." Novelist James Fenimore Cooper; actor Gary Cooper.
Coop

Corbett Lat. "Dark as a raven." Most common in the 19th century. Actor Corbin Bernsen.
Corbet, Corbie, Corbin, Corbit, Corbitt, Cory

Corcoran Ir. Gael. "Ruddy."
Cork

Cordell OF. Occupational name: "Rope maker."

Corey Ir. Gael. Place name: "The hollow." Transferred to a surname and occasionally used as a first name for either sex. Also diminutive for "Cor-" names.
Correy, Corrie, Corry, Cory, Currie, Curry

Cormick Gael. "Chariot driver."
Cormac, Cormack

Corliss OE. "Benevolent, cheery."
Corley

Cornelius Lat. "Like a horn." Comes from a famous Latin clan name, and was often used under the Roman Empire. Railroad millionaire Cornelius Vanderbilt.
Con, Connie, Cornall, Cornelious, Cornell, Cornelus, Corney, Cornilius, Neel, Neil, Neely

Cornell Fr. Var. **Cornelius**.
Cornall, Cornel, Corney

Cornwallis OE. "Man from Cornwall." Surname transferred to a first name in the 19th century. Famous English general in the Revolutionary War, George Cornwallis.

Cort OG. "Brave."
Corty, Kort

Corwin OE. "Heart's friend or companion."
  Corwyn, Corwynn
Corydon Gk. "Battle-ready."
  Coridon, Coryden, Coryell
Cosgrove Ir. Gael. "Victorious champion."
  Cosgrave
Cosmo Gk. "Orderliness, organization." Saint Cosmas, a martyr, was patron saint of the Italian city of Milan, and the name was further spread there by the fame of Cosimo de'Medici, Grand Duke of Tuscany. His friend the Duke of Gordon took the name to Britain in the 17th century, but it was never widely used.
  Cosimo, Cosmé, Kosmo
Coulson Surname derived from **Nicholas** (Gk. "people of victory"), mostly 19th-century use.
  Colson
Courtland OE. Place name: "Land of the court."
  Cortland, Cortlandt, Courtlandt
Courtney OE. "Court-dweller." Surname transferred to first name; usually feminine in U.S. Immensely popular for girls in the late eighties, which will probably limit its use as a boys' name in the future. Actor Tom Courtenay.
  Cortney, Courtenay, Courtnay, Curt
Covell OE. Place name: "Slope with the cave."
Cowan Ir. Gael. Place name: "Hollow in the hill."
  Coe
Coyle Ir. Gael. "Follows the battle."
Craddock Welsh. "Love." Anglicization of a Welsh name, more common as a surname.
  Caradoc, Caradog
Craig Gael. "Rock." Surname that has become very popular since its introduction as a first name only 50 years ago.
Crandall OE. Place name: "Valley of cranes."
  Crandal, Crandell
Cranley OE. Place name: "Meadow with the cranes."
  Cranlee, Cranleigh, Cranly
Cranston OE. Place name: "Settlement of cranes." U.S. Senator Alan Cranston.

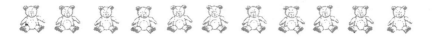

Craven OE. Last name, formerly place name, of unclear meaning. As an adjective, however, the usual definition is "cowardly." Mostly 19th-century use.

Crawford OE. Place name: "Ford of the crows." Particularly well used in Scotland, as both a surname and a given name.

Creighton OE. Place name: "Rocky spot."
Crayton, Crichton

Cresswell OE. Place name: "Well where watercress grows."
Carswell

Crispin Lat. "Curly-haired." Saint Crispin, supposedly a 3rd-century martyr (though there is some doubt about his legend), is patron of shoemakers, and Henry V fought the battle of Agincourt on his feast day, October 25. The name was somewhat popular in Britain in the 17th and 18th centuries, and was revived in the 1960s, but has not spread to the U.S. in significant numbers.
Crepin, Crispino, Crispo, Crispus

Crofton OE. "Settlement of the cottages."

Cromwell OE. Place name: "Winding stream." Limited use as a first name, probably out of admiration for 17th-century English reformer Oliver Cromwell.

Crosby Scan. Place name: "At the cross." Singer Bing Crosby.
Crosbey, Crosbie

Crosley OE. Place name: "Meadow of the cross."
Croslea, Crosleigh, Crosly, Crosslee, Crossley, Crosslie

Crowther OE. Occupational name: "Fiddler."

Cullen Ir. Gael. "Handsome." Poet William Cullen Bryant.
Cullan, Cullin

Culley Ir. Gael. Place name: "The woods."
Cully

Culver OE. "Dove."
Colver, Cully

Cunningham Ir. Gael. "Village of the milk pail."
Conyngham

Curran Ir. Gael. "Hero."
Currey, Currie, Curry

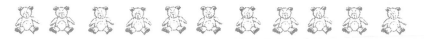

Curt Dim. **Courtney, Curtis, Conrad**. Most common in the U.S.
Kurt
Curtis OF. "Polite, courteous." Surname used as first name, notably in the U.S. since the 1950s. General Curtis Le May.
Curcio, Curt, Curtice, Curtiss, Kurtis
Cuthbert OE. "Famous, brilliant." Saint Cuthbert was a much-loved 7th-century English bishop. He was most famous in northern England and Scotland, and his name was most common there, though it fell out of favor after the 1930s. Never popular in America.
Cutler OE. Occupational name: "Knife maker."
Cyprian Gk. "From Cyprus." Steadily used in Britain until the 17th century, but never transferred to the U.S.
Cipriano, Ciprien, Cyprien
Cyrano Gk. "From Cyrene." Use is bound to recall Edmond Rostand's popular play *Cyrano de Bergerac* (1897), based on the life of the 17th-century author and swashbuckler of that name.
Cyril Gk. "The lord." Popularity confined to Britain, from the turn of the century to the 1930s. Actor Cyril Ritchard.
Ciril, Cirilio, Cyrill, Cyrille, Cirillo, Cyrillus, Cirilo, Kiril, Kyril
Cyrus Per. "Sun or throne." Famous Persian emperor who appears in the Old Testament; he allowed exiled Jews to rebuild Jerusalem. Puritan use brought it to the U.S., where it was somewhat popular, but faded in modern times. Inventor Cyrus McCormick; former Secretary of State Cyrus Vance.
Ciro, Cy

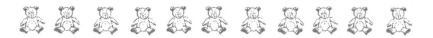

Dacey Ir. Gael. "from the south". Lat. "from Dacia," an area that is now Romania. The form Dacian enjoyed a burst of popularity in the 1970s along with other "-ian" names like Damian and Dorian.

Dacian, Dacy, Daicey, Daicy

Dag Scan. "Daylight." In Norse mythology the god Dag is the son of light. Diplomat and author Dag Hammarskjöld.

Dagny

Dagan Heb. "Grain, the earth."

Dagon

Dagwood OE. Place name: "Shining forest." Virtually preempted by a character from the popular comic strip *Blondie*. Dagwood is the harassed husband of a dizzy blonde.

Dalbert OE. "Bright-shining one."

Delbert

Dale OE. Place name: "Valley." Originally a surname meaning "one who lives in the valley." The term "dale" is still used in parts of England. Most famous as a first name in the 1930s. Success guru Dale Carnegie.

Daley, Dayle

Dallas Scot. Gael. Place name of a village in northeastern Scotland, used as a first name since the 19th century, and apparently unrelated to Dallas, Texas, which was named for a U.S. vice president.

Dal, Dallis

Dalton OE. Place name: "The settlement in the valley."

Dallton, Dalten

Daly Ir. Gael. "Assembly." Common Irish surname, used since the 1940s as a first name. Decathlon champion Daley Thompson.

Daley, Dawley

Dalziel Scot. Gael. Place name: "The small field."

Damek Slavic. Var. **Adam**. "Son of the red earth."

Adamec, Adamek, Adamik, Adamok, Adham, Damick, Damicke

Damian Gk. Meaning not clear: possibly "to tame," although the Greek root is also close to the word for "spirit." The name was revived in various forms (Da-

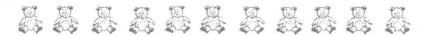

mon, Damien) in the 1950s, having been neglected since the Middle Ages. Auther Damon Runyon.

Daemon, Daimen, Daimon, Daman, Damen, Dameon, Damian, Damiano, Damien, Damion, Damon, Damyan, Damyen, Damyon

Dan Dim. **Daniel**. Heb. "God is my judge." Used from time to time on its own. Actors Dan Ackroyd, Dan Blocker.

Dana OE. "From Denmark." Also possibly a place name referring to an English river. Surname first used as a boy's name in the 19th century, but now almost exclusively a girl's name, and a specifically American one. Artist Charles Dana Gibson.

Dane, Danie

Daniel Heb. "God is my judge." In the famous Old Testament story, Daniel is thrown into a den of lions because he insists on praying to his God while a captive in Babylon; he was, of course, rescued by the same God. The name has been used with moderate frequency until a spurt of popularity in the late 1950s, which endured until the early 1980s. Today's parents may have fond memories of the TV-inspired "Daniel Boone" coonskin hats they wore in the 1960s. Novelist Daniel Defoe; entertainers Danny Thomas, Danny Kaye; Senator Daniel Patrick Moynihan; actors Daniel Day-Lewis, Danny De Vito, Danny Aiello.

Dan, Danal, Dane, Daneal, Dani, Danial, Daniele, Dannel, Dannie, Danny, Danyal, Danyel

Dante Lat. "Lasting, enduring." Actually a nickname, since Italian poet Dante Alighieri's full name was Durante, and modern use of the name almost always refers to him. English artist Dante Gabriel Rossetti.

Darby OE. Place name: "Park with deer." Derived from Derby, a surname used as a first name. Darby is occasionally used for girls.

Darbie, Derby

Darcy Ir. Gael. "Dark." Also Norman place name, "from Arcy." In Britain, more likely to be a boy's name, but in the U.S., more likely to be feminine.

D'Arcy, Darcey, Darsey, Darsy

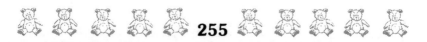

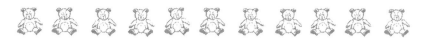

Darius Gk. "Rich." Darius the Great was a renowned emperor of Persia in the 5th century B.C.
Dario, Derry

Darnell OE. Place name: "The hidden spot."
Darnall

Darrel Transferred surname, possibly originated as a French place name, like Darcy. There are many forms, of which Darryl is the favorite by a nose. In fact, that spelling, and the popularity of the name in the 1950s, may stem from the fame of film producer Darryl Zanuck. Baseball star Darryl Strawberry; musician Daryl Hall.
Darral, Darrell, Darrill, Darrol, Darryl, Daryl, Derril, Deryl, Deryll

Darren Ir. Gael. "Great." Originally a surname, first used as a given name in this century. Its popularity was probably influenced by the TV series "Bewitched," in which the rather hapless leading man was named Darren.
Daren, Darin, Daron, Darran, Darrin, Darron, Darryn, Derron

Darton OE. Place name: "Settlement of the deer."

Darwin OE. "Dear friend." Naturalist Charles Darwin.
Darwyn, Derwin, Derwynn

David Heb. "Dear one." In the Old Testament, the young David used his slingshot to kill the mighty giant Goliath, and went on to become King of Israel and author of the Psalms. He has been a favorite subject of artists, notably sculptors of the Italian Renaissance, like Michelangelo and Donatello. Saint David is the patron saint of Wales, so the name is popular there, and in Scotland, where David was a royal name. In the U.S. the name is used by Jewish and Christian families alike, and has been in the top ten boys' names for the last forty years. Explorer David Livingstone; actor David Niven; baseball star Dave Winfield; TV host David Letterman; musician David Bowie.
Dafydd, Dai, Dave, Davey, Davidde, Davide, Davidson, Davie, Davin, Davis, Daven, Davon, Davy

Davis OE. "David's son." Contraction of surname that cropped up in the Middle Ages. Confederate President Jefferson Davis, actor Brad Davis.
Dave, Davidson, Davies, Davison, Davy

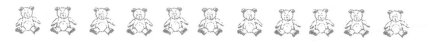

Dawson OE. "David's son." Another form of the medieval surname.

Dean OE. Place name, "valley," or occupational name, "church official." Surname used as a first name, mostly since the 1950s. Actor Dean Martin, U.S. Secretaries of State Dean Acheson, Dean Rusk.
Deane, Deen, Dene, Deyn, Dino

Dearborn OE. Place name: "Brook of the deer."
Dearbourn, Dearburne, Deerborn

Decimus Lat. "Tenth," as in tenth child. In the 1990s, opportunities for use seem negligible.

Declan Ir. Unknown meaning: name of a saint, popular in Ireland.

Dedrick Var. **Theodoric**. OG. "The people's ruler." Also the source for the better-known **Derek**.
Dedric, Diederick

Deems OE. "Judge's child."

Delaney Ir. Gael. "Offspring of the challenger."
Delaine, Delainey, Delainy, Delane, Delany

Delano OF. Surname of unclear origin: possibly "night-time" *(de la nuit)* or "nut tree" *(de la noix)*. It would be merely one of those odd family names if it had not been made famous by U.S. President Franklin Delano Roosevelt.

Delbert OE. "Day-bright."
Bert, Bertie, Dalbert

Delling ONorse. "Scintillating."

Delmore OF. "Of the sea." The more familiar form, at least as a place name, is the Spanish Delmar. Use is American only. Poet Delmore Schwartz.
Delmar, Delmer, Delmor

Delroy Fr. "The king." More common forms are Elroy and Leroy.
Delroi

Delwin OE. "Proud friend" or "bright friend."
Dalwin, Dalwyn, Delavan, Delevan, Dellwin, Delwyn, Delwynn

Demetrius Gk. "Follower of Demeter." Little used in English-speaking countries, though its Greek and Russian

forms are well-known in those countries. Composer Dimitri Shostakovich.

Demetri, Demetris, Dhimitrios, Dimetre, Dimitri, Dimitrios, Dimitry, Dmitri, Dmitrios, Dmitry

Demos Gk. "The people." Also possibly homage to Greece's most famous orator, Demosthenes. Rare, even in Greece.

Demas

Dempsey Ir. Gael. "Proud." Boxer Jack Dempsey.

Dempsy

Dempster OE. "One who judges."

Denby Scan. Place name: "The Danes' village."

Danby, Denbey, Denney, Dennie, Denny

Denham OE. Place name: "Village in a valley."

Denholm Scot. Place name. In the public eye currently because of the English actor Denholm Elliott.

Denley OE. Place name: "Meadow near the valley."

Denlie, Denly

Denman OE. Surname derived from place name: "Man who lives in the valley."

Dennis Gk. "Follower of Dionysius." Dionysos was the classical Greek god of wine, but the name also appears in the New Testament. Saint Denis is the patron saint of France. The name has had alternating centuries of favor and disfavor (16th out, 17th in), reaching the height of its 20th-century popularity around 1920. Actors Dennis Quaid, Dennis Christopher, Dennis Hopper.

Den, Denies, Denis, Dennes, Dennet, Denney, Dennie, Dennison, Denny, Dennys, Denys, Deon, Dion, Dionisio, Dionysius, Dionysus

Dennison OE. "Son of Dennis."

Den, Denison, Dennyson, Tennyson

Denton OE. Place name: "Settlement in the valley."

Denny, Dent, Denten, Dentin

Denver OE. Place name: "Green valley." Singer John Denver.

Denzil Cornish place name, used as a first name almost exclusively in Britain. Actor Denzel Washington.

Denzel, Denzell, Denziel, Denzill, Denzyl

Derek OG. "The people's ruler." Most common of the

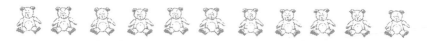

many anglicized forms of **Theodoric**, popular starting around 1890, peaking in the 1930s.

Darrick, Dereck, Deric, Derick, Derik, Derk, Derreck, Derrek, Derrick, Derrik, Derryck, Derryk, Deryk, Deryke, Dirk, Dirke, Dyrk

Dermot Ir. Gael. "Without envy."

Dermott, Diarmid, Diarmuid

Derry Ir. Gael. Place name: City in Northern Ireland formerly known as Londonderry. Also short form of Derek, Dermot, etc.

Derrie

Derward OE. "Deer keeper."

Durward

Derwin OE. "Dear friend."

Darwin, Darwyn, Derwyn, Derwynn, Durwin

Desmond Ir. Gael. "From South Munster." Munster was an ancient kingdom in Ireland. Used in England since 1900, and briefly popular around 1920, but unusual now. South African cleric and activist Bishop Desmond Tutu.

Desmund

Deverell OE. Place name: "Bank of the river."

Devin Ir. Gael. "Bard, poet."

Dev, Devon

Devine Ir. Gael. "Ox."

Devlin Ir. Gael. "Fierce courage."

Devland, Devlen, Devlyn

Devon English and American place name. More common for girls than for boys.

Devin, Devonn, Devyn

Dewey Welsh. Var. **David**. People may remember the Dewey Decimal System, invented by Melvil Dewey in 1876 and the organizing principle for the majority of American libraries until the Libary of Congress got in on the act and changed all the numbers.

Dewi, Dewie

DeWitt Flem. "Blond." Early American statesman De Witt Clinton.

Dewitt, Dwight, Witt

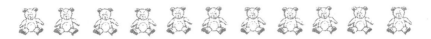

Dexter Lat. "right-handed" or OE. "woman dyer." Modern use, more common in Britain.
　　Dex

Diamond OE. "Bright guardian." Also, for girls, a jewel name. Actor Lou Diamond Phillips.

Dick dim. **Richard** OG. "dominant ruler"; also **Frederick** OG. "peaceful ruler." Actor Lou Diamond Phillips.

Diego Sp. Var. **James**. Heb. "he who supplants."

Dieter OG. "Army of the people."

Dietrich Ger. form of **Theodoric** OG. "People's ruler." See **Derek**.
　　Dedrick, Derek, Deke, Diederick, Dirk

Didier Fr. "Much-desired." Male form of Désirée; currently popular in France.

Digby ONorse. "Town by the ditch." Like many English surnames adapted from place names, became a first name in the late 19th century without ever becoming very widespread.

Dillon Ir. Gael. "Loyal." Often confused with its homonym, the Welsh Dylan. Actor Matt Dillon.
　　Dillan, Dilon, Dyllon, Dylon

Dinsmore Ir. Gael. Place name: "The hill fortress."

Dirk Var. **Derek**

Dixon OE. "Son of Dick." Scottish surname transferred to first name.
　　Dickson

Doane OE. Place name: "Low, rolling hills."

Doherty Ir. Gael. "Harmful." Surname common in Ireland, transferred occasionally to first-name status.
　　Docherty, Dougherty, Douherty

Dolan Ir. Gael. "Black-haired."

Dolph Dim. **Adolph**.
　　Dolf, Dolphus

Dominic Lat. "Lord." Possibly because of the fame of Saint Dominic, founder of an important monastic order, a name popular among Catholic families, though its use has spread since the 1950s. Still more common in Britain than the U.S. Clever for a child born on Sunday, "the Lord's day."
　　Demenico, Demingo, Dom, Domenic, Domenico,

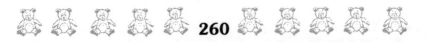

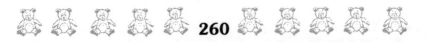

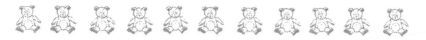

Domingo, Domini, Dominick, Dominie, Dominik, Dominique, Nick

Donahue Ir. Gael. "Dark fighter." TV host Phil Donahue.
Donohoe, Donohue

Donald Scot. Gael. "World mighty." Common in Scotland for centuries, and popular elsewhere for some 50 years, peaking in 1925 but less and less popular since the 1950s, perhaps because Disney preempted the name by giving it to a cartoon duck. Actor Donald Sutherland; real estate tycoon Donald Trump; singer Donny Osmond.
Donal, Donall, Donalt, Donaugh, Donnel, Donnell, Donny

Donato Lat. "Given."

Donnelly Ir. Gael. "Brown-haired fighter."
Donnell

Donovan Ir. Gael. "Dark." Surname become first name or, in the case of the pop singer who recorded "Mellow Yellow" in the late 1960s, only name.
Donavon, Donevin, Donevon, Donoven, Donovon

Dooley Ir. Gael. "Dark hero."

Doran Ir. Gael. "Fist" or "stranger, exile."
Dore, Dorian, Doron, Dorran, Dorren

Dorian Gk. Place name: "From Doris," an area in Greece. Introduced by Oscar Wilde in *The Picture of Dorian Gray*; the hero of the tale is a beautiful young man who succumbs to a life of vice. Notwithstanding this discouraging precedent, the name has had some popularity in the U.S.
Dorien, Dorrian, Dorryen

Dougal Celt. "Dark stranger." Most common in Scotland.
Doyle, Dougall, Dugal, Dugald, Dugall

Douglas Scot. Gael. Place name: "Black water." Though it was originally a girl's name, by the 19th century Douglas was used for boys. Its period of great popularity, which peaked in the 1950s, seems to have been inspired by the actors Douglas Fairbanks, father and son. Since the 1970s, its eclipse has been fairly complete. Gen. Douglas MacArthur.
Douglass, Dugaid

Dow Ir. Gael. "Dark-haired."

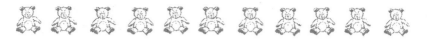

Doyle Ir. Gael. "Black stranger." Var. **Dougal**.

Drake Middle English. This is an unusually specific name, for it derives from the word *draca*, which was the medieval term for "dragon." Originally Drake designated the man who kept the inn with the dragon trademark, or the "Sign of the Dragon." It followed the usual route of becoming a surname, and thence a first name. English explorer Sir Francis Drake.

Drew Welsh. "Wise." Dim. **Andrew**. Used as an independent name since the 1960s.
Dru

Drummond Celt. Meaning unclear. Use as a first name is concentrated in Scotland.

Drury OF. "Loved one." Drury Lane is a famous street in London's theater district, and also the home of the Muffin Man in a well-known children's song.

Dryden OE. Place name: "Dry valley." Poet John Dryden.

Duane Ir. Gael. "Swarthy." Used primarily since the 1940s, predominantly in the U.S.
Dewain, Dewayne, Duwain, Duwayne, Dwain, Dwayne

Dudley OE. Place name: "People's field." Aristocratic family name in England, used as a first name since the 19th century. The absurd Canadian Mountie Dudley Doright was a staple character in the 1960s "Rocky and Bullwinkle Show." Actor Dudley Moore.

Duff Gael. "Swarthy." There are many English surnames turned first names that derive from the Gaelic *dubh*, which means dark. They may describe places (i.e., Douglas), or personal characteristics, as in this case.
Duffey, Duffy

Dugan Ir. Gael. "Swarthy."
Doogan, Dougan, Douggan, Duggan

Duke Lat. "Leader." Last name transferred to first name, or possibly an abbreviation of the highly unusual Marmaduke. Current use is probably inspired either by John Wayne (who was nicknamed "Duke"), or the great jazz musician Duke Ellington.

Duncan Scot. Gael. "Brown fighter." A royal name in early Scotland: There was a King Duncan in 11th-century Scotland whose cousin Macbeth murdered him. Shake-

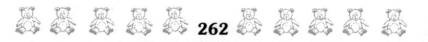

speare later picked up the tale in his tragedy *Macbeth*. The name disappeared until a spell of 19th-century use in Scotland and a flurry of mostly English popularity in the 1950s and 1960s. Never a big hit in the U.S. Cabinetmaker Duncan Phyfe.

    Dunn

Dunham Gael. "Brown man."

Dunley OE. Place name: "Meadow with the hill."

Dunlop Scot. Gael. Place name: "Muddy hill."

Dunmore Scot. Gael. Place name: "Big fortress on the hill."

Dunn Gael. "Brown." Writers Dominick and John Gregory Dunne.

    Dunne

Dunstan OE. Place name: "Brown hill with stones." Name of an English saint who was Archbishop of Canterbury in the 10th century. Rarely used, even in Britain.

Dunton OE. Place name: "Hill settlement."

Durant Lat. "Enduring." Much more common as a last name. Dante is an abbreviated version. The 19th-century historians Will and Ariel Durant; American painter Asher Durand; entertainer Jimmy Durante.

    Dante, Durand, Durante

Durward OE. Occupational name: "Warder at the gate."

    Derward

Durwin OE. "Dear friend."

    Derwin, Derwyn, Durwyn

Dustin OG. "brave warrior," or OE. place name: "Dusty area." Use of the name is almost certainly influenced by the fame of actor Dustin Hoffman.

    Dustan, Duston, Dusty

Dwight Flemish. "White or blond." Var. **De Witt**. Some sources claim Dwight is a contraction of a surname derived from Dionysius. Given fame in the U.S. by two Yale University presidents, and by President Dwight Eisenhower. Its moderate use as a first name was probably inspired by him, and had trailed off by the 1970s. Baseball star Dwight Gooden.

Dyer OE. Occupational name: "Dyer." Curiously enough, Dexter refers to a female dyer.

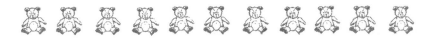

Dylan Welsh. "Son of the sea." Welsh legend tells of a sea-god named Dylan, but modern use of the name, which has spread well beyond Wales, is probably homage to poet Dylan Thomas. The best-known example of this tribute is singer Bob Dylan, whose last name was originally Zimmerman.

Dyson OE. Last name that is probably a contraction of Dennison. Transferred to first-name use in the 19th century.

Eamon Ir. Var. **Edmund**. OE. "Wealthy protector." Irish President Eamon de Valera may have been the inspiration behind the spurt of popularity between the 1950s and the 1970s. The name is rare in America.
Eamonn

Earl OE. "Nobleman, leader." The most popular of the English titles of nobility to be used as a first name, though Baron and Duke also occur. In the democratic U.S. it is probably a transferred surname rather than an allusion to the hereditary aristocracy. Author Erle Stanley Gardner; actor Errol Flynn; basketball star Earl ("the Pearl") Monroe; musician Earl Scruggs; Chief Justice of the U.S. Supreme Court Earl Warren.
Earle, Earlie, Early, Erl, Erle, Errol, Erroll, Erryl, Rollo

Eaton OE. Place name: "Settlement on the river."
Eatton, Eton, Eyton

Ebenezer Heb. "Rock of help." In the Old Testament, Samuel created a memorial to his victory over the Philistines, and called the stone Ebenezer. The name came to America with the Puritans, and was, improbably enough, at one point almost as popular a name as John. It was fading by the 19th century, and Ebenezer Scrooge in Charles Dickens's *A Christmas Carol* probably hastened its disappearance.

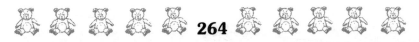

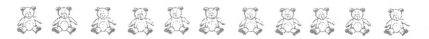

Eb, Ebbaneza, Eben, Ebeneezer, Ebeneser, Ebenezar, Eveneser

Eberhard OG. "Courage of a boar." Var. **Everett**. Pencil magnate Eberhard Faber.

Eberhardt, Everard, Everhardt, Evrard

Edbert OE. "Wealthy and bright."

Edel OG. "Noble." Unusual as a name in itself, but the first syllable of many combined forms such as **Adalric** and **Adelaide**. Biographer Leon Edel.

Adel

Eden Heb. "Pleasure, delight." It is a short step from the Hebrew meaning of the word to its general association with Paradise. The name is used for girls as well as boys. English statesman Sir Anthony Eden.

Eaden, Eadin, Edin, Edyn

Edgar OE. "Wealthy spearman." A royal name in Anglo-Saxon England which, like Edmund, endured through the Norman invasion and the resulting influx of Norman names. In Shakespeare's *King Lear*, Lear's son is called Edgar. Revived, like many Anglo-Saxon names, at the turn of the century, but the revival was short-lived. Poet Edgar Allan Poe; puppeteer Edgar Bergen; artist Edgar Dégas; author Edgar Rice Burroughs.

Ed, Eddie, Edgard, Edgardo, Ned, Neddy, Ted, Teddie

Edison OE. "Son of Edward." Inventor Thomas Edison.

Eddison, Eddy, Edson

Edmund OE. "Wealthy protector." A popular, and sainted, king of the East Angles in the 9th century gave the name enough popularity to survive the Norman Conquest. Astronomer Edmund Halley; poet Edmund Spenser; explorer Sir Edmund Hillary; Governor Edmund "Pat" Brown; Senator Edmund Muskie.

Eadmund, Eamon, Eamonn, Ed, Eddie, Edmon, Edmond, Edmonde, Edmondo, Ned, Neddie, Ted, Teddy

Edric OE. "Wealthy ruler." Anglo-Saxon name that was pushed out of fashion by the Normans in the 11th century but revived briefly at the end of the 19th.

Edrick

Edsel OE. Place name: "Wealthy man's house." Linked in most minds to automotive pioneer Edsel Ford, and the

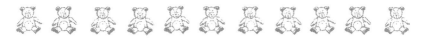

ill-fated car named after him. The name is still used in the Ford family.

Edward OE. "Wealthy defender." A name with long-lasting popularity throughout the English-speaking world. Used by kings of England (including the saint Edward the Confessor) since before the Norman Conquest, and still a staple in the royal family. Though less of an obvious choice since the 1930s, it is still popular. Photographer Edward Steichen; ballet dancer Edward Villella; U.S. Senator Edward Kennedy; poet Edward Lear; artist Edouard Manet; Edward, Duke of Windsor.
Ed, Eddie, Eddy, Edik, Edouard, Eduard, Eduardo, Edvard, Ewart, Lalo, Ned, Neddie, Ted, Teddie

Edwin OE. "Wealthy friend." Anglo-Saxon name revived at the end of the 19th century, and used with some frequency since then. Astronaut Edwin "Buzz" Aldrin; Attorney General Edwin Meese III.
Eadwinn, Ed, Eddy, Edlin, Eduino, Edwyn, Ned, Neddy, Ted

Efrem Var. **Ephraim.** Actor Efrem Zimbalist, Jr.

Egan Ir. Gael. "Burning." Irish use predominates.
Egann, Egon

Egbert OE. "Brilliant sword." Another 19th-century Anglo-Saxon revival, now little heard.

Egerton OE. Place name and surname that occurs in the English aristocracy. Transferred to first-name use mostly in Britain.
Edgerton

Egidio It. "Kid, young goat." The anglicized version is Giles.

Eginhard Ger. "Sword power."
Eginhardt, Egon, Einhard, Einhardt, Enno

Egor Rus. "Farmer." Currently popular in Russia, but very exotic in English-speaking countries.
Igor, Ygor

Einar ONorse. "Battle leader." Refers to the heroes of Valhalla, in the Old Norse legends.
Ejnar, Inar

Eion Ir. Var. **John** Heb. "the Lord is gracious," by way of Ian.
Ean

Elbert Var. **Albert**. OE. "Highborn/shining." The long form is Ethelbert, but it is virtually obsolete.

Elchanan Heb. "God is gracious."
Elhanan, Elhannan

Elden Var. **Alden**. OE. "Old friend." Also possibly "valley of the elves." Surname changed to first name.
Eldin, Eldon, Eldwin, Eldwyn, Elton

Elder OE. Place name: "Elder trees." Also, in U.S., may denote a forebear who had high standing in one of the Protestant churches that are governed by councils of elders.

Eldon OE. Place name: "Sacred hill." Used since the 19th century.

Eldred OE. "Old counsel." Anglo-Saxon name lost in the onslaught of Norman names, and brought back in the 19th-century craze for the picturesque remnants of the past.
Aldred, Eldrid

Eldridge Ger. "Sage ruler." Civil rights activist Eldridge Cleaver.
Eldredge, Eldrege, Eldrige

Eleazer Var. **Lazarus**. Heb. "The Lord will help." The 19th-century fondness for obscure biblical names (Eleazer among them) tends to confirm the stereotype of the repressed religious Victorians. If nothing else, they must have read their Bibles carefully to come up with these names.
Elazar, Eleasar, Eleazaro, Eli, Elie, Eliezer, Ely

Eli Heb. "On high." In the Old Testament, Eli was Israel's high priest. This was a very holy name to the Hebrews. The Puritans used it freely, and it persisted through the 19th century but faded after the 1930s. American inventor Eli Whitney; author Elie Wiesel; actor Eli Wallach.
Elie, Eloi, Eloy, Ely

Elias Gk. Var. **Elijah**. Most common in the 17th century.
Elice, Ellice, Ellis, Elyas

Elihu Heb. "God, the Lord." Like **Eleazer**, occasionally used in the 19th century.

Elijah Heb. "The Lord is my God." A great prophet in the

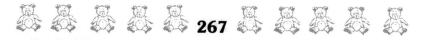

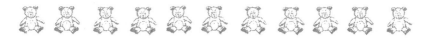

Old Testament. Felix Mendelssohn, reputedly Queen
Victoria's favorite composer, wrote an oratorio about
him in 1846. The name was most popular in the early
19th century. Film director Elia Kazan.
**Eli, Elia, Elias, Elie, Elihu, Eliot, Eliyahu, Elliot, Ellis, Ely,
Elyot, Elyott**

Elisha Heb. "The Lord is my salvation." The successor to
Elijah, as recounted in the Old Testament. Puritan name
in the 17th century, a bit more widespread in the 19th,
and all but obsolete now.
Eli, Elisee, Eliseo, Elisher, Lisha

Elkanah Heb. "God has made." A man's name in the Old
Testament, but occasionally used for girls as well.
Elkana

Ellard OG. "Noble and valorous."
Allard, Allerd

Ellery OE. Place name: "Island with elder trees." Some
sources propose a relationship to Hilary. The famous fictional detective Ellery Queen is probably the best-known
user of the name.
Ellary, Ellerey

Elliot Anglicization of **Elijah** or **Eli**. Surname first used as
a given name in modern Scotland. Most popular in the
U.S. Poet T. S. Eliot; actor Elliott Gould; Attorney General Elliot Richardson.
Eliot, Eliott, Elliott, Elyot, Elyott

Ellis Anglicization of **Elias**. Surname transferred to first
name. Ellis Bell was the pseudonym used by Emily
Brontë; when they first began publishing, each of the
Brontë sisters chose a name that could be considered
masculine. Anne was Acton Bell, and Charlotte was Cur-
rer Bell.

Ellison OE. "Son of Ellis." Author Ralph Ellison.
Elison, Ellson, Ellyson, Elson

Ellsworth OE. "Nobleman's estate."
Ellswerth, Elsworth

Elmer OE. "Highborn and renowned." Anglo-Saxon
name that has been much more popular in the U.S. than
in Britain, especially in the late 19th century. Sinclair
Lewis's well-known novel *Elmer Gantry*, published in

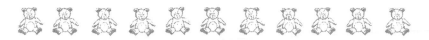

1927, was about a compelling charlatan of a minister. It was shocking, successful, and discouraging to parents who were considering Elmer as a name for their babies. Cartoon character Elmer Fudd.

Aylmar, Aylmer, Aymer, Ellmer, Elmir

Elmo Lat. from Gk. "amiable" or It. "godly helmet." Var. **Anselm**. Saint Elmo is the common name for Saint Erasmus, a 4th-century bishop-martyr who is patron saint of sailors. Saint Elmo's fire (also the name of a popular movie in the early 1980s) refers to the electrical discharges occasionally sighted at the top of a ship's mast. Parents who already have children may know Elmo as a furry red toddler-monster featured on "Sesame Street."

Elmore OE. Place name: "Moor with elm trees." Author Elmore Leonard.

Elroy Var. **Leroy**. Fr. "King."

Elsdon OE. Place name: "Hill of the nobleman."

Elston OE. Place name: "Settlement of the nobleman."
   Ellston

Elton OE. Place name: "Old Settlement" or "Ella's town." Musician Elton John.
   Alton, Eldon, Ellton

Elvin OE. "Elf friend" or "highborn friend." Var. **Alvin**.

Elvio Sp. from Lat. "Blond, fair."

Elvis Scan. "All-wise." Variants are rare, since use, as in the case of singer Elvis Costello (né Declan Patrick McManus), is almost always influenced by the fame of Elvis Presley.
   Alvis, Alvys, Elvys

Elwell OE. Place name: "Old well."

Elwin Var. **Elvin**.
   Elvin, Elvis, Elvyn, Elwin, Win, Wynn

Elwyn Welsh. "Fair brow." Easily confused with Elwin, but more likely to be found in Wales, where it has a different meaning altogether.
   Elwin, Elwynn

Elwood OE. Place name: "Old wood."
   Ellwood, Woody

Ely OE. Place name (a river in South Wales and a cathe-

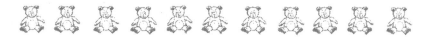

dral and town in Cambridgeshire) turned surname. Or, more likely, a variant of **Eli**.

Emerson OG. "Emery's son." First-name use may be tribute to Ralph Waldo Emerson, the transcendentalist philosopher and "sage of Concord."

Emery OG. "Home ruler." Saw 19th-century use as a first name, predominantly American rather than British.
Amerigo, Amery, Amory, Emeri, Emerich, Emmerich, Emmery, Emory

Emil Lat. "Eager to please." The French form, Emile, took root slightly earlier in English-speaking countries. Used only since the mid–19th century, without any great period of popularity. French author Emile Zola; actor Emilio Estevez.
Aymil, Emelen, Emile, Emilian, Emilio, Emilion, Emilyan, Emlen, Emlin, Emlyn

Emlyn Welsh place name given some prominence by playwright and actor Emlyn Williams.

Emmanuel Heb. "God is among us." Used in both the Old and the New Testaments, and as another name for Jesus. Slight use in the 17th century grew gradually right through the 19th, then tailed off. In the U.S. Manuel is fairly common among Catholics of Hispanic descent, who also use Jesus quite freely. Fashion designer Emmanuel Ungaro; pianist Emmanuel Ax.
Eman, Emanual, Emanuel, Emanuele, Immanuel, Immanuele, Manny, Manual, Manuel, Manuelo

Emmett Various derivations are possible, including OG. "energetic, powerful," OE. "an ant," or even a last name relating to Emma. Famous clown Emmett Kelly.
Emmet, Emmit, Emmot, Emmott

Engelbert OG. "Angel-bright." Entertainer Engelbert Humperdinck (whose original name, less memorable if more euphonious, was Arnold Dorsey).
Bert, Berty, Engelbert, Ingelbert, Inglebert

Ennis Var. **Angus**. Ir. Gael. "Sole or only choice."

Enoch Heb. "Vowed, dedicated." Old Testament name for the father of Methuselah. Briefly popular from the 1860s to 1880s, inspired by Tennyson's famous and sentimental poem "Enoch Arden." Now scarce.
Enock

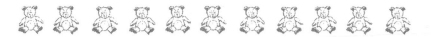

Enos Heb. "Man." Old Testament name for one of Adam and Eve's great-grandsons. Mildly revived, not by the Puritans, but in the 19th century. Obscure in this century.

Enrico It. Var. **Henry**. OG. "Estate ruler." Use by English-speaking families probably reflects the fame of operatic tenor Enrico Caruso.

Enzo It. Var. **Henry**. OG. "Estate ruler."

Ephraim Heb. "Fertile, productive." Old Testament name used mostly in the 18th and 19th centuries.
Efraim, Efrayim, Efrem, Efren, Ephream, Ephrem, Ephrim

Erasmus Gk. "Loved, desired." The 16th-century Dutch humanist philosopher Geert Geerts wrote as Desiderius Erasmus. (Desiderius is the Latin form of Erasmus.) He may have been thinking of Saint Erasmus, who is more popularly known as Saint Elmo. Use of the name was greatest in the latter half of the 19th century, and probably refers to the philosopher rather than the saint.
Erasme, Erasmo, Ras

Erastus Gk. "Beloved."
Eraste, Rastus

Ercole It. "Splendid gift."

Erhard OG. "Strong resolve."
Erhardt, Erhart

Eric Scan. "All-ruler." In spite of the renown of Viking explorer Eric the Red (who colonized Iceland around A.D. 985) and his son Leif Ericsson, who reputedly discovered North America half a millennium before Columbus, Eric was little used until the turn of the 19th century. It caught on, however, becoming fashionable in Britain in the 1920s, in the U.S. some 50 years later. Author Erich Segal; musician Eric Clapton.
Erek, Erich, Erick, Erik, Errick, Eryk, Rick, Rikky

Erin Ir. Gael. Name for Ireland. Mostly used by girls, and not in Ireland itself.

Erland OE. "Noble's land."

Erling OE. "Noble's son."

Ernest OE. "Sincere." Its great popularity at the turn of

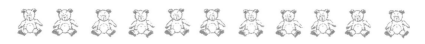

the 20th century was only confirmed by Oscar Wilde's play, *The Importance of Being Earnest*. Fell out of use after the 1930s. Author Ernest Hemingway; actor Ernest Borgnine; entertainer Ernie Kovacs.

Earnest, Ernesto, Ernestus, Ernie, Ernst

Errol Origin unclear, though most sources consider it a variation of Earl. It may also derive from a Scottish place name; there have been Scottish Earls of Erroll for more than 600 years. The most famous modern Errol was dashing movie actor Errol Flynn.

Erroll, Erryl, Rollo

Erskine Scot. Gael. Place name: "High cliff." Transference from last name to first occurred only in this century. Novelist Erskine Caldwell.

Ervin Scot. Gael. Place name, or "beautiful." Var. **Irving.** OE. "Sea friend." General Erwin Rommel.

Ervine, Ervyn, Erwin, Erwyn, Erwynn, Irvin

Esteban Sp. Var. **Stephen**.

Esau Heb. "Hairy." In the Old Testament the story is told how Esau came out of the womb covered with hair, while his twin brother, Jacob, was hairless. The name was used somewhat in the 19th century.

Esmé Fr. "Esteemed." Originally a male name brought to Scotland by a French cousin of James VI. Now scarce, even for girls.

Esmond OE. "Protected by grace." Survived the Norman Conquest as a last name, but was not rediscovered as a first name until the late 19th century, and was never widely used.

Ethan Heb. "Firmness, steadfastness." An Old Testament name given fame in the U.S. by Revolutionary War leader Ethan Allen, who captured Fort Ticonderoga with only 83 men.

Etan

Etienne Fr. Var. **Stephen**.

Ethelbert OE. "Highborn, shining." The original form of Albert. A 6th-century king of Kent whom Saint Augustine converted to Christianity. The name was revived in the 19th century but is now extremely scarce.

Ethelwin OE. "Highborn friend." Anglo-Saxon name that

followed the same cycle of 19th-century revival and 20th-century disuse.

Ethelwyn, Ethelwynne

Ettore It. "loyal."

Eugene Gk. "Wellborn." In use since the early Christian era, and chosen by four popes. After centuries of disuse, it was dusted off in the 19th century and became very popular in the U.S. No longer in the first rank, but still occurs. Senator Eugene McCarthy; playwrights Eugene O'Neill, Eugène Ionesco; artist Eugène Delacroix.

Eugen, Eugenio, Eugenius, Evgeny, Gene

Eusebius Gk. "Devout." Name of a number of saints, the best-known of whom was a 4th-century Italian bishop.

Eustace Gk. "Fertile." Brought to Britain with the Normans, but never hugely popular there. Most common in the late 19th century, little used in the U.S. The last names Stacey and Stacy come from Eustace. (As girls' names, they are diminutives of Anastasia.)

Eustache, Eustachius, Eustachy, Eustashe, Eustasius, Eustatius, Eustazio, Eustis, Eustiss

Evan Welsh. Var. **John**. Most common in Wales, but well-known in all English-speaking countries ever since the mid–19th century.

Euan, Euen, Evans, Even, Evin, Evyn, Ewan, Ewen, Owen

Evelyn Surname transferred to first name, and more common for girls than boys. Author Evelyn Waugh's first wife was also called Evelyn.

Evelin

Everard OE. "Boar hardness." Norman name more common as a surname, but revived in the 19th century. German form is **Eberhard**. Now rare.

Eberhard, Everardo, Evered, Everhart, Evrard, Evraud

Everett OE. "Boar hardness." Surname deriving from **Everard**, used as a first name in the 19th century. Senator Everett Dirksen.

Eberhard, Eberhardt, Everard, Evered, Everet, Everitt, Evrard, Eward, Ewart

Everley OE. Place name: "Boar meadow." Singing group Everly Brothers.

Everly

Everton OE. Place name: "Boar settlement." Used as a first name only in this century.

Ewald OE. "Law-powerful."
Evald

Ewan Scot. Gael. Unclear origin: perhaps "young man" or a variant of **Eugene**. Use confined to Scotland until the mid–20th century, but now spreading.
Euan, Euen, Ewen

Ewert OE. Occupational name: "Shepherd." Literally, "ewe-herder."
Ewart

Ewing OE. "Law-friend." Unusual, though some families may have been inspired to use it in the 1980s by the Ewing family on the popular TV series "Dallas."
Ewin, Ewynn

Ezekiel Heb. "Strength of God." An important Old Testament prophet. Since the end of the 19th century, all but obsolete.
Ezechiel, Eziechiele, Eziequel, Zeke

Ezra Heb. "Helper." Old Testament prophet. The Puritans brought the name to America, where it was most used in the 19th century. Poet Ezra Pound.
Azariah, Azur, Esdras, Esra, Ezer, Ezri

Fabian Lat. Clan name, possibly meaning "one who grows beans." Name of a 3rd-century saint/pope, and latterly of a 1960s pop star. Not much used in the intervening 1700 years.
Fabe, Fabek, Faber, Fabert, Fabianno, Fabiano, Fabien, Fabio, Fabius, Fabiyus, Fabyan, Fabyen, Faybian, Faybien

Fabrice Fr. from Lat. "Works with the hands."
Fabrizio, Fabrizius

Fabron Fr. "Young blacksmith."
Fabre, Fabroni

Fagan Ir. Gael. "Little ardent one." The wily con artist Fagin in Dickens's *Oliver Twist* has probably put an indelible stamp on this name, particularly given the fame of the musical and movie versions.
Fagin

Fairfax OE. "Blond."

Faisal Arab. "Resolute."
Faysal

Falkner OE. Occupational name: "Falcon trainer." Author William Faulkner.
Falconer, Falconner, Faulconer, Faulconner, Faulkner, Fowler

Fane OE. "Happy, joyous."

Farley OE. Place name: "Meadow of the sheep" or "meadow of the bulls." Surname transferred occasionally to first name. Actor Farley Granger.
Fairlay, Fairlee, Fairleigh, Fairlie, Farlay, Farlee, Farleigh, Farlie, Farly, Farrleigh, Farrley, Lee, Leigh

Farnell OE. Place name: "The fern hill." Originally a surname.
Farnall, Fernald, Furnald

Farnham OE. Place name: "Meadow with ferns." Common surname with a little spurt of late–19th-century use as a first name.
Farnam, Farnum, Fernham

Farnley OE. Place name: "Field with ferns."
Farnlea, Farnlee, Farnleigh, Farnly, Fernleigh, Fernley

Farold OE. "Mighty voyager."

Farouk Arab. "Discerning truth from falsehood."
Faruq, Faruqh

Farquhar Scot. Gael. "Very dear one." First-name use is occasional, and mostly Scottish.
Farquharson, Farquar, Farquarson

Farr OE. "Voyager."

Farrell Ir. Gael. "Hero, man of courage."
Farrel, Farrill, Farryll, Ferrel, Ferrell, Ferrill, Ferryl

Faust Lat. "Fortunate, enjoying good luck." Very rare as a first name, no doubt owing to the literary connotations, for the legendary Faust sells his soul to the devil. His

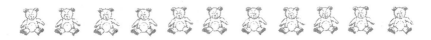

story was retold by Marlowe, Goethe, Wagner, and Thomas Mann, among others.

Faustino, Fausto, Faustus

Favian Lat. "Man of wisdom."

Fay Ir. Gael. "Raven." Extremely rare as a boy's name, though somewhat popular for girls.

Fayette

Fedor Ger. Var. **Theodore.** Gk. "Gift from God."

Feodor, Fyodor

Felipe Sp. Var. **Philip.** Gk. "Lover of horses."

Filip, Filippo, Fillip, Flip, Lippo, Pip, Pippo

Felix Lat. "Happy, fortunate." Not common in America, possibly because of a strong association with Felix the Cat and, more recently, "The Odd Couple's" Felix Unger. American physicist Felix Bloch.

Fee, Felic, Felice, Felicio, Felike, Feliks, Felizio, Felyx

Felton OE. Place name: "Settlement on the field."

Felten, Feltin

Fenton OE. Place name: "Settlement on the marsh." First used as a given name in the 19th century, but never widespread.

Ferdinand OG. "Bold voyager." A name that has always been more popular in Southern Europe than in the English-speaking countries. Explorers Ferdinand Magellan, Hernando Cortez. Former Philippines president Ferdinand Marcos.

**Ferd, Ferdie, Ferdinando, Ferdo, Ferdynand, Fernand,
Fernando, Hernando, Nando**

Fergus Ir. Gael. "Highest choice." Mostly Scottish use.

**Fearghas, Fearghus, Feargus, Fergie, Ferguson,
Fergusson**

Fermin Sp. "Strong."

Firmin

Fernley OE. Place name: "Fern meadow." Used since the late 19th century as a first name for children of both sexes, though primarily in Britain.

**Farnlea, Farnlee, Farnleigh, Farnley, Fernlea, Fernlee,
Fernleigh**

Ferrand OF. "Gray-haired."

Farand, Farrand, Farrant, Ferrant

Ferris Ir. Gael. Possibly derived from Fergus, or else, via Pierce, an Irish variant of Peter.
Farris, Farrish, Ferriss

Fidel Lat. "Faithful." The Puritans named boys Faithful, but Fidel is the modern form. However, since Fidel Castro's rise in Cuba, it is unlikely to be used by today's parents.
Fidele, Fidelio, Fidelis, Fido

Fielding OE. Place name: "The field."
Feilding

Filbert OE. "Very brilliant." Saint Philibert was a 7th-century monk who gave his name to a nut, since his feast day falls at the time when the nuts are ripe. In the U.S. filberts are more usually known as hazelnuts. The name is uncommon in any of its forms.
Bert, Filberte, Filberto, Philbert, Philibert, Phillbert

Filmore OE. "Very famous." Historically best-known under the presidency of Millard Fillmore (1850–53), but nostalgic rock fans may also remember the famous rock and roll venue in San Francisco.
Fillmore, Filmer, Fylmer

Finian Ir. Gael. "Fair." Perhaps familiar from the 1968 film *Finian's Rainbow* (Fred Astaire's last musical), but little used as a first name.
Finnian, Fionan, Fionn, Phinean, Phinian

Finlay Ir. Gael. "Fair-haired courageous one." Most often used in Scotland, where it is a common last name.
Findlay, Findley, Finlea, Finlee, Finley, Finn, Finnlea, Finnley, Lee, Leigh

Finn Ir. Gael. "fair" or OG. "from Finland."
Fin

Finnegan Ir. Gael. "Fair." Common Irish surname. Given some prominence by James Joyce's last novel, *Finnegan's Wake*.
Finegan

Fiorello It. "Little flower." Would be almost unknown in the U.S. without the fame of New York mayor Fiorello La Guardia.

Fisk Middle English. "Fish." Probably an occupational name, indicating an ancestor who was a fishmonger.
Fiske

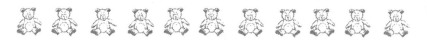

Fitch Middle English. Animal name: A fitch is a mammal related to the ferret or ermine. Use as a name probably goes back to an ancestor who hunted or kept fitches, rather than relating to the late–19th-century fashion for nature names.

Fitz OF. "Son of . . ." Usually short for one of the "Fitz-" names below. Derives from the Norman *filz* or "son."

Fitzgerald OF./OG. "Son of the spear-ruler." In the U.S., famous as the middle name of John F. Kennedy, and the last name of his grandfather, who was known as "Honey Fitz."

Fitzhugh OF./OG. "Son of intelligence." American painter Fitzhugh Lane.

Fitzpatrick OF./Lat. "Son of the nobleman."

Fitzroy OF. "Son of the king."

Flaminio Sp. "Roman priest."

Flann Ir. Gael. "Ruddy, red-haired."
Flannery

Flavian Lat. "Yellow hair." Originally a Latin clan name, and common enough in the Roman Empire, but never revived in an English-speaking country.
Flavel, Flavelle, Flavien, Flavio, Flavius, Flawiusz

Fleming OE. "Man from the Lowlands." Author (and James Bond creator) Ian Fleming.
Flemming, Flemmyng, Flemyng

Fletcher Middle English. Occupational name: "Arrow-maker."
Flecher, Fletch

Flint OE. Place name: "Stream." Denotes an ancestor who lived near a stream. In the U.S., "flint" is a kind of stone.
Flynt

Florent OF. "In flower." Impresario Florenz Ziegfeld.
Fiorentino, Florentin, Florentino, Florenz, Florinio, Florino

Florian Lat. "Blooming." Most common in Middle European countries.
Florien, Florrian, Floryan

Floyd Welsh. "Gray-haired." Anglicization of Lloyd. Boxing star Floyd Patterson.

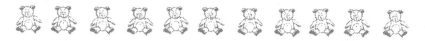

Flynn Ir. Gael. "Son of the ruddy man."
Flin, Flinn, Flyn

Folke Scand. "People's guardian."
Folker, Volker, Vollker

Forbes Scot. Gael. "Field." Used mostly in Scotland. Magazine founder Malcolm Forbes.

Ford OE. Place name. "River crossing." Most Americans will automatically associate the name with the car. Author Ford Madox Ford; automotive pioneer Henry Ford.

Forest OF. Occupational name, "woodsman," or place name, "woods." Most common in the U.S., spelled with two *r*s. Novelist E. M. Forster.
Forester, Forrest, Forrester, Forster, Foster

Fortune OF. "Lucky."
Fortunato, Fortunatus, Fortune, Fortunio

Foster OE. Occupational name: "Woodsman." Var. **Forest**.

Fowler OE. Occupational name: "Bird trapper."

Franchot Fr. Var. **Francis**. Actor Franchot Tone.

Francis Lat. "Frenchman." France was originally the Kingdom of the Franks. Saint Francis of Assisi gave the name its first fame; though he was named John, he had been nicknamed Francis because his father had him taught French as a boy. The name traveled to England via France, and was popular in the 17th and 19th centuries. Frank is more often used now probably owing to the rise of the feminine version and homonym, Frances. Philosopher Sir Francis Bacon; composer Franz Josef Haydn; King Francois I of France; playwright Ferenc Molnar; French president François Mitterrand; film director Francis Ford Coppola; "Star Spangled Banner" author Francis Scott Key.
Chico, Ferenc, Feri, Fran, Franco, Francesco, Franchot, Francisco, Franciskus, Francois, Franio, Frank, Frankie, Franko, Frann, Frannie, Frans, Fransisco, Frants, Franz, Franzel, Franzen, Franzin, Frasco, Frascuelo, Frasquito, Paco, Pacorro, Panchito, Pancho, Paquito

Frank Dim. **Francis** or **Franklin**. Used as an independent name since the 17th century, and very popular at the turn of the 20th century right through the 1930s. Now

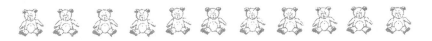

out of fashion, despite the durable popularity of its most famous bearer, Frank Sinatra. Astronaut Frank Borman; actor Frank Langella; architect Frank Lloyd Wright; musician Frank Zappa.

Franklin Middle English. "Free landholder." Surname transferred to first name, popular in the U.S., especially in the 1930s and 1940s as homage to President Franklin Delano Roosevelt. President Franklin Pierce apparently made less of an impression, as his term (1853–57) did not inspire a surge of infant Franklins.
Francklin, Francklyn, Frank, Franklinn, Franklyn, Franklynn

Frazer Derivation unclear, possibly OE. "curly hair" or an old French place name. (Relationship to the French *fraise* [charcoal] is debated.) Used mostly in Scottish families.
Fraser, Frasier, Frazier

Frayne Middle English. "Foreign."
Fraine, Frayn, Frean, Freen, Freyne

Frederick OG. "Peaceful ruler." Taken by the Hanoverian kings to Britain, where it began a steady ascent to great popularity that only faded in the 1930s. No longer fashionable, but sufficiently common so that it doesn't sound outlandish. Actor Fred MacMurray; dancer Fred Astaire; cartoon character Fred Flintstone; children's TV personality Fred Rogers; composer Frédéric Chopin; abolitionist Frederick Douglass; philosopher Friedrich Nietzsche.
Eric, Erich, Erick, Erico, Erik, Eryk, Federico, Federigo, Fred, Fredd, Freddie, Fredek, Frederic, Frederich, Frederico, Frederigo, Frederik, Fredi, Fredric, Fredrick, Fredrik, Friedel, Friedrich, Friedrick, Fridrich, Fridrick, Fritz, Fritzchen, Fritzi, Fritzl, Fryderyk, Ric, Rick, Ricky, Rik, Rikki

Freeborn OE. Use of the descriptive term. May date back to slave days, or to the era of widespread serfdom, when to be born free was worthy of commemoration.

Freedom Use of the word as a given name is more common than one might think.

Freeman OE. See **Freeborn.**
Freedman, Freeland, Freemon, Friedman, Friedmann

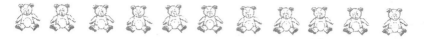

Fremont OG. "Protector of freedom." Explorer John Fremont.

Frewin OE. "Free friend."
Frewen

Frick OE. "Brave man." Industrialist and philanthropist Henry Clay Frick.

Fridolf OE. "Peaceful wolf."
Freydolf, Freydulf, Fridulf

Fritz Ger. Dim. **Frederick**. Film director Fritz Lang.

Fulbright OG. "Very bright." See **Filbert**.
Fulbert, Philbert, Philibert, Phillbert

Fuller OE. Occupational name: "One who shrinks cloth." The woolen fabric that was such a staple of the medieval English economy needed to be treated by fullers before it was made into clothes. The surname was most often used as a first name in the 19th century.

Fulton OE. Place name: "Settlement of the fowl" or "people's estate." Surname used as first name: in the U.S., possibly a compliment to Robert Fulton, inventor of the steamboat. Catholic bishop Fulton J. Sheen.

Fyfe Scot. Gael. Place name: Fifeshire is an area of Scotland. American cabinetmaker Duncan Phyfe.
Fife, Fyffe, Phyfe

Fyodor Rus. from Gk. "Divine gift." Var. **Theodore**. Author Fyodor Dostoyevsky.
Fedor, Feodor, Fyodr

G

Gable OF. Dim. **Gabriel**. When used, is probably influenced by the fame of actor Clark Gable, who was often known by just his last name.

Gabriel Heb. "Hero of God." Gabriel is an archangel who appears in Christian, Jewish, and Muslim texts. The name has been uncommon in English-speaking countries, except for a spell of use in the 18th and 19th centuries. Musician Peter Gabriel.

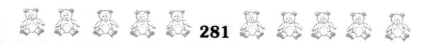

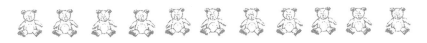

Gabby, Gabe, Gabi, Gabie, Gabriele, Gabrielli, Gabriello, Gabrielo, Gaby, Gavriel, Gavril, Gavrilo

Gadiel Arab. "God is my fortune."

Gaetan It. Place name: Gaeta is a region in Southern Italy; the Gulf of Gaeta is just north of Naples.

Gaetano, Kajetan

Gage OF. "Oath."

Gair Ir. Gael. "Small one."

Gaer, Geir

Galbraith Ir. Gael. "Foreign Briton." In Ireland, the name would have been used most commonly to describe a Scot. Economist John Kenneth Galbraith.

Galbrait, Galbreath

Gale Ir. Gael. "Foreigner"; OE. "cheerful, happy." Much more common now as a girl's name, when it is usually a diminutive of Abigail.

Gael, Gail, Gaile, Gayle

Galen Gk. "Healer" or "tranquil." A 2nd-century Greek physician named Galen was for centuries the only authority on the emergent practice of medicine.

Gaelan, Galeno, Galin, Gaylen, Gaylin, Gaylinn, Gaylon

Gallagher Ir. Gael. "Foreign helper."

Galloway Old Gael. "Foreign Gael." Another name for a Scot. The Irish population include a strong Scottish strain.

Gallway, Galway

Galton OE. "Owner of a rented land."

Gallton

Galvin Ir. Gael. "Sparrow" or "brilliantly white."

Gallven, Gallvin, Galvan, Galven

Gamal Arab. "Camel."

Gamali, Jamal, Jammal, Jemaal, Jemal

Gamaliel Heb. "Recompense of God." An obscure biblical name probably brought to the U.S. by the Puritans. Little used since the 19th century. President Warren Gamaliel Harding.

Gamble ONorse. "Old."

Gannon Ir. Gael. "Fair-skinned."

Gardner Middle English. Occupational name: "Gardener." In the eastern U.S., reminiscent of two

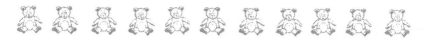

distinguished families, known as the "blind" Gardners (the name has no *i*) or the "sighted" Gardiners. The former are famous for the Isabella Stewart Gardner Museum in Boston; the latter for Gardiner's Island on Long Island Sound.

Gardener, Gardie, Gardiner

Gareth Welsh. "Gentle." The name of one of King Arthur's knights. Used in Britain since the 1930s, but rare elsewhere.

Garith, Garreth, Garyth

Garfield OE. "Spear field." Use as a first name probably honored President James Garfield, though indignation at his untimely death outweighed admiration for his skills, since his term lasted only a few months before he was assassinated in 1881. More recently the president has been upstaged by a fat orange cartoon cat who has made the name his own.

Garland OE. Place name: "Land of the spear." OF. "Wreath."

Garlan, Garlen, Garllan

Garman OE. "Spearman."

Garmann, Garrman

Garner Middle English. "To gather grain." Possibly a place name or occupational name originally, denoting an ancestor who lived near a granary, or who helped harvest grain.

Garnier

Garnett OE. "spear" or OF. "Red like a pomegranate." Although the girl's name is more likely to be a jewel name in the tradition of Pearl or Ruby, for boys, Garnet is usually a transferred last name. In England, boys may have been named for a famous Victorian soldier, Sir Garnet Wolseley.

Garnet

Garnock Old Welsh. Place name: "River of alder trees."

Garrett Var. **Gerard** dating from the Middle Ages.

Gareth, Garrard, Garret, Garritt, Garrot, Garrott, Garyth, Jarret, Jarrett, Jarrot, Jarrott

Garrick OE. "Spear-rule." English actor David Garrick; newscaster Garrick Utley.

Garek, Garreck, Garrik, Garryck, Garryk

Garroway OE. "Spear-fighter."
> **Garraway**

Garson OE. "Gar's son." Gar in this case may be a diminutive of Garrett, Gareth, Garland, etc.

Garth Scan. Occupational name: "Keeper of the garden." Used as a first name in this century, but never widely. Illustrator Garth Williams.

Garton OE. Place name: "Triangle-shaped settlement."

Garvey Ir. Gael. "Rough peace."
> **Garrvey, Garrvie, Garvie, Garvy**

Garvin OE. "Spear-friend."
> **Garvan, Garven, Garvyn, Garwen, Garwin, Garwyn, Garwynn**

Garwood OE. Place name: "Wood with fir trees."
> **Garrwood, Woody**

Gary OE. "Spear." Popularized by film idol Gary Cooper, whose name was originally Frank. From the 1950s to the 1970s, very fashionable, now dormant. Cartoonists Garry Trudeau, Gary Larson.
> **Gari, Garey, Garrie, Garry**

Gaspar Var. **Caspar.** Possibly Persian "he who guards the treasure."
> **Caspar, Casper, Gaspard, Gasparo, Gasper, Jasper, Kaspar, Kasper**

Gaston Fr. "Man from Gascony." Gascony is a region in the south of France whose inhabitants are reputed to be hot-tempered.
> **Gascon**

Gauthier Teut. "Strong ruler." Fashion designer Jean-Paul Gaultier.
> **Galtero, Gaultier, Gautier, Gualterio, Gualtiero**

Gavin Welsh. "White falcon" or "little falcon." As Gawain, this was the name of one of King Arthur's knights. The Scottish form, Gavin, has spread from Scotland to broad acceptance in Britain, especially in the last 30 years. Still rare in the U.S.
> **Gavan, Gaven, Gavyn, Gavynn, Gawain, Gawaine, Gawayn, Gawayne, Gawen, Gwaine, Gwayn**

Gaylord OF. "Lively, high-spirited."

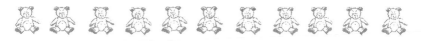

Gaillard, Gallard, Gay, Gayelord, Gayler, Gaylor

Gaynor Ir. Gael. "Son of the fair-skinned one." From a different root than the feminine version; for male children, this is strictly a transferred last name, and unusual at that.

Gainer, Gainor, Gay, Gayner, Gaynnor

Geary Middle English. "Variable."

Gearey, Gery

Gene Dim. **Eugene.** Gk. "Well-born." Used as an independent name since the late 19th century, especially in America. Actors Gene Kelly, Gene Wilder, Gene Hackman.

Genio, Geno, Jeno

Geoffrey Var. **Jeffrey.** OG. Unclear, something to do with "peace." Norman name popular through the Middle Ages in Britain, and revived in the mid–19th century after a 350-year rest. The peak of its popularity was the 1970s in the U.S., and it is no longer a favorite. Performer Geoffrey Holder; medieval poet Geoffrey Chaucer; fashion designer Geoffrey Beene.

Geoff, Geoffery, Geoffroy, Geoffry, Geofrey, Jefery, Jeff, Jefferey, Jefferies, Jeffery, Jeffree, Jeffrey, Jeffry, Jeffrie, Jeffries, Jefry, Jeoffroi

George Gk. "Farmer." The popularity of the dragon-killing Saint George (patron of Boy Scouts, soldiers, and England) is undimmed by the fact that little proof of his existence can be found. George was a royal name in England, and admiration for George Washington in the U.S. gave the name a parallel popularity in the renegade colonies from the 18th century until the middle of the 20th. Now less common. Rock star George Michael; fashion designer Giorgio Armani; comedians George Burns, George Carlin; baseball legend George "Babe" Ruth; U.S. President George Bush.

Egor, Georas, Geordie, Georg, Georges, Georgi, Georgie, Georgios, Georgy, Giorgio, Giorgios, Goran, Gyorgy, Gyuri, Igor, Jiri, Jorgan, Jorge, Jorgen, Jurgen, Jurek, Jurik, Yurik, Ygor

Geraint Lat. "Old." A Sir Geraint figures in certain Ar-

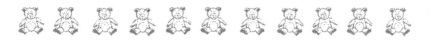

thurian legends; the name is sparingly used in Britain in this century.

Gerald OG. "Spear ruler." Old name revived in the 19th century. Most popular in the middle of this century, but now less common. U.S. President Gerald Ford.

Garald, Garold, Gary, Gearalt, Geralde, Geraldo, Gerard, Geraud, Gerek, Gerhard, Gerik, Gerold, Gerrald, Gerrard, Gerri, Gerrild, Gerrold, Gerry, Geryld, Giraldo, Giraud, Girauld, Jerald, Jerold, Jerri, Jerrold, Jerry

Gerard OE. "Spear brave." Closely related to Gerald, and its use follows a similar pattern, though it is still increasing. Particularly popular in Ireland. Poet Gerard Manley Hopkins.

Garrard, Garrat, Garratt, Garrett, Gearard, Gerardo, Geraud, Gerhard, Gerhardt, Gerrard, Gerri, Gerry, Gherardo

Geremia It. Var. **Jeremiah.** Heb. "The Lord exalts."

Germain Fr. "From Germany." There were several early saints called "Germanus" for their national origin, the most famous of whom gave his name to a church in Paris, Saint Germain-des-Prés. Singer Jermaine Jackson.

Germaine, German, Germane, Germano, Germayn, Germayne, Jermain, Jermaine, Jermane, Jermayn, Jermayne

Geronimo It. Var. **Jerome.** Gk. "sacred name." Famous as the name of an Apache Indian chief and also as the cry with which American parachutists in World War II would leap from airplanes. Nobody knows why.

Hieronimo, Hieronymus

Gershom Heb. "Exile." Old Testament name, appearing, appropriately enough, in Exodus. The Puritans adopted it and brought it to the U.S., where it is rare, but like many Hebrew names, kept alive by Orthodox Jewish families.

Gersham, Gershon, Gerson

Gervase OG. Meaning unclear; possibly "with honor." Because of the popularity of a Saint Gervase, the name has been steadily used by English Catholics, but is otherwise unusual.

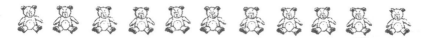

Garvey, Gervais, Gervaise, Gervaso, Gervayse, Gerwazy, Jarvey, Jarvis, Jervis

Giacomo It. Var. **Jacob**. Heb. "he who supplants."

Gibson OE. "Son of Gilbert."

Gibb, Gibbons, Gibbs, Gillson, Gilson

Gideon Heb. "Feller of trees." A biblical judge and hero who, with an army of only 300 men, liberated the Israelites from the Midianites. The latter-day Gideons are the group responsible for placing Bibles in hotel bedrooms. The name is only occasionally used, but seems ripe for a revival.

Gideone, Hedeon

Gifford OE. Either "brave giver" or "puffy-faced." It is astonishing how rarely the derivations of names mean anything negative; this exception to that rule is used as a first name from time to time. Sports figure Frank Gifford.

Giffard, Gifferd

Gilad Arab. "Hump of a camel."

Gilead

Gilbert OG. "Shining pledge." Norman name much used in the Middle Ages, but use tapered away to mostly local favor in Scotland and Northern England. Very unusual in the U.S. Author Gilbert Chesterton.

Bert, Bertie, Burt, Gib, Gibb, Gil, Gilberto, Gilburt, Gill, Giselbert, Giselberto, Giselbertus, Guilbert

Gilby ONorse. "estate of the hostage"; Ir. Gael. "blond boy."

Gilbey, Gillbey, Gillbie, Gillby

Gilchrist Ir. Gael. "Christ's servant."

Giles Gk. "Kid, young goat." The link with a shield or shield-bearer (sometimes the translation given for Giles) probably comes from the kidskin ancient shields were made of. In modern times the name, a particular favorite in Scotland, was popular in Britain in the 1970s.

Egide, Egidio, Egidius, Gide, Gil, Gilles, Gyles

Gillean Ir. Gael. "Servant of Saint John." Related to **Gilchrist, Gillespie, Gilmore,** etc., which all use the "Gil-" particle, meaning "servant."

Gillan, Gillen, Gillian

Gillespie Ir. Gael. "Son of the bishop's servant."
  Gillis
Gillett OF. "Young Gilbert." Poet Gelett Burgess.
  Gelett, Gelette, Gillette
Gilmer OE. "Renowned hostage."
Gilmore Ir. Gael. "Servant of the Virgin Mary."
  Gillmore, Gillmour, Gilmour
Gilroy Ir. Gael. "Servant of the redhead."
  Gilderoy, Gildray, Gildroy, Gillroy
Gino It. Dim. **Ambrogino** Gk. "ever-living" or **Luigino** or possibly Eugene. Gk. "well-born."
Giovanni It. Var. **John**. Heb. "The Lord is gracious." Artist Giovanni Bellini; author Giovanni Boccaccio.
  Gianni, Giannino
Girvin Ir. Gael. "Small rough one."
  Girvan, Girven, Girvon
Giulio It. Var. **Julius**. Lat. "Youthful."
  Giuliano
Giuseppe It. Var. **Joseph**. Heb. "The Lord increases." Composer Giuseppe Verdi.
Giustino It. Var. **Justin**. Lat. "Just, fair."
  Giusto
Gladwin OE. "Lighthearted friend."
  Gladwinn, Gladwyn, Gladwynne
Glanville OF. Place name: "Settlement of oak trees."
Glen Ir. Gael. Place name: "Glen." A glen is a narrow valley between hills. As a surname, Glen would indicate an ancestor who lived in such a valley. Singer Glen Campbell; band leader Glenn Miller.
  Gleann, Glenn, Glennie, Glenny, Glin, Glyn, Glynn
Glendon Scot. Gael. Place name: "Settlement in the glen."
  Glenden, Glendin, Glenton
Glenville Gael. Place name that has been used occasionally as a first name. Along with Glendon, it has probably gained legitimacy from the popularity of Glen as a given name.
Goddard OG. "God-hard."
  Godard, Godart, Goddart, Godhart, Godhardt, Gothart, Gotthard, Gotthardt, Gotthart
Godfrey OG. "God-peace." Popular medieval name that

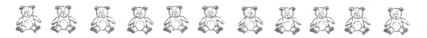

faded very gradually to its near-disuse today. The fact that it was the name of a valet in the 1936 film *My Man Godfrey* might indicate that there was something indefinably buffoonish about the name by that date.
Godefroi, Godfry, Godofredo, Goffredo, Gottfrid, Gottfried

Godwin OE. "Friend of God" or "good friend." Anglo-Saxon name that, though it did outlast the Norman Conquest in England, did not benefit from the 19th century revival that resuscitated many ancient names, so it is almost unknown in the U.S.
Godewyn, Godwinn, Godwyn, Goodwin, Goodwyn, Goodwynn, Goodwynne

Golding OE. "Little golden one."

Goldwin OE. "Golden friend." Film pioneer Samuel Goldwyn.
Goldewin, Goldewyn, Goldwinn, Goldwyn, Goldwynn

Goliath Heb. "Exile." Though babies are frequently named for David, the Old Testament bard, very few are given the name of the giant he killed with his slingshot. Even Cain, the first assassin, has inspired more parents. Nevertheless, the name is used from time to time.
Golliath

Gomer OE. "Famous battle" or "good fight." Also an Old Testament name. Grown-up fans of the goofy marine depicted by Jim Nabors in the 1960s TV series "Gomer Pyle" may have trouble taking the name seriously.

Gonzalo Sp. "Wolf." Tennis star Pancho Gonzales.
Goncalve, Gonsalve, Gonzales

Gordon OE. Meaning unclear, possibly a place name meaning "hill near meadows" or "triangular hill." Historically associated with Scotland, but principal use has been 20th century. Balladeer Gordon Lightfoot.
Gordan, Gorden, Gordie

Gore OE. "Spear" or "wedge-shaped object." "Gore" is also an old term for a small, triangular-shaped piece of land, so this may be considered a place name, denoting an ancestor who lived on or near such a piece of land. Author Gore Vidal.

Gorman Ir. Gael. "Small blue-eyed one."

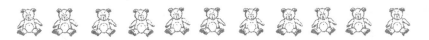

Gower Old Welsh. "Pure."

Grady Ir. Gael. "Renowned."
   Gradea, Gradee, Gradey, Graidey, Graidy

Graham OE. "Gray homestead." Mostly Scottish name that was popular in Britain in the 1950s, without ever being much used in America. Author Graham Greene; inventor Alexander Graham Bell.
   Graeham, Graeme, Grahame

Granger Middle French. "Farmer."
   Grainger, Grange

Grant Fr. "Tall, big." Another Scottish name, but one that has been more popular in the U.S. as a first name, probably inspired by President Ulysses S. Grant. Painter Grant Wood.
   Grantham, Grantley

Grantland OE. Place name: "The large fields," or possibly "Granta's fields."
   Grantleigh, Grantley, Grantly

Granville OF. Place name: "Big town." Though never frequent, use of the name has diminished since the 1960s, possibly because its slightly aristocratic sound has seemed too undemocratic for the age of equality.
   Granvil, Granvile, Granvill, Grenville

Gray OE. "Gray-haired."
   Grey

Grayson OE. "Son of the gray-haired man."
   Graydon, Greydon, Greyson

Greeley OE. Place name: "Gray meadow." American use of the name (which is far from widespread) may reflect admiration for 19th-century journalist and politician Horace Greeley.
   Greelea, Greeleigh, Greely

Greenwood OE. Place name: "Green wood."

Gregory Gk. "Watchful, vigilant." A staple name in the Middle Ages, used by 16 popes and ten saints. Modern popularity dates from the 1940s, which means it is probably linked to actor Gregory Peck's rise to stardom. Like most names that were very fashionable in the 1950s, it is now a bit out of style. Cyclist Greg LeMond; musician Gregg Allman.

Graig, Greer, Greg, Greger, Gregg, Greggory, Gregoire, Gregoor, Gregor, Gregorio, Gregorius, Gregos, Grigor, Grigorios, Grzegorz

Gresham OE. Place name: "Village surrounded by pasture."

Greville OF. Place name used occasionally in Britain.
Grevill

Griffin Lat. "Hooked nose." The name of a mythical beast, usually half eagle (hence the hooked nose), half lion. Use as a name may be connected to the frequent heraldic use of the animal. Actor Griffin Dunne.
Griff, Griffon, Gryphon

Griffith Welsh. "Strong chief." Used most often as a first name in the 16th through 18th centuries. This is the kind of slightly nostalgic name that seems ripe for revival, except that it's hard to say in a hurry.

Grimshaw OE. Place name: "Dark woods."

Griswold OF. Ger. Place name: "Gray woods."

Grosvenor OF. "Great hunter." Grosvenor is the last name of one of the richest families in Britain. Their stake in London real estate is commemorated in names like Grosvenor Square.

Grover OE. Place name: "Grove of trees." American use was probably inspired by President Grover Cleveland, but has faded since mid–20th century. Parents of "Sesame Street" viewers are more likely to be reminded of the self-proclaimed "cute, furry, lovable little monster" Grover.

Guido It. Var. **Guy**.

Guildford OE. Place name: "Ford with yellow flowers."
Gilford, Guilford

Guillaume Fr. Var. **William**. OG. "Will-helmet." Poet Guillaume Apollinaire.
Guglielmo, Guilherme, Guillermo, Gwillym, Gwilym

Gunther Scan. "Warrior." Author Günter Grass.
Guenter, Guenther, Gun, Gunnar, Gunner, Guntar, Gunter, Guntero, Gunthar

Gus Dim. **Augustus**, Lat. "Worthy of respect."
Gustav

Gustave Scan. "Staff of the gods." A royal name in Sweden, used elsewhere in Europe in the 17th century, and

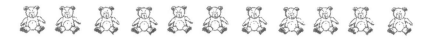

in England in the 19th century. American use (which is uncommon) tends to harken back to Scandinavian ancestry. Composer Gustav Mahler; writer Gustave Flaubert.

Gus, Gustaf, Gustaff, Gustaof, Gustav, Gustavo, Gustavus, Gustus, Gusztav

Guthrie Ir. Gael. Place name: "Windy spot." Folk singer Woody Guthrie.

Guthry

Guy Unclear origin, though some sources make a case for French "guide" or Old German "warrior." Made infamous in 1605 by Guy Fawkes, scapegoat of a plot to blow up the Houses of Parliament; in Britain November 5th is still Guy Fawkes Day, when a dummy was traditionally burned in effigy. The English shunned the name for two hundred years, but it became acceptable again by the mid–19th century, and use was increasing by the 1950s. To Americans, it is still a very English-sounding name.

Guido

Gwynn Old Welsh. "Fair."

Gwin, Gwyn

Habib Arab. "Loved one."

Hackett OF./Ger. Occupational name: "Little hewer" (of wood).

Hacket, Hackit, Hackitt

Hackman OF./Ger. Occupational name: "Hewer, hacker" (of wood). Actor Gene Hackman.

Hadden OE. Place name: "Hill of heather."

Haddan, Haddon, Haden, Hadon

Hadley OE. Place name: "Heather meadow." Interior designer Albert Hadley.

Hadlea, Hadlee, Hadleigh, Hadly, Leigh

Hadrian Var. **Adrian.** Lat. "From Adria." Adria was a

north Italian city. A Roman Emperor Hadrian was responsible for the building of a vast wall across northern Britain, parts of which still stand.

Adrian, Adriano, Adrien, Hadrien

Hadwin OE. "Friend in war."

Hadwinn, Hadwyn, Hadwynne

Hagen Ir. Gael. "Youthful one."

Hagan, Haggan

Hagley OE. Place name: "Enclosed meadow."

Haglea, Haglee, Hagleigh, Hagly

Haig OE. Place name: "Enclosed with hedges."

Hakeem Arab. "Wise, all-knowing."

Hakim

Hakon Scan. "Of the highest race." A royal name in Norway, but little used in English-speaking countries.

Haaken, Haakin, Haakon, Hakan, Hako

Hal Dim. most commonly of **Henry**. In Shakespeare's plays about Henry IV, his son (to become Henry V) is affectionately known as "Prince Hal." Actors Hal Holbrook, Hal Linden.

Halbert OE. "Shining hero."

Halburt

Haldan Scan. "Half-Danish." The name takes on a certain significance when you consider that in ancient Britain, the Danes were fierce and frequent invaders.

Haldane, Halden, Halfdan, Halvdan

Hale OE. Either place name "from the hall," or "healthy hero." Revolutionary War hero Nathan Hale.

Hal, Hayle

Haley OE. Place name "hay meadow" or Ir. Gael. "ingenious, clever." The use of Hayley as a girl's name probably spells the end of its use as a boy's name.

Hailey, Haily, Haleigh, Hayleigh, Hayley

Halford OE. Place name: "Valley ford."

Hallford

Hall OE. Occupational name: "Worker at the hall." In this case, the hall would signify a large house or manor.

Hallam OE. Place name: "The valley."

Halley OE. Place name "meadow near the hall" or OE. "holy." This is a different name from the homonym Ha-

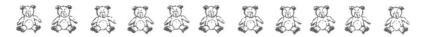

ley, but will probably also be discarded as a boy's name. Astronomer Edmund Halley.

Halliwell OE. Place name: "Holy well."
Hallewell, Hellewell, Helliwell

Hallward OE. Occupational name: "Guardian of the hall." Like many of these Anglo-Saxon names, it is unusual as a first name.
Halward

Halsey OE. Place name: "Hal's island."
Hallsey, Hallsy, Halsy

Halstead OE. Place name: "The manor grounds."
Halsted

Halton OE. Place name: "Estate on the hill."

Ham Heb. "Heat." Old Testament name, one of the sons of Noah. Little used; the names of Noah's other two sons, Shem and Japheth, are even more rare.

Hamal Arab. "Lamb."

Hamar ONorse. "Hammer."

Hamilton OE. Place name of several possible meanings such as "home-lover's estate" or "hill with grass." It was the surname of several aristocratic British families, and made the transition to a first name in the early 19th century. U.S. statesman Alexander Hamilton.
Hamel, Hamelton, Hamil, Hamill

Hamill OE. "Scarred." May refer to the facial characteristic of a distant ancestor. Actor Mark Hamill.
Hamel, Hamell, Hammill

Hamish Scot. Var. **James**. Heb. "He who supplants." Almost unknown outside of Scotland.

Hamlet OG./Fr. "Village: home." This name, like Hamlin, derives from a German root that means "home." Hamlet was a common first name until the beginning of the 19th century, but now its use would inevitably recall Shakespeare's tortured Danish prince. Author Dashiell Hammett.
Hammet, Hammett, Hammond, Hamnet, Hamnett

Hamlin OG. "Little home-lover." Actor Harry Hamlin.
Hamblin, Hamelin, Hamlen, Hamlyn

Hanford OE. Place name: "High ford."

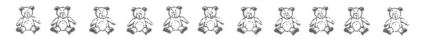

Hank Dim. **Henry**. OE. "Estate ruler." Usually a nickname rather than a given name. Baseball star Hank Aaron.

Hanley OE. Place name: "High meadow."
Handlea, Handleigh, Handley, Hanlea, Hanlee, Hanleigh, Hanly, Henlea, Henlee, Henleigh, Henley

Hans Scan. Var. **John**. Heb. "The Lord is gracious." Writer Hans Christian Andersen.

Hanson Scan. "Son of Hans."
Hansen, Hanssen, Hansson

Harbin OF./Ger. "Little bright warrior."

Harcourt OF. "Fortified farm."
Harcort

Harden OE. Place name: "Valley of the hares."
Hardin

Harding OE. "Son of the courageous one." This name is closely related to **Hardy**. U.S. President Warren G. Harding.

Hardwin OE. "Courageous friend."
Hardwinn, Hardwyn, Hardwynn

Hardy OG. "Bold, brave." Writer Thomas Hardy; Fashion designer Hardy Amies.

Harford OE. Place name: "Ford of the hares." Like many place names turned surnames, this was used as a first name in the nineteenth century.

Hargrove OE. Place name: "Grove of the hares." In modern times it seems curious that ancient names took such close note of the whereabouts of rabbits, but they might have constituted a significant portion of the average man's diet in those days.
Hargrave, Hargreaves

Harkin Ir. Gael. "Dark red."
Harkan, Harken

Harlan OE. Place name: "Army land."
Harland, Harlen, Harlenn, Harlin, Harlyn, Harlynn

Harley OE. Place name: "The long field." Familiar to most people as half of the name of a great motorcycle, the Harley-Davidson.
Arlea, Arleigh, Arley, Harlea, Harlee, Harleigh, Harly

Harlow OE. Place name: "Army hill."
Arlo

Harmon Var. **Herman**. OG. "Army man." Actor Mark Harmon.

Harold Scan. "Army ruler." An Anglo-Saxon name revived to great popularity in the mid–19th century. It was greatly in vogue until the turn of the century, but is now rare. British Prime Minister Harold Macmillan; playwright Harold Pinter.

Araldo, Aralt, Aroldo, Arry, Garald, Garold, Hal, Harald, Haralds, Haroldas, Harry, Herold, Herrold, Herrick, Herryck

Harper OE. "Harp player."

Harrison OE. "Son of Harry." Harrison is the more popular version of this name, but neither it nor Harris has been used much as a first name in the latter part of this century. Actor Harrison Ford.

Harris, Harriss

Harry Dim. **Henry**. OE. "Home ruler." Since about 1920, Harry has been used as an independent name about as frequently as Henry. In the U.S. this may have something to do with admiration for President Harry S. Truman. Actor Harry Belafonte; U.S. Supreme Court Justice Harry A. Blackmun; magician Harry Houdini.

Hart OE: "Stag." Poet Hart Crane; actor Hart Bochner.

Hartford OE. Place name: "Stag ford."

Hartley OE. Place name: "Stag meadow."

Hartlea, Hartlee, Hartleigh, Hartly

Hartman OG. "Hard, strong man."

Hartmann

Hartwell OE. Place name: "Well of the stags."

Harwell, Harwill

Harvey OF. "Burning for battle" or "strong and ardent." Norman name revived in the 19th century, but now uncommon. Many people may recall the Jimmy Stewart movie *Harvey* in which he was upstaged by a giant invisible rabbit.

Herve, Hervey

Harwood OE. Place name: "Wood of the hares."

Hashim Arab. "Crusher of evil."

Hasheem

Haskel Heb. "Intellect."

Haskell

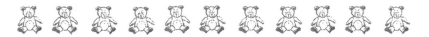

Haslett OE. Place name: "Headland with the hazel trees." Literary critic William Hazlitt.
Hazel, Hazlett, Hazlitt

Hassan Arab. "Handsome."
Hasan

Hastings OE. "Son of the austere man."
Hastie, Hasty

Havelock Scan. "Sea competition."

Haven OE. Place name: "Sanctuary, safe harbor."
Hagan, Hagen, Havin, Hogan

Hawley OE. Place name: "Hedged meadow."
Hawleigh, Hawly

Hawthorne OE. Place name: "Where hawthorn trees grow." Use in the U.S. may reflect admiration for the novelist Nathaniel Hawthorne.
Hawthorn

Hayden OE. Place name: "Hedged valley." Most commonly used in Wales.
Haden, Haydn, Haydon

Hayes OE. Place name: "Hedged area." U.S. President Rutherford B. Hayes.

Hayward OE. Occupational name: "Keeper or guardian of the hedged enclosure."

Haywood OE. Place name: "Hedged forest." Writer Heywood Broun.
Heywood, Woody

Heath Middle English. Place name: "Heath." In Britain "heath" is the name for a large, open space that's not under cultivation.

Heathcliff Middle English. Place name indicating a cliff near a heath. Most parents today would automatically associate it with the passionate hero of Emily Brontë's *Wuthering Heights.*

Heber Heb. "Togetherness." An Old Testament name used by the Puritans but rare in this century.
Hebor

Hector Gk. "Holds fast." One of the great heroes of the Trojan war, though today the verb form "to hector" means to bully or browbeat.
Ettore

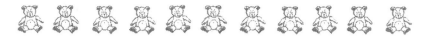

Hedley OE. Place name: "Heathered meadow." Used in Britain in the late 19th century, but rare in the U.S.
Headley, Headly, Hedly

Hedeon Rus. Var. **Gideon**. Heb. "Feller of trees."

Helmut Middle French. "Helmet." Photographer Helmut Newton.

Henderson OE. "Son of Henry."
Hendrie, Hendries, Hendron, Henryson

Henley OE. Place name: "High meadow." Variant of Hanley, but made famous by the English town that hosts an annual worldwide crew regatta.

Henry OG. "Estate ruler." Norman name that took root in Britain and became a royal name used by eight kings and, most recently, for the younger son of the Prince of Wales. This exposure may give new popularity to a name that was extremely common until the first quarter of this century. Explorer Henry Hudson; actor Henry Fonda; author Henry James; poet Henry Wadsworth Longfellow; artists Henri Matisse, Henri de Toulouse-Lautrec, Henri Rousseau; playwright Henrik Ibsen.
Arrigo, Enrico, Enrikos, Enrique, Enzio, Hal, Hank, Harry, Heike, Heindrick, Heindrik, Heiner, Heinrich, Heinrick, Heinrik, Heinz, Hendrick, Hendrik, Henerik, Henning, Henri, Henrik, Henrique, Henryk, Hinrich

Herbert OG. "Bright army" or "bright warrior." Norman name that faded in the Middle Ages, to be revived enthusiastically in the 19th century. Now unusual. U.S. President Herbert Hoover.
Bert, Bertie, Erberto, Harbert, Hebert, Herb, Herbie, Heribert, Heriberto

Hercules Gk. Meaning not quite clear: Possibly "glorious gift" or "glory of Hera." The legendary Greek hero who exhibited incredible strength. In modern times his physical strength might have been rivaled by the intellectual power of his namesake, Agatha Christie's fictional detective Hercule Poirot.
Herakles, Hercule, Herculie

Herman OG. "Army man." Another 19th-century revival

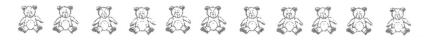

of a Norman name, this one especially a U.S. favorite. Uncommon since the turn of the century. Authors Herman Hesse; Herman Melville.

Armand, Armando, Armin, Ermanno, Ermano, Ermin, Harman, Harmon, Hermann, Hermie, Hermon

Hernando Sp. Var. **Ferdinand**. OG. "Bold voyager."

Herrick OG. "War ruler." The 17th-century poet Robert Herrick.

Herrik, Herryck

Hershel Heb. "Deer." Football star Herschel Walker; actor Herschel Bernardi.

Hersch, Herschel, Herschell, Herzl, Hirsch, Hirschel

Hesperos Gk. "Evening or evening star." The Greeks referred to Italy as Hesperia, since the sun set and the evening star rose there.

Hespero

Hewett OF. Dim. **Hugh**. Ger. "Small intelligent one."

Hewet, Hewie, Hewitt, Hewlett, Hewlitt

Hewson OE. "Hugh's son."

Hezekiah Heb. "God gives strength." Old Testament name little used since the 19th century.

Hieremias Gk. Var. **Jeremiah**. Heb. "Jehovah lifts up."

Hieronymos Gk. Var. **Jerome**. Heb. "Sacred name." Painter Hieronymus Bosch.

Hierome, Hieronim, Hieronimos, Hieronymus

Hilary Gk. "Cheerful, happy." The name comes from the same root as the word "hilarious." Although it was used for boys (including a pope and a saint) until the 17th century, it was revived at the turn of the 20th century as a girl's name.

Hilaire, Hilarie, Hilario, Hilarion, Hilarius, Hillary, Hillery, Hilliary, Ilario, Illario

Hildebrand OG. "Battle sword."

Hillard OG. "Hard warrior."

Hillier, Hillyer

Hillel Heb. "Greatly praised." Sometimes used in honor of the celebrated 1st century Jewish scholar Rabbi Hillel.

Hilliard OG. "battle guard" or OE. Place name "yard on a hill."

Hiller, Hillierd, Hillyard, Hillyer, Hillyerd

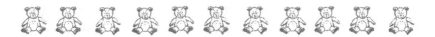

Hilton OE. Place name: "Hill settlement." Hotelier Conrad Hilton.
Hylton

Hippolyte Gk. Meaning not entirely clear, but alludes to horses. The Hippolytus in Greek legend, son of Theseus, was dragged to death by his bolting chariot-horses. Extremely rare.
Hippolit, Hippolitos, Hippolytus, Ippolito

Hiram Heb. Meaning not clear, possibly "most noble." Old Testament name little used in the 20th century, though fairly popular in the 19th.
Hi, Hirom, Hy, Hyrum

Hobart A particularly American (though unusual) variant of Hubert.
Hobard, Hobie, Hoebart

Hobson OE. "Son of Robert."

Hodgson OE. "Son of Roger."

Hogan Ir. Gael. "Youth."

Holbrook OE. Place name: "Stream near the hollow." Actor Hal Holbrook.
Brook, Holbrooke

Holcomb OE. "Deep valley." "Combe" is a term, sometimes used in England, for a deep, narrow valley.

Holden OE. Place name: "Hollow valley."

Hollis OE. Place name: "near the holly bushes" or "holly-tree grove." Used as a girl's name with some frequency as well.

Holmes Middle English. Place name: "Islands in the river." Arthur Conan Doyle's fictional detective Sherlock Holmes.

Holt OE. Place name: "Woods, forest."

Homer Gk. "Security, pledge." The name of the classical poet, author of the *Iliad* and the *Odyssey*. More popular in the U.S. than elsewhere, especially in the 19th century. Artist Winslow Homer.
Homere, Homeros, Homerus, Omero

Honoré Lat. "Honored one." Familiar because of a fashionable neighborhood and a shopping street in Paris called the Faubourg Saint Honoré.
Honorius, Honoratus

Horace Lat. Clan name, possibly meaning "timekeeper." Late 19th-century use may have been inspired in part by the famous Roman poet Horace. British Admiral Horatio Nelson; journalist Horace Greeley.
Horacio, Horatio, Horatius, Horaz, Oratio, Orazio

Horst OG. "A thicket." Photographer Horst P. Horst.

Horton OE. Place name: "Gray settlement." Dr. Seuss character Horton of *Horton Hears a Who*.
Horten, Orton

Hosea Heb. "Salvation." Name of an Old Testament prophet, but less popular, even in the 19th century, than other prophets' names like Joel or Amos.
Hoseia

Houghton OE. Place name: "Settlement on the headland."

Houston OE. Place name: "Settlement on the hill" or "Hugh's town." Sam Houston was the first president of the republic of Texas, before Texas entered the United States.
Huston, Hutcheson, Hutchinson

Howard OE. Meaning unclear, possibly occupational name indicating a watchman of some kind. Millionaire Howard Hughes; sportscaster Howard Cosell.
Howie, Ward

Howe OG. "lofty one" or Middle English place name "Hill."

Howell Welsh. "Eminent, remarkable." The anglicized version of Hywel, a name mostly used in Wales.

Howland OE. Place name: "Land with hills."
Howlan, Howlen

Hubbard Var. **Hubert**.

Hubert OG. "Bright or shining intellect." An old European name that was popular around the turn of the century, but is now rare. U.S. Vice President Hubert Humphrey.
Bert, Hobard, Hobart, Hubbard, Hube, Huberto, Hubie, Humberto, Ulberto

Hudson OE. "Hugh's son." Explorer Henry Hudson.

Hugh OG. "Mind, intellect." Popular medieval name, steadily used (though at a diminishing rate) in the modern era. Its widespread use in the Middles Ages resulted

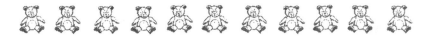

in spin-off names like Hudson, Hewson, and Houston. Film director Hugh Hudson; *Playboy* founder Hugh Hefner; U.S. Supreme Court Justice Hugo Black.

Hew, Hewe, Huey, Hughes, Hughie, Hugo, Hugues, Huw, Ugo

Hulbert OG. "Bright grace."

Bert, Hulbard, Hulburd, Hulburt

Humbert OG. "Renowned Hun." Made famous by the narrator of Vladimir Nabokov's *Lolita*, Humbert Humbert. Italian author Umberto Eco.

Umberto

Humphrey OG. Meaning unclear, but alludes to peace. In the Middle Ages, the form Humfrey was used in England, but Humphrey was the usual form from 1700 on. Never immensely popular, especially since the 1960s. Actor Humphrey Bogart.

Humfrey, Humfrid, Humfried, Humfry, Humph, Humphery, Humphry, Hunfredo, Onfre, Onfroi, Onofredo, Onofrio

Hunt OE. The word as a name, perhaps originally a shortening of **Hunter** or **Huntington**.

Hunter OE. Occupational name: "Hunter." Mostly Scots use. Journalist Hunter Thompson.

Huntington OE. Place name: "Hunter's settlement."

Huntingdon

Huntley OE. Place name: "Meadow of the hunter."

Huntlea, Huntlee, Huntleigh, Huntly

Hurlbert OE. "Shining army."

Hurlburt, Hurlbutt

Hurley Ir. Gael. "Sea tide."

Hurlee, Hurleigh, Hurly

Hurst Middle English. Place name: "Thicket of trees." Sometimes occurs as a place name in combination with the tree name, as in Elmhurst or Pinehurst.

Hearst, Hirst

Hussein Arab. "Small handsome one."

Husain, Husein

Hutton OE. Place name: "Settlement on the bluff." Actor Timothy Hutton.

Hutten

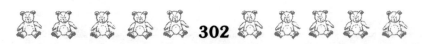

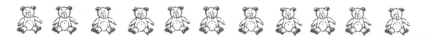

Huxford OE. Place name: "Hugh's ford."

Huxley OE. Place name: "Hugh's meadow." Author Aldous Huxley.
Huxlea, Huxlee, Huxleigh, Huxly

Hyacinthe Fr. "Hyacinth." Owing to the English-speaking tradition of flower names for girls, unlikely to be used as a boy's name, despite its origin as a male name.

Hyatt OE. Place name: "Lofty gate."

Hyde OE. Place name referring to a "hide," a measure of land current in the early Middle Ages. It amounted to about 120 acres.

Hyman Anglicized variant of **Chaim**. Heb. "Life."
Hayim, Hayyim, Hymie, Mannie

Iago Sp. Var. **James**. Heb. "He who supplants." The Spanish name for Saint James, Santiago, was given to a number of geographical features (rivers, lakes, mountains) in South America, as well as being the capital city of Chile. Still, most English-speaking parents will remember the treacherous villain of Shakespeare's *Othello*.
Jago

Ian Scot. Var. John. Heb. "God is gracious." One of the few Scottish names that has achieved really broad popularity since the beginning of this century. James Bond's creator Ian Fleming; actor Ian McKellen.
Ean, Eann, Iain

Ib Dan. "Baal's pledge." Baal was an ancient god of the Semites. Dancer Ib Andersen.

Ibrahim Arab. Var. **Abraham**. Heb. "Father of many." This form of the name is more common in Moslem countries.

Ichabod Heb. "The glory is gone." An Old Testament name brought to the U.S. by the Pilgrims and given fame by Washington Irving, who named a character Ichabod Crane in *The Legend of Sleepy Hollow*.

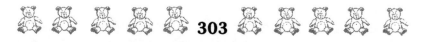

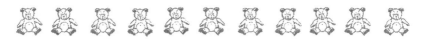

Idris Welsh. "Eager lord." Mostly used in Wales around the turn of the century.

Ignatius Meaning unclear, though some sources suggest Latin "ardent, burning." The most famous Ignatius is Saint Ignatius of Loyola, founder of the Society of Jesus, popularly known as the Jesuits. The name is rare in English-speaking countries.
Iggie, Ignac, Ignace, Ignacio, Ignacius, Ignatious, Ignatz, Ignaz, Ignazio, Inigo

Igor Rus. Var. **Ingvar**. Scan. "Ing's soldier." Composer Igor Stravinsky.
Inge, Ingemar, Ingmar

Ilario It. Var. **Hilary**. Gk. "Cheerful, merry."

Ilias Gk. Var. **Elijah**. Heb. "The Lord is my God."

Imad Arab. "Support, mainstay."

Immanuel Var. **Emmanuel**. Heb. "God is among us."

Ince Hung. "Innocent."

Ingemar Scan. "Ing's son." Ing, in Norse mythology, was a powerful god of fertility and peace. His name is an element in several modern names. Film director Ingmar Bergman.
Ingamar, Ingemur, Ingmar

Inglebert Var. **Englebert** OE. "Angel-bright."
Ingelbert

Ingram OE. "Raven of Anglia." A first name until the 17th century, now more commonly a surname that is occasionally transferred.
Ingraham, Ingrim

Ingvar Scan. "Ing's soldier."
Ingevar

Inigo OE. Var. **Ignatius**. In modern times, likely to be homage to the great English architect Inigo Jones.

Innis Scot. Gael. Place name: "Island."
Innes, Inness, Inniss

Innocenzio It. "Innocent."
Innocenty, Inocencio

Ioakim Rus. Var. **Joachim**. Heb. "God will judge."
Ioachime

Ira Heb. "Watchful." Old Testament name revived in the

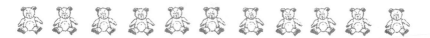

19th century, but never very popular. Lyricist Ira Gershwin.

Irving OE. "Sea friend." Also a Scottish place name. Used as a first name since the middle of the last century. Composer Irving Berlin, author Irving Stone.
Earvin, Erv, Ervin, Irv, Irvin, Irvine

Irwin OE. "Boar friend." Revived from roughly 1860 to 1940s, but little used since. Author Irwin Shaw.
Erwin, Erwinn, Erwyn, Irwinn, Irwyn

Isaac Heb. "Laughter." In the Old Testament, Abraham's son, born when his father was 100 years old. The Puritans used the name enthusiastically, and it remained popular through the 18th century, fading very gradually. Less fashionable in the last 50 years. Scientist Isaac Newton; angler Izaak Walton; authors Isaac Bashevis Singer, Isaac Asimov.
Ike, Ikey, Ikie, Isaak, Isac, Isacco, Isak, Itzak, Izaak, Izak, Izik, Izsak, Yitzhak, Zack, Zak

Isaiah Heb. "The Lord helps me" or "salvation of God." Like so many Old Testament names, popular with the Puritans in the 17th century, brought to America, and revived by the Victorians. Now rare.
Isa, Isaia, Isia, Isiah, Issiah

Isham OE. Place name: "Home of the iron one."

Ishmael Heb. "The Lord will hear." Old Testament name immortalized in the first line of Herman Melville's *Moby Dick*: "Call me Ishmael."

Isidore Gk. "Gift of Isis." Isis was the principal goddess of ancient Egypt, and Isidore was a popular name among the ancient Greeks. There are several saints named Isidore, but the name is probably most famous in its feminine form, Isadora.
Dore, Dorian, Dory, Isador, Isadore, Isidor, Isidoro, Isidro, Issy, Izidor, Izydor, Izzy, Ysidro

Ismail Arab. Name of a Moslem prophet.

Israel Heb. Meaning unclear, though some sources suggest "wrestling with the Lord," for this was the name given **Jacob** in the Old Testament after his three-day bout with his Lord. Came to be synonymous with the Jewish people, and was consequently used as the name

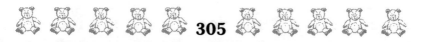

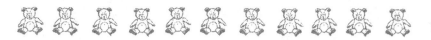

for the new Jewish state founded in 1948. Author Israel Shenker.
Yisrael

Istvan Hung. Var. **Stephen**. Gk. "Crowned." Film director Istvan Szabo.

Ivan Rus. Var. **John**. Heb. "God is gracious." Used in English-speaking countries for the last hundred-odd years. Tennis star Ivan Lendl.

Ivo OG. "Yew wood." Since yew wood was used for bows, the name may have been an occupational one meaning "archer." The most famous form is probably Ives from the old nursery rhyme "As I was going to St. Ives/I met a man with seven wives..." Uncommon nevertheless.
Ivar, Iven, Ives, Ivon, Yves, Yvo

Ivor Norse, meaning unclear. Possibly related to **Ivo** or to **Ingvar**. Used now and then in Britain, scarce in the U.S.
Ifor, Iver, Yvor

J

Jabez Heb. "Borne in pain." Old Testament name that lasted fairly well until around 1930.
Jabes, Jabesh

Jabir Arab. "Consolation."

Jacinto Sp. from Gk. **Hyacinth** (flower name). There was a 3rd-century Saint Hyacinth, and the name has been used for both sexes. In Greek legend, Apollo loved a beautiful youth of the name; the hyacinth flower sprang up from his blood when he died.
Giacintho, Giacinto, Jacindo

Jack Familiar form of **John** Heb. "the Lord is gracious" or, less often, **Jacob** Heb. "he who supplants." Used as an independent name from the 1850s to the 1920s, then subsided. Currently experiencing a flutter of stylishness, possibly because of its slightly rugged, down-home aura.

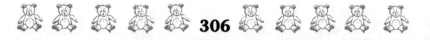

Actors Jackie Gleason, Jack Nicholson; comedian Jack Benny; exercise guru Jack LaLanne.

Jackie, Jacko, Jacky

Jackson OE. "Son of Jack." May indicate an ancestor's admiration for U.S. President Andrew Jackson or, in Southern families, Civil War General Stonewall Jackson. Artist Jackson Pollock; singer Jackson Browne.

Jack, Jackie, Jacky, Jakson

Jacob Heb. "He who supplants." In the Old Testament, Jacob, Esau's brother, impersonates his brother at his blind father's deathbed by covering his hands with a goatskin ("for Esau was a hairy man"), securing the blessing meant for the elder son. The name is unusual now, having been used with some steadiness in the last two centuries. Senator Jacob Javits.

Cob, Cobb, Cobby, Giacamo, Giacobo, Giacomo, Giacopo, Hamish, Iacopo, Iacovo, Iago, Iakob, Iakobos, Iakov, Jaco, Jacobo, Jack, Jackie, Jacko, Jacky, Jacques, Jacquet, Jago, Jaime, Jake, Jakie, Jakob, Jakov, Jakub, James, Jamesie, Jamey, Jamie, Jamsey, Jay, Jayme, Jim, Jimmie, Seamus, Shamus, Yakov

Jacques Fr. Var. **James** via **Jacob**. Familiar from the well-known song "Frère Jacques." Undersea explorer Jacques Cousteau.

Jacot, Jaques

Jael Heb. "Mountain goat." Also used for girls, although rare in either case.

Yael

Jaime Sp. Var. **James**.

Jaimey, Jaimie, Jayme, Jaymie

Jake Dim. **Jacob**. Used independently since the 1960s.

Jamal Arab. "Handsome." Very popular in the U.S. among black or Muslim families. TV star Malcolm-Jamal Warner.

Jamaal, Jamahl, Jamall, Jameel, Jamell, Jamil, Jamill, Jammal

James English variant of **Jacob**. In the New Testament there are two apostles known as James, though the Old Testament version of the name is always Jacob. The apostles are known a bit unfairly as James the Greater

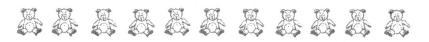

and James the Less. The name was popularized by the Stuart kings James I and II, and has been a stable favorite ever since. Writer James Joyce; actors James Mason and Jimmy Stewart; entertainer Jimmy Durante; five U.S. presidents: James Buchanan, James Garfield, James Madison, James Polk, Jimmy Carter.

Diego, Giacomo, Giamo, Hamish, Iago, Jacques, Jago, Jaime, Jaimes, Jaimey, Jaimie, Jameson, Jamesie, Jamesy, Jamey, Jamie, Jamison, Jaymes, Jaymie, Jim, Jimmie, Jimmy, Seamus, Shamus

Jameson OE. "Son of James."
Jamieson, Jamison

Jamie Dim. **James**. Mostly Scottish, but its current popularity for girls may limit its future as a boy's name.
Jaime, Jaimie, Jamey, Jayme

Jan Dutch. Var. **John**. Painters Jan Van Eyck, Jan Vermeer.
Hans, Janek, Janos

Janson Scan. "Jan's son." Used as a first name only in this century.
Jansen, Jantzen, Janzen, Jenson, Jensen

Japheth Heb. "He expands." Along with Ham and Shem, one of Noah's sons. Little used, except by the Puritans.

Jareb Heb. "He will struggle."

Jared Heb. "He descends." Old Testament name used by the Puritans, and suddenly, inexplicably popular in the 1960s.
Jarad, Jarid, Jarrad, Jarred, Jarrid, Jarrod, Jerad, Jerrad

Jarman OG. "German."
Jerman

Jarek Slavic. "January."
Janiusz, Januarius

Jaroslav Slavic. "Beauty of spring." A popular name in Czechoslovakia. Historian Jaroslav Pelikan.

Jarrett Var. **Garrett**. OE. "Spear-brave."
Jarret, Jarrot, Jarrott

Jarvis Var. **Gervase**. OG. Meaning unclear: possibly "with honor."
Jarvey, Jervey, Jervis

Jason Heb. "The Lord is salvation." The name is actually

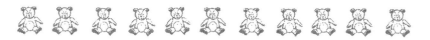

a variation of Joshua, formed by biblical translators. Jason was a legendary Greek hero who, after many adventures, recovered the Golden Fleece from an enemy kingdom. The name was phenomenally popular in the 1970s after centuries of sporadic use. Now on the wane. Actor Jason Robards.
Jaisen, Jaison, Jase, Jasen, Jasin, Jasun, Jay, Jayson

Jasper Eng. Var. **Caspar**. Possibly Persian "he who guards the treasure." Jasper is also a strikingly colorful variety of quartz. Painter Jasper Johns.
Jaspar

Javier Sp. Var. **Xavier**. Meaning obscure, but refers to Saint Francis Xavier.

Jay Lat. "Jaybird." A medieval name that has survived in a small way, especially in the U.S., where it is given to boys and girls alike. Its use may be inspired by a great early American jurist, John Jay. Financier Jay Gould.
Jae, Jaye

Jean Fr. Var. **John**. Author and artist Jean Cocteau; playwright Jean Molière.

Jed Dim. **Jedidiah**. Lent a certain rustic aura by Jed Clampitt, a character on the popular 1960s TV show "The Beverly Hillbillies."
Jedd, Jedediah

Jedidiah Heb. "Beloved of the Lord." Old Testament name that was used by the Puritans in the 17th century.
Jedd, Jedediah

Jeff Dim. **Jefferson, Jeffrey**. Used as an independent name in this century. Actors Jeff Daniels, Jeff Goldblum.

Jefferson OE. "Son of Jeffrey." Surname used as a first name. A sterling example of this use is president of the Confederacy Jefferson Davis, who was born in 1808, during the presidency of Thomas Jefferson.
Jeff, Jeffey, Jeffie

Jeffrey OG. Meaning unclear, but refers to "peace." Norman name popular through the Middle Ages in Britain and revived in the mid–19th century after a 350-year rest. The peak of its popularity was the 1970s in the U.S., with this form preferred to Geoffrey.
Geoff, Geoffrey, Geoffroy, Geoffry, Geofrey, Geofry,

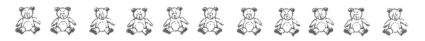

Godfrey, Godfry, Gottfried, Jefery, Jeff, Jefferey, Jefferies, Jeffery, Jeffree, Jeffries, Jeffry, Jeffy, Jefry, Jeoffroi

Jem Dim. **James** or **Jeremiah**. Rare as nickname or independent name.

Jenkin Flemish. "Little John." A name as popular and well used as John has naturally produced numerous last names as well, some of which find their way back to first-name status.

Jenkins, Jenkyn, Jenkyns, Jennings

Jens Scan. Var. **John**.

Jensen, Jenson

Jeremiah Heb. "The Lord exalts." Old Testament prophet who lived in Jerusalem when it fell to the Babylonians. The Book of Jeremiah is so relentlessly gloomy in outlook that "jeremiad" has become the term for a lengthy denunciatory complaint. The Puritans used Jeremiah somewhat, but Jeremy has eclipsed it in modern times.

Dermot, Dermott, Diarmid, Geremia, Jem, Jemmie, Jereme, Jeremia, Jeremias, Jeremija, Jeremiya, Jeremy, Jerry

Jeremy Modern form of **Jeremiah**. One source suggests that the modern penchant for Jeremy was sparked by a 1960s TV series called "Here Come the Brides." This may be true, since the Jeremy on the show had brothers named Jason and Joshua, names that were simultaneously fashionable. The vogue for all three is fading. Actor Jeremy Irons.

Jem, Jemmie, Jemmy, Jeramee, Jeramey, Jeramie, Jere, Jereme, Jeremie, Jeromy, Jerry

Jermaine Var. **Jarman**. OG. "German." Made famous by Michael Jackson's older brother, Jermaine.

Jerome Gk. "Sacred name." The 5th-century Saint Jerome was responsible for a Latin translation of the Bible. He is often portrayed with a lion, from the legend that he removed a thorn from the lion's pad and the beast rewarded him with lifelong fidelity. The name has been best used in the 16th and 19th centuries. Songwriter Jerome Kern; choreographer Jerome Robbins.

Gerome, Geronimo, Gerrie, Gerry, Hierome, Hieronim,

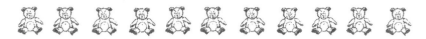

Hieronimo, Hieronimos, Hieronymos, Hieronymus, Jeroen, Jeromo, Jeronimo, Jerrome, Jerry

Jerry Dim. **Jeremy, Gerald**, etc.

Jerzy Pol. Var. **Goerge**. "Farmer." Writer Jerzy Kozinski.

Jesse Heb. "The Lord exists." The biblical father of King David. In America the formidable athlete Jesse Owens (whose success at the 1936 Olympics chagrined the Nazis) has given the name great resonance for black families; the fame of politician Jesse Jackson may continue to do so. Outlaw Jesse James.

Jess, Jessie

Jesus Heb. "The Lord is salvation." Used mostly by families of Latin American origin, but Joshua, from the same Hebrew derivation, occurs more often.

Jethro Heb. "Preeminence." Old Testament name that occurred from time to time until the late 19th century. A flicker of modern use may have been inspired by the rock group Jethro Tull.

Jeth

Jim Dim. **James**. Used occasionally as an independent name.

Jimi, Jimmee, Jimmey, Jimmie, Jimmy

Joab Heb. "Praise Jehovah."

Joachim Heb. "God will judge."

Akim, Ioakim, Joacheim, Joaquim, Joaquin

Job Heb. "The afflicted." In the Old Testament, the Book of Job recounts the trials of an innocent man who was sorely tried by his God but remained faithful: hence "the patience of Job." Revived by the Puritans and used fairly steadily since the 17th century.

Joab, Jobe

Jock Familiar var. **Jacob** or **John**. A slang term for a Scotsman, probably because the local accent turns Jack into Jock. Not actually used in Scotland, and in the U.S. avoided because it is a slightly derogatory term for an athlete. Sportsman Jock Whitney.

Jocko

Jody Familiar var. **Joseph**. In Marjorie Kinnan Rawlings's Pulitzer Prize-winning novel *The Yearling*, the young

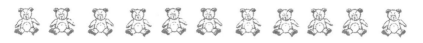

hero is called Jody, but the name is more likely to be used for a girl.

Jodey, Jodi, Jodie

Joe Dim. **Joseph.** Sometimes given as an independent name.

Joel Heb. "Jehovah is the Lord." Along with Amos, the most common of the Old Testament prophets' names, though Hosea also occurs. For some reason the parents of the late 20th century who have scoured the Old Testament for names have had a strong predilection for those beginning with *J.* Actor Joel McCrea.

John Heb. "The Lord is gracious." Given a sound foundation by two crucial saints, John the Baptist and John the Evangelist. The name has been used by 25 popes, an English king, and endless numbers of parents all over the world. In the English-speaking countries it was the most popular boy's name for over 400 years, losing ground only in the 1950s. Now some of its variants, like Ian and Sean, are gaining. Actors John Gielgud, John Barrymore, John Wayne; four U.S. presidents: John F. Kennedy, John Tyler, John Adams, John Quincy Adams; poet John Donne; Beatle John Lennon; composer Johannes Bach.

Anno, Ean, Evan, Ewan, Ewen, Gian, Giannes, Gianni, Giannis, Giannos, Giovanni, Hannes, Hanno, Hans, Hanschen, Hansel, Hansl, Iain, Ian, Ioannes, Ioannis, Ivan, Ivann, Jack, Jackie, Jacky, Jan, Jancsi, Janek, Janko, Janne, Janos, Jean, Jeannot, Jehan, Jens, Joao, Jock, Jocko, Johan, Johann, Johannes, Johnie, Johnnie, Johnny, Jon, Jona, Jonnie, Juan, Juanito, Sean, Seann, Shane, Shaughn, Shaun, Shawn, Vanek, Vanko, Vanya, Yanni, Yanno, Zane

Johnson OE. "Son of John." Mostly 19th-century use. Playwright Ben Jonson.

Jonson, Johnston

Jonah Heb. "Dove." Jonah is the biblical hero who was swallowed alive by a whale, in whose belly he lived for three days. He had been thrown overboard by sailors from the ship he was traveling on in order to calm a stormy sea; by extension, the term "Jonah" means some-

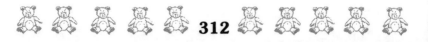

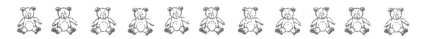

one who brings bad luck. The name, nevertheless, has been used with some frequency, though never immense popularity.

Jonas

Jonathan Heb. "Gift of Jehovah." Related to Nathan, rather than to John. In the Old Testament, the great friend of King David. Used in the 17th century, then neglected from the 18th until the 1940s. Some of its current steady use probably comes about because it resembles John. English author Jonathan Swift; actor Jon Voight.

Johnathan, Johnathon, Jon, Jonathon

Jones Surname derived from **John**. Particularly popular in Wales.

Jordan Heb. "Descend." Named after the River Jordan. First used in the Middle Ages by Crusaders returning from the Holy Land. Revived slightly in the 19th century. Unusual now (though used for both sexes), but a good candidate for revival in the 1990s quest for the unusual.

Giordano, Jared, Jarred, Jerad, Jerred, Jordaan, Jordao, Jordon, Jori, Jory, Jourdain, Jourdan

Jorge Sp. Var. **George**. Lat. "Farmer."

Jorgen Dan. Var. **George**. Lat. "Farmer."

Jeorg, Jerzy, Jorg, Jori, Joris, Jurgen, Juri

Jose Sp. Var. **Joseph**.

Joseito, Pepe, Pepito

Joseph Heb. "Jehovah increases." Name that occurs for principal figures in both the Old and the New Testaments of the Bible. It has been much less widely used than **John** and has many fewer international variants. Actor Josef Sommer; writers Joseph Conrad, Joseph Wambaugh; revolutionary Che Guevara.

Che, Giuseppe, Giuseppino, Iosep, Jo, Jodi, Jodie, Jody, Joey, Joop, Joos, Jose, Josef, Joseito, Josep, Josip, Josif, Josephe, Josephus, Joszef, Jozef, Osip, Pepe, Pepito, Peppi, Pino, Pipo, Sepp, Seppi, Yousef, Yusif, Yusuf, Yusup, Yuszef

Joshua Heb. "The Lord is salvation." An Old Testament hero, Moses' successor. Passed over by the Puritans, re-

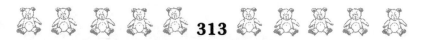

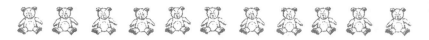

vived in the 18th century, and currently immensely fashionable in the U.S.

Josh, Joshuah, Josua, Josue, Jozua

Josiah Heb. "The Lord supports." An Old Testament king of Judah. Most common in the 18th century, now rare. Porcelain entrepreneur Josiah Wedgwood.

Josia, Josias

Juan Sp. Var. **John**.

Judah Heb. "Praise." **Jude** is the more common form.

Jud, Judas, Judd, Jude

Jude Lat. Var. **Judah**. Very unusual, probably because of the traitorous apostle Judas Iscariot. There was, however, another apostle named Jude who now enjoys some popularity as the patron saint of lost causes.

Jud, Judah, Judas, Judd

Jules Fr. Var. **Julius**. Author Jules Verne; playwright Jules Feiffer.

Julian Lat. Var. **Julius**. First took hold in the 18th century, and became fashionable in the 1950s through 1970s. Musician Julian Lennon.

Jolyon, Julien

Julius Lat. Clan name: "Youthful." Common in Christian Rome and revived in the 19th century, but now out of use. Singers Julio Iglesias, Julius La Rosa.

Giulio, Jolyon, Jule, Jules, Julio

Juri Slavic. Var. **George**. Lat. "Farmer."

Jaris, Yuri

Justin Lat. "Fair, righteous." Another name well used by Roman Christians, but unusual elsewhere until very recently. It is now quite fashionable, especially in the U.S.

Giustino, Giusto, Justen, Justinas, Justinian, Justinius, Justino, Justinus, Justis, Justo, Justus, Justyn

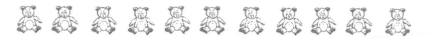

Kaiser Var. **Caesar.** Lat. Possibly "hairy." The connotations, of course, are of imperial rule, as in Germany's Kaiser Wilhelm.

Kalil Arab. "Friend." Writer Kahlil Gibran.
Kahlil, Kaleel, Khaleel, Khalil

Kamal Arab. "Perfection, perfect."
Kameel, Kamil

Kane Welsh. "beautiful" or Ir. Gael. "warrior's son." Surname transferred occasionally to first name in this century.
Cahan, Cain, Kahan, Kain, Kaine, Kayne, Keane

Kareem Arab. "Highborn, generous." Basketball star Kareem Abdul-Jabbar.
Karim

Karl OG. "Man." Var. **Charles.** The Germanic form of the name; as Carl, it was fairly well used in the U.S. 1850–1950. *K* spellings are not as readily adopted for boys' names as they are for girls'. Fashion designer Karl Lagerfeld; economist Karl Marx.
Carl, Kale, Karel, Karlan, Karlens, Karli, Karol, Karoly

Kaspar Var. **Caspar.** Possibly Per. "He who guards the treasure." Originally Jasper. Traditionally one of the Three Kings (perhaps the one carrying the gold) was named Caspar.
Kasper

Kavan Ir. Gael. "Handsome."
Cavan

Kavanagh Ir. Gael. "Follower of Kevin." Principally an Irish surname.
Cavanagh, Cavanaugh, Kavanaugh

Kay Old Welsh. "Rejoicing." Ancient name borne, in legend, by one of the knights of the Round Table. Now all but obliterated as a male name by the women's name Kay, which is a diminutive of Katherine.

Kazimierz Var. **Casimir.** Slavic. "Bringing peace." Associated with Poland for her famous 11th-century king who brought peace to the nation.
Kazimir, Kazmer

Keane OE. "Sharp." As in a "keen wit" or a "keen eye." Actor Edmund Kean.
Kean, Keen, Keene

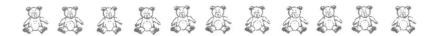

Kearney Var. **Carney**. Ir. Gael. "The winner."
Karney, Karny, Kearny
Kedar Arab. "Powerful."
Kadar
Keefe Ir. Gael. "Handsome; lovable, loved."
Keegan Ir. Gael. "Small and ardent."
Keelan Ir. Gael. "Small and slim."
Keeley Ir. Gael. "Handsome." Also possibly a variant of
Kelly (Ir. Gael. "eager for battle").
Kealey, Kealy, Keelie, Keely
Keenan Ir. Gael. "Small and ancient."
Keen, Keenen, Kienan, Kienen
Keir Gael. "Dark-skinned, swarthy." Actor Keir Dullea.
Keith Scot. Gael. "Forest." Originally a place name,
adopted as a first name for non-Scots in the 19th century.
Peaked in the 1960s in the U.S., and now on the wane.
Baseball player Keith Hernandez; Rolling Stone Keith
Richard; actor Keith Carradine.
Kelby ONorse. Place name: "The farm near the spring."
Kelbey, Kelbie, Kellby
Kell ONorse. Place name: "Spring."
Kelly Ir. Gael. "Warrior." Originally a very common Irish
last name, and very popular as a girl's first name from the
1950s. Use for boy babies has diminished accordingly.
Kelley, Kellie
Kelsey OE. Place name, incorporating a word particle that
means "island." Mostly recent usage, for boys as well as
girls.
Kelsie, Kelsy
Kelton OE. Place name: "Town of the keels." Probably
originally referred to a town where ships were built.
Keldon, Kelten, Keltonn
Kelvin Meaning and origin unclear: possibly OE. "keel
friend" (keel, in this case, standing in for ship) or a place
name alluding to a river. Brief spurt of use in the 1920s
was mostly British.
Kelvan, Kelven, Kelvyn, Kelwin, Kelwyn
Kemp Middle English. "Fighter, champion."
Kempton Middle English. Place name: "From the war-
rior's settlement."

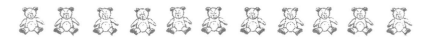

Ken Dim. **Kenneth** and other "Ken-" names. Used independently, but parents who played with Barbie dolls in the 1960s may be hard put to name a baby after Barbie's boyfriend Ken.
Kennie, Kenny

Kendall OE. Place name: "The valley of the Kent," a river in western England. Some sources also suggest "the bright river valley." In either case, a transferred surname used as a first name since the 19th century.
Kendal, Kendell, Kenny

Kendrick OE. "Royal ruler." Revived as a first name in the 19th century, but unusual.
Kendricks, Kendrik, Kendryck, Kenric, Kenrick, Kenricks, Kenricks, Kenrik

Kenelm OE. "Brave helmet."

Kenley OE. Place name: "The king's meadow."
Kenlea, Kenlee, Kenleigh, Kenlie, Kenly

Kenn Welsh. "Bright water."

Kennard OE. "Brave and strong."
Kennaird

Kennedy Ir. Gael. Some sources suggest "helmet/head," while "ugly/head" is also offered, which would make this one of the rare names to refer to negative characteristics or habits possessed by ancestors. Use of Kennedy as a first name may be inspired by President John F. Kennedy.
Canaday, Canady, Kennedey

Kenneth Ir. Gael. "Handsome" or "sprung from fire." Originally a favorite Scottish name that spread starting in the late 19th century. Very popular in the U.S. in the 1950s and 1960s, but now out of favor. Art historian Kenneth Clark; actor Kenneth Branagh.
Ken, Kennet, Kennett, Kennith, Kenny

Kent OE. Place name: a county in England. Familiar as a surname, and used in the U.S. as a first name. In the 1930s and 1940s monosyllabic names (Clark, Burt, Kirk) seemed to project a manly aura and enjoyed a consequent burst of popularity.

Kenton OE. Place name: "The royal settlement." In use as a first name since the 1950s.

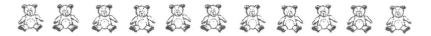

Kenward OE. "Brave or royal guardian."

Kenway OE. "Brave or royal fighter."

Kenyon Ir. Gael. "Blond."

Kermit Ir. Gael. "Without envy." A variant of **Dermot**, made famous (and virtually unusable) by the popular green Muppet Kermit the Frog.

Kern Ir. Gael. "Small swarthy one."

Kernaghan Ir. Gael. "Victorious."
   Carnahan, Kernohan

Kerr Scan. Place name: "The swampy place." Used basically in Scotland as a first name.
   Carr, Karr

Kerry Irish place name: Kerry is a county in southwestern Ireland. Also, according to some sources, "dark-haired." Used more often for girls.
   Kearie, Keary, Kerrey, Kerrie

Kerwin Possibly OE. "swamp friend" or Ir. Gael. "little dark one."
   Kervin, Kervyn, Kerwinn

Kevin Ir. Gael. "Handsome" (a meaning that certainly applies to two famous Kevins, actors Kline and Costner). Originally an Irish name that spread to wider use in the 20th century. Most popular in the 1960s, now fading.
   Kevan, Keven, Kevon, Kevyn

Khalid Arab. "Never-ending."

Kieran Ir. Gael. "Dark, swarthy." Becoming popular in Ireland, and showing some signs of spreading further afield.
   Keiran, Keiron, Kernan, Kiernan, Kieron

Kidd Middle English. "Kid, young goat." Probably an occupational name, possibly indicating an ancestor who kept goats. Pirate Captain William Kidd.

Killian Ir. Gael. "Small and fierce." From the same root as **Kelly**.

Kim Dim. "Kim-" names like **Kimball** and **Kimberly**. Also the title of a famous Kipling novel, but the days when children were named for Kipling characters is long since past.

Kimball OE. "Bold war-leader."
   Kimbal, Kimbell, Kimble

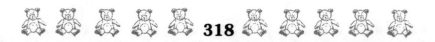

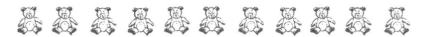

Kimberly OE. Place name: The "-ly" suffix indicates a meadow. *The Facts on File Dictionary of First Names* traces the masculine use of the name to the Boer War, when many English soldiers were fighting in the South African town of Kimberley. It has been virtually taken over by girls, however, and was a great favorite in the 1960s.
Kimberleigh, Kimberley

Kincaid Celt. "Battle leader."

King OE. "King." A last name since the Middle Ages. Modern use may be homage to Martin Luther King.

Kingman OE. "King's man." U.S. Ambassador Kingman Brewster.

Kingsley OE. Place name: "King's meadow." Surname transferred to first name, particularly in Britain. Novelist Kingsley Amis; actor Ben Kingsley.
Kingslea, Kingslie, Kingsly, Kinslea, Kinslee, Kinsley, Kinslie, Kinsly

Kingston OE. Place name: "King's settlement."

Kingswell OE. Place name: "King's well."

Kinnard Ir. Gael. Place name: "The tall hill."
Kinnaird

Kinnell Ir. Gael. Place name: "Top of the cliff."

Kipp OE. Place name: "Pointed hill."
Kip

Kirby OE. Place name: "Church village." Mostly 19th-century use.
Kerbie, Kerbey, Kirbey, Kirbie, Kirkby

Kiril Gk. "The Lord." As Cyril, used in Britain around the turn of the century.
Cyril, Kirillos, Kyril

Kirk ONorse. "Church." Some 19th-century use in Britain, but it was really brought into circulation by actor Kirk Douglas.
Kerk

Kirkley OE. Place name: "Church meadow." Like the following names, this became a last name after being a place name, and is only occasionally used as a first name.
Kirklea, Kirklee, Kirklie, Kirkly

Kirkwell OE. Place name: "Church spring."

Kirkwood OE. Place name: "Church forest." Author James Kirkwood.

Kit Dim. **Christopher**. Gk. "Bearer of Christ." A nickname for Christopher long before Chris was thought of. Christopher Columbus named the Caribbean island of Saint Kitts for himself and Saint Christopher, the patron of travelers.

Klaus Var. **Claus** (dim. **Nicholas**: Gk. "Victorious people"). Even spelled with the more anglicized *C*, unusual in English-speaking countries. Actor Klaus Maria Brandauer.
Klaas, Klaes

Klemens Var. **Clement**. Lat. "Mild, giving mercy."
Klemenis, Klement, Kliment

Konrad Var. **Conrad**. OG. "Courageous advice." Despite occasional increases in numbers, a name that has never been widely popular in English-speaking countries. Anthropologist Konrad Lorenz.
Kord, Kunz

Konstantin Var. **Constantine**. Lat. "Steadfast." The form Constant was popular among the Puritans (as a virtue name) and was revived in the 19th century to occasional modern use. Constantine, the Latin form, was the name of the first Christian Roman emperor, and a royal name in Greece.
Konstant, Konstantio, Konstanty, Konstanz, Kostas

Kornel Var. **Cornelius**. Lat. "Like a horn." Comes from a Latin clan name and, as Cornelius, was often used under the Roman Empire. Painter Kees Van Dongen.
Kees, Kornelisz

Knox OE. Place name: "Hills." Last name occasionally pressed into use as a first name.

Knute Var. **Canute**. Scan. "Knot." Brought to Britain by 11th-century King Canute of Denmark, who became king of England in 1016. Very rare, except in those of Scandinavian descent. Football coach Knute Rockne.
Knud, Cnut, Knut

Krispin Var. **Crispin**. Lat. "Curly-haired." Saint Crispin, supposedly a 3rd-century martyr, is patron of shoemakers. The name was somewhat popular in Britain in the

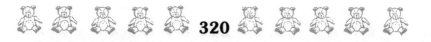

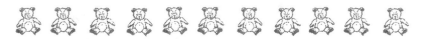

17th and 18th centuries, and was revived in the 1960s, but has not spread to the U.S. in any significant numbers.

Kristian Var. **Christian**. Gk. "Anointed, Christian." A girl's name that (contrary to the usual movement) became a male name, possibly after the huge success of John Bunyan's *Pilgrim's Progress* (1684), whose hero is called Christian.

Krist

Kristofer Var. **Christopher**. Gk. "Carrier of Christ." The much-loved story of Saint Christopher is that he lived alone by a river, carrying travelers across the ford on his back. A child whom he was carrying became almost too heavy to bear, and proved afterward to be the Christ child. Actually the tale has little basis in fact, and probably springs from the literal translation of the name, which originally alluded to carrying Christ in one's heart. Actor Kris Kristofferson.

Kristoffer, Kristofor, Kristopher, Kristophor, Krzysztof

Kurt Ger. Var. **Conrad**. OG. "Courageous advice." Actor Kurt Russell; author Kurt Vonnegut; U.N. Secretary General Kurt Waldheim.

Kyle Scot. Place name: "Narrow spit of land." Well-traveled parents may have crossed the Kyle of Lochalsh to reach the Isle of Skye. Used more often for boys than for girls. Actor Kyle MacLachlan.

Laban Heb. "White." Old Testament name revived by the Puritans. Has appeared sporadically since.

Lachlan Scot. Gael. Either "belligerent" or "from the fjord-land," which would refer to Norway, thus indicating a Viking ancestor. The name is unusual, even in Scotland.

Lacy OF. Place name of obscure meaning, used as a boy's

name in the 19th century and only occasionally for either sex today.

Lacey

Ladd Middle English. "Manservant or young man." Most likely to be a transferred surname.

Lad, Laddey, Laddie, Laddy

Laird Scot. "Lord of the land."

Lamar OG. "Land famous." Plutocrat Lamar Hunt.

Lamarr, Lemar, Lemarr

Lambert OG. "Land brilliant." Medieval and Renaissance use was encouraged by veneration for the Belgian martyr Saint Lambert, but in the more secular times since, nothing has occurred to save it from neglect.

Bert, Lamberto, Lambirt, Landbert

Lamont Scan. "Man of law." Mostly U.S. use around the 1940s.

Lammond, Lamond, Lemond

Lance Var. **Lancelot**. Mildly popular on its own in the middle of this century. Parents may have erroneously thought it referred to the medieval jousting weapon.

Lantz, Lanz, Launce

Lancelot OF. "Servant." Most famous, of course, for the knight of the Round Table who seduced King Arthur's wife, Guinevere. Used as a first name in the romantic 19th century, rare since the middle of this century.

Launcelot

Lander Middle English. Occupational name: Possibly "laundry-man" or "landowner." More probably the latter, since the laundering trade, in medieval Britain, was unlikely to provide much of a career.

Landers, Landor

Landon OE. Place name: "Grassy plain."

Landan, Landen, Landin

Lane Middle English. Place name. More common for boys than for girls, though still unusual for both. This is the kind of name that is likely to be a mother's maiden name transferred to a first name.

Laine, Layne

Lang ONorse. "Tall one."

Lange

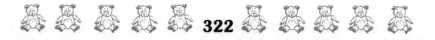

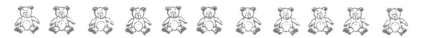

Langdon OE. Place name: "Long hill."
  Landon, Langden
Langford OE. Place name: "Long ford." Many English place names are just compounds of familiar elements that still exist in our spoken language.
Langley OE. Place name: "Long meadow."
  Langlea, Langlee, Langleigh, Langly
Langston OE. Place name: "Long town" or "tall man's town." The "Lang-" element could have two meanings in this instance. Author Langston Hughes.
  Langsden, Langsdon
Langward OE. Descriptive/occupational name: "Tall guardian."
Langworth OE. Place name: "Long paddock."
Lanny Dim. **Roland**. OF. "Famous land." More common as a nickname.
Larkin Ir. Gael. "Rough, fierce."
Larrimore OF. "Armorer."
  Larimore, Larmer, Larmor
Larry Dim. **Lawrence**. Given as an independent name in this century.
Lars Scan. Var. **Lawrence**.
  Larson, Larsson
Laszlo Hung. "Famous ruler."
  Laslo, Lazlo
Latham Scan. Place name: "The barn."
Lathrop OE. Place name: "Farmstead with barns."
Latimer Middle English. Occupational name: "Interpreter." Possibly one who could translate into Latin.
  Latymer
Lawford OE. Place name: "The hill-ford." Actor Peter Lawford.
Lawler Ir. Gael. "Mutterer."
  Lawlor, Loller, Lollar
Lawrence Lat. "From Laurentium." Laurentium was a city south of Rome known for its numerous laurel trees. Though the place no longer exists, the name endures, at first given staying power by the popularity of Saint Lawrence (who was martyred by being grilled alive). Brought to Britain with the Norman Conquest, and after

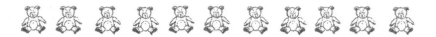

an eventual 19th-century decline, was soundly revived in the U.S. in this century. Popularity began to tail off after the 1970s. Actor Laurence Olivier; band leader Lawrence Welk.

Larrance, Larrey, Larry, Lars, Laurance, Lauren, Laurence, Laurens, Laurent, Laurentios, Laurentius, Laurenz, Laurie, Laurits, Lauritz, Lawrance, Lawrey, Lawrie, Lawry, Lenci, Lon, Lonny, Lorant, Loren, Lorenc, Lorencz, Lorens, Lorenzo, Lorin, Loritz, Lorry, Lowrance

Lawson OE. "Son of Lawrence." Used as a first name mostly since 1850.

Lawton OE. Place name: "Hill-town." Actor Charles Laughton.

Laughton

Lazarus Heb. "The Lord will help." Biblical name: Lazarus was the man whom Jesus raised from the dead. Little used, perhaps since in the Middle Ages it became a synonym for "leper."

Eleazer, Lazar, Lazare, Lazaro, Lazzaro

Leander Gk. "Lion-man." The mythical Greek Leander swam across the Hellespont to visit his beloved, Hero. This was a saint's name as well, but has never been very widely used.

Ander, Leandre, Leandro, Leandros, Lee, Leo

Lee OE. Place name: "Pasture or meadow." One of the few truly unisex names. Usually a name becomes exclusively feminine once it is used for girls (Ashley, Leslie). The tenacious masculine hold on Lee may have been helped by tough-guy actor Lee Marvin. U.S. use seems to have been sparked by admiration for Confederate General Robert E. Lee. Peaked in the 1950s. Chrysler chairman Lee Iacocca; actor Lee Majors.

Leigh

Leggett OF. "One who is sent; delegate."

Legate, Leggitt, Liggett

Leif Scan. "Loved." Explorer Leif Ericsson.

Lief

Leighton OE. Place name: "Meadow settlement." Used as a first name starting in the 19th century.

Layton, Leyton

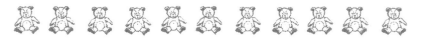

Leith Scot. Gael. "Broad river."

Leland OE. Place name: "Meadow land." Philanthropist Leland Stanford.
Le, Leeland, Leighland, Leyland

Lemuel Heb. "Devoted to God." Old Testament name passed over in the wholesale Puritan revival of biblical names, but given new life from around 1840 into the 1930s. Currently extremely rare.
Lem, Lemmie

Lennon Ir. Gael. "Small cloak or cape."

Lennox Scot. Gael. "With many elm trees."
Lenox

Leo Lat. "Lion." Common in Roman times, and the name of 13 popes, but little used in the 18th and early 19th centuries. Perhaps it was the historical appeal of the name that made it more popular at the turn of the century. Astrological appeal notwithstanding, it is not much in fashion today. Author Leo Tolstoy; actor Leo G. Carroll.
Lee, Leon, Leontios, Lev, Lion, Lyon

Leon Gk. Var. **Leo**. Very popular in the U.S. 1870–1890. Has not been revived, however. Author Leon Uris.

Leonard OG. "Lion-bold." Name of a saint who was much venerated in the Middle Ages (as patron of prisoners, among others), but did not inspire many parents until the 18th century. Use grew gradually to 1930, has diminished since. Artist Leonardo Da Vinci; composer Leonard Bernstein; actor Leonard Nimoy.
Lee, Len, Lenard, Lennard, Lennerd, Lennie, Lenny, Leo, Leon, Leonardo, Leonerd, Leonhard, Leonid, Leonidas, Leonides, Lonnard, Lonny

Leopold OG. "People brave." Use mainly British and European. The fact that it has been a royal or aristocratic name in Belgium, Austria, and Britain has not increased its sparse use.
Leo, Leupold

Leroy OF. "The king." Occupational name: one of the servants or pages of a king. Revived in the late 19th century, especially in America, but use today is minimal.
Elroi, Elroy, Lee, Leeroy, Leroi, Roy

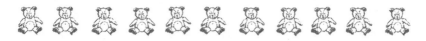

Leslie Scot. Gael. Place name: Some sources suggest "the gray castle." Became a last name, then (in the 18th century) a first name used for boys and girls. Boys' use has been tied to admiration for actor Leslie Howard, and is more common in Britain. Not much used now. Actor Leslie Nielsen.
Leslea, Leslee, Lesley, Lesly, Lezly

Lester OE. Place name: "From Leicester," an area in central England. First-name use dates from the mid–19th century, and its popularity lasted about 100 years. Georgia governor Lester Maddox.
Leicester, Les

Lev Rus. Var. **Leo.**

Leverett OF. "Baby rabbit." May indicate an ancestor who hunted or trapped rabbits.
Leveret, Leverit, Leveritt

Leverton OE. "From the rush-farm."

Levi Heb. "Joined, attached." In the Old Testament, one of Jacob's sons, whose descendants (known as the Levites) were Israel's tribe of priests. After its revival by the Puritans, the name has been steadily used.
Levey, Levin, Levon, Levy

Lewis Anglicization of **Louis**. Briefly popular in the late 19th century, but now takes a back seat to Louis, which is not particularly fashionable. Author Lewis Carroll.
Lew, Lewes, Lou, Louis

Liam Ir. Var. **William.** OG. "Will–helmet." Actor Liam Neeson.

Liberio Port. "Freedom."

Lidio Port. "From Lydia." Lydia was an area of Asia famous for its two rich kings, Midas and Croesus. The female form, Lydia, is more common than the male.

Lincoln OE. Place name: "Town by the pool." Surname transferred occasionally to a first name. The fame of Abraham Lincoln did not, surprisingly enough, encourage parents to use the name widely, and it is not a favorite today.
Linc, Link

Lindberg OG. Place name: "Linden tree mountain."

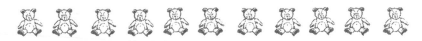

Would probably be unknown as a first name without the career of flier Charles Lindbergh. Very scarce.

Lindbergh, Lindburg, Lindy

Lindell OE. Place name: "Linden tree valley."

Lindall, Lindel, Lyndall, Lyndell

Lindley OE. "Linden tree meadow."

Lindlea, Lindlee, Lindleigh, Lindly

Lindsay OE. Place name: "Island of linden trees." Originally a surname, used for boys until the middle of this century, but now quite popular as a girl's name. Film director Lindsay Anderson.

Lind, Lindsee, Lindsey, Lindsy, Linsay, Linsey, Lyndsay, Lyndsey, Lyndsie

Linford OE. Place name: "Linden tree ford" or "flax ford." The elements meaning flax ("Lin-") and linden tree ("Lind-") are so similar that they have probably been confused over the years.

Lynford

Linley OE. Place name: "Flax meadow."

Linlea, Linlee, Linleigh, Linly

Linton OE. Place name: "Flax settlement."

Lintonn, Lynton, Lyntonn

Linus Gk. "Flax." May have originated as a descriptive name, applied to someone with flaxen or extremely pale hair. This description does not apply to today's best-known Linus, the famous *Peanuts* character who is lost without his blanket.

Lionel Lat. "Young lion." Used in the Middle Ages and never resoundingly revived beyond a twinge of popularity in the 1920s and 1930s. Actor Lionel Barrymore; pop star Lionel Richie.

Lionello

Litton OE. Place name: "Settlement on the hill." Author Lytton Strachey.

Lytton

Livingston OE. Place name: "Leif's settlement."

Livingstone

Llewellyn Welsh. "Resembling a lion." This is the generally accepted meaning, though some scholars think the

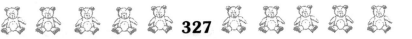

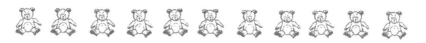

origin relates to an element meaning "leader." Rare outside of Wales in any case.

Lew, Llewellen

Lloyd Welsh. "Gray" or "sacred." One of the most common Welsh names in general use, perhaps because it is one of the simplest. Particularly widespread in the 1940s. Actor Lloyd Bridges; Senator Lloyd Bentsen.

Floyd, Loyd

Locke OE. Place name: "Woods" or "fortified place."

Lock, Lockwood

Logan Ir. Gael. Place name: "Small hollow." Author Logan Pearsall Smith.

Lombard Lat. "Long-bearded." May also have origins as a place name: Lombardy is an area in northern Italy. Very rare as a first name.

Lon Dim. **Alonso**. OG. "Ready for battle." Mostly associated with sinister film actor Lon Chaney.

Lonnie, Lonny

Loren Var. **Lawrence** via **Lorenzo**. A purely modern form, in use since the 1940s but not common.

Lorin, Lorren, Lorrin

Lorimer Lat. Occupational name: "Harness maker."

Lorrimer

Loring OG. "Renowned warrior's son." Related to **Louis**.

Lorring

Lorne Var. **Lawrence**. Also a Scottish place name, and more common in Scotland. Actor Lorne Green; TV producer Lorne Michaels.

Lorn

Louis OG./Fr. "Renowned warrior." The German form is Ludwig, and an early French variant was Clovis, a name borne by several Frankish kings. The later French kings (18 of them) who chose Louis as their name were no doubt harking back to those early monarchs, one of whom included the 13th-century saint. Lewis was the more common form in Britain until a mid–19th-century revival of Louis, which was very popular in the U.S. until the depression era. Musician Louis Armstrong; scientist Louis Pasteur; archaeologist Louis Leakey; author Louis L'Amour; actor Lou Gossett, Jr.

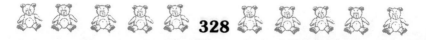

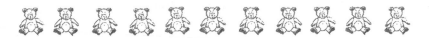

Aloysius, Lew, Lewes, Lewis, Lodovico, Lou, Louie, Lucho, Ludovic, Ludovicus, Ludvig, Ludvik, Ludwig, Luigi, Luis

Lowell OF. "Young wolf." Mostly 19th-century use. Poet Robert Lowell.

Lovel, Lovell, Lowe, Lowel

Lucas Var. **Luke**. Generally a transferred last name, but gaining popularity in Britain as a first name.

Lucian Lat. "Light." More unusual form of **Lucius,** which itself is quite rare. Artist Lucian Freud; opera star Luciano Pavarotti.

Luciano, Lucianus, Lucien, Lucio, Lucjan, Lukianos, Lukyan

Lucius Lat. "Light." Used by the Romans, but extremely scarce in the 20th century.

Luca, Lucas, Luce, Lucias, Lucio, Lukas, Luke

Ludlow OE. Place name: "Ruler's hill."

Ludlowe

Ludwig Ger. "Renowned in battle." Very unusual in English-speaking countries, where Louis or Lewis are used instead. Composer Ludwig van Beethoven.

Luke Gk. "From Lucanus," a region of southern Italy. Not, strictly speaking, a nickname for Lucius and Lucian, though it may be used that way. The most famous Luke is, of course, the author of the Gospel and of Acts. He was a physician, and is patron saint of doctors and artists. After medieval use, rather neglected, but a recent strong surge of interest in Britain may spark a revival in the U.S.

Loukas, Luc, Lucas, Lucian, Lucien, Lucio, Lucius, Luck, Lucky, Lukacs, Lukas

Lundy Scot. Place name "grove near the island," or possibly Fr. "Monday's child." Generally a transferred surname.

Lunn Ir. Gael. "Strong, warlike."

Lon, Lonn

Luther OG. "Army people." Generally homage to Martin Luther, the German religious reformer, or to Martin Luther King, Jr., the civil rights activist. Botanist Luther Burbank.

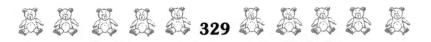

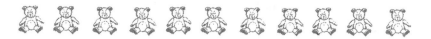

Lotario, Lothair, Lothar, Lothario, Lutero

Lyle OF. Place name: "The island." First-name use was mostly in the middle of this century.

Lisle, Lyall, Lyell, Lysle

Lyman OE. "Meadow-dweller."

Leaman, Leyman

Lynch Ir. Gael. "Mariner." One of the most common Irish last names, occasionally transferred for first-name use. Film director David Lynch.

Lyndon OE. Place name: "Linden tree hill." First-name use coincides with the 19th-century fondness for transferred surnames, but has been given extra renown by President Lyndon Baines Johnson.

Lin, Linden, Lindon, Lindy, Lyn, Lynden

Lysander Gk. "Liberator."

Mac Scot. Gael. "Son of." Also used as a nickname for given names that begin with "Mac-," many of which are transferred last names.

Mack, Mackey, Mackie

Macadam Scot. Gael. "Son of Adam." The 19th-century engineer John McAdam gave his name to a method of paving roads that became very widespread.

MacAdam, McAdam

Macallister Ir. Gael. "Son of Alistair." Alistair is the Scottish version of Alexander.

MacAlister, McAlister, McAllister

Macardle Ir. Gael. "Son of great courage."

MacArdell, McCardell

Macbride Ir. Gael. "Son of the follower of Saint Brigid,"who was an influential 5th-century Irish nun.

Macbryde, McBride

Maccoy Ir. Gael. "Son of Hugh." The phrase "the real Mc-

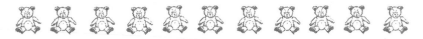

Coy" came from Scotland, where it referred to something of the highest quality.
MacCoy, McCoy

Maccrea Ir. Gael. "Son of grace." Actor Joel McCrea.
MacCrae, MacCray, MacCrea, Macrae, McCrea

Macdonald Scot. Gael. "Son of Donald." The McDonalds were a powerful Scottish clan.
MacDonald, McDonald

Macdougal Scot. Gael. "Son of Dougal." Since Dougal means "dark foreigner," this may refer to an ancestor who was a Viking invader (not all of whom were blond).
MacDougal, MacDowell, McDougal, McDowell

Macgowan Ir. Gael. "Son of the blacksmith."
MacGowan, Magowan, McGowan

Mackenzie Ir. Gael. "Son of the wise ruler."
McKenzie

Mackinley Ir. Gael. "Learned ruler." U.S. President William McKinley.
McKinley

Macmahon Ir. Gael. "Son of the bear." TV host Ed McMahon.
MacMahon, McMahon

Macmurray Ir. Gael. "Son of the seafarer." Actor Fred McMurray.
MacMurray, McMurray

Macy OF. Place name: "Matthew's estate." Department store founder R. H. Macy.
Macey

Maddock Old Welsh. "Benevolent, charitable."
Madoc, Madock, Madog

Maddox Anglo-Welsh. "Benefactor's son." A contracted form of "Maddock's son." Novelist Ford Madox Ford.
Madox

Madison OE. "Son of the mighty warrior." More common than many of these "son of" names, possibly because of admiration for U.S. President James Madison.
Maddison, Maddy, Madisson

Magee Ir. Gael. "Son of Hugh."
MacGee, MacGhee, McGee

Magnus Lat. "Great." Appropriately enough, a royal

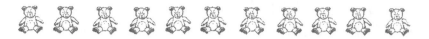

name in Norway and Denmark. It was transferred from Scandinavia to Scotland, where it is used somewhat.
Magnes, Manus

Maguire Ir. Gael. "Son of the beige one."
MacGuire, McGuire, McGwire

Major Lat. "Greater." Use (which is sparing) probably harks back to the military title used in the British and American armies.
Majer, Mayer, Mayor

Makarios Gk. "Blessed."
Macario, Macarios, Maccario, Maccarios

Malachi Heb. "Angel, messenger." Name of one of the minor prophets in the Old Testament, but not widely used. Author Malachi Martin.
Malachie, Malachy, Malechy

Malcolm Scot. Gael. "Devotee of St. Columba." The name of the prince of Scotland who became king after Macbeth murdered his father, Duncan. Shakespeare's play was based on historical fact. The name has been used primarily in Scotland, but spread more widely in the middle of the 20th century. Black families may use it in honor of Malcolm X. Publisher Malcolm Forbes.
Malcolum, Malkolm

Malik Arab. "Master." Actor Art Malik.
Maliq

Malin OE. "Little strong warrior."
Mallin, Mallon

Mallory OF. "Unhappy, unlucky." Literally, *malheureux*. Originally a nickname, transferred to a last name and thus to a first name. Poet Sir Thomas Malory.
Mallery, Mallorie, Malory

Maloney Ir. Gael. "Pious, disciple of Sunday worship."
Malone, Malony

Malvin Var. **Melvin**. Could come from a number of sources: possibly Ir. Gael. "Polished chief," OE. "council-friend," or an adaptation of **Melville**.
Malvinn, Malvyn

Mandel Ger. "Almond."
Mandell

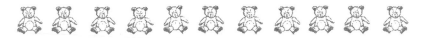

Manfred OE. "Man of peace." Seldom found in real life, but used by Byron for an antihero in an epic poem.
Manfrid, Manfried, Mannfred, Mannfryd

Manley OE. Place name: "Man's meadow." Or originally a descriptive term meaning "masculine." Poet Gerard Manley Hopkins.
Manlea, Manleigh, Manly

Manning OE. "Son of the man."

Mansel OE. "From the manse." A manse is a house occupied by a clergyman.
Mansell

Mansfield OE. Place name: "Field by the little river."

Manton OE. Place name: "Man's or hero's town."
Manten, Mannton

Manuel Dim. **Emanuel**. Heb. "God be with us." Most widely used in Spanish-speaking countries. Shoe designer Manolo Blahnik.
Mano, Manolo

Manville OF. Place name: "Great town."
Mandeville, Manvile, Manvill

Marcel Fr. Dim. **Marcellus**. Lat. "Little warrior." One of the less common of a group of names that all have their root in the Roman god of war, Mars. Author Marcel Proust; pantomime artist Marcel Marceau.
Marceau, Marcelin, Marcellin, Marcellino, Marcello, Marcellus, Marcelo, Marcely

Marcus Lat. "Warlike." The root of such names as Mark and Marcel, and based on the name of the Roman war god, Mars. Common enough in Roman times, but unknown in English-speaking countries until the 19th century. When Mark was hugely popular in the 1970s, Marcus also crept up the charts possibly boosted by the hit TV series "Marcus Welby, M.D."
Marc, Marco, Marko, Markus

Marden OE. Place name: "The valley with the pool."

Mario It. Var. **Mark**.
Marius

Marion Fr. Var. **Mary**. Heb. "Bitter or rebellious." Almost always a girl's name, and likely to cause some confusion if given to a boy. The most famous male Marion, Marion

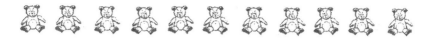

Morrison, chose the unmistakably masculine "John Wayne" when he changed his name.

Mariano

Mark Lat. "Warlike." The anglicized version of Marcus. In spite of the automatic exposure given the name by the evangelist Saint Mark, it was not popular in the Middle Ages, nor indeed was it really common until a sudden inexplicable flurry of use in the 1950s. The popular author Mark Twain (whose real name was Samuel Clemens) took his pseudonym from the call of Mississippi River boatmen: "Mark twain!" meant that the water they were navigating was two fathoms deep. Explorer Marco Polo; choreographer Mark Mitchell; New York governor Mario Cuomo; swimmer Mark Spitz.

Marc, Marco, Marcos, Marcus, Mario, Marius, Marko, Markos, Markus

Marland OE. Place name: "Land near the lake."

Marley OE. Place name: "Meadow near the lake." Musician Bob Marley.

Marlea, Marleigh, Marly

Marlon OF. "Little hawk." Current use is inspired by the career of actor Marlon Brando.

Marlin

Marlow OE. Place name: "Hill near the lake." Rare as a first name, though classic film lovers might be reminded of Humphrey Bogart as Philip Marlowe in *The Big Sleep*. English playwright Christopher Marlowe.

Marlowe

Marmion OF. "Tiny one." Extremely rare, though used by Sir Walter Scott in a popular narrative poem of that title.

Marmyon

Marsden OE. Place name: "Swampy valley." Painter Marsden Hartley.

Marsdon

Marsh OE. Place name: "Swamp or marsh." Like Marsden and Marston, more generally a last name, occasionally used as a first name. Nineteenth-century parents were particularly fond of transferring surnames as given names.

Marshall OF. Occupational name: "Horse-keeper." Also a

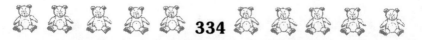

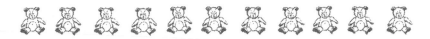

military title of great honor, as in "field marshal." As a last name, common in Scotland, and used rather widely as a first name since the early 19th century. Department store founder Marshall Field; media theorist Marshall McLuhan.

Marschal, Marsh, Marshal, Marshell

Marston OE. Place name: "Town by the marsh."

Martin Lat. "Warlike." Like Marcus and its variants, Martin originates with the Roman war god, Mars. The 4th-century Saint Martin (most famous for dividing his cloak in two and giving half to a beggar) was much venerated, making his name popular in the Middle Ages. The influence of Protestant reformer Martin Luther may have added to the name's appeal, since it was used very steadily right into the 19th century. The pattern since then has been of growing disuse, except for a spurt of popularity in the 1950s. U.S. President Martin Van Buren; civil rights activist Martin Luther King, Jr.; film director Martin Scorsese.

Marinos, Mart, Martel, Martell, Marten, Martie, Martijn, Martinien, Martino, Martinos, Martinus, Marton, Marty, Martyn

Marvin Origin obscure, though many sources suggest OE. "sea lover," while others claim that it is Welsh. Popular in America starting in the 19th century, peaking in the 1920s, and now unusual. Actor Lee Marvin; songwriter Marvin Hamlisch; singer Marvin Gaye.

Marve, Marven, Marwin, Marwynn, Mervin, Mervyn, Merwin, Merwyn, Murvin, Murvynn

Marwood OE. Place name: "Lake near the woods."

Maslin OF. "Little Thomas."

Maslen, Masling

Mason OF. Occupational name: "Stoneworker." Transferred from surname status starting in the mid–19th century. Actor James Mason.

Mather OE. "Powerful army." The surname of a dynasty of 17th- and 18th-century Massachusetts theologians, Richard, Increase, and Cotton Mather.

Matthew Heb. "Gift of the Lord." Like Mark, Luke, and John, given great exposure by the author of one of the

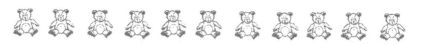

four Gospels. In more religious eras, parents would hear these names over and over again in the course of a year. Matthew began to be neglected in the 19th century and was little used early in the 20th until an enthusiastic revival at midcentury. Popularity is beginning to ebb again. Actors Matthew Broderick, Matthew Modine; photographer Mathew Brady; poet Matthew Arnold; tennis star Mats Wilander.

Mat, Mata, Mateo, Mateusz, Mathé, Matheu, Mathew, Mathian, Mathias, Mathieu, Matias, Mats, Matt, Mattaeus, Mattaus, Matteo, Matthaus, Mattheus, Matthias, Matthiew, Mattias, Mattie, Mattieu, Matty, Matvey, Matyas, Matz

Matthias Ger. Var. **Matthew.**

Mathias, Mattias

Maurice Lat. "Dark-skinned, Moorish." Roman name brought to Britain by the Normans and widely used into the 17th century. A 19th-century revival faded around the end of that century, and it is now largely neglected. Actor Maurice Chevalier; writer Maurice Sendak; composer Maurice Ravel.

Mauricio, Maurids, Maurie, Maurise, Maurits, Maurizio, Maury, Maurycy, Morey, Morice, Moricz, Moris, Moritz, Moriz, Morrel, Morrey, Morrice, Morrill, Morris, Morriss, Moss

Max Dim. **Maxwell, Maximilian.** Appeared at the turn of the 20th century, fashionable by the 1930s, then faded, but parents of the late 1980s were showing interest in it again. Writer Max Beerbohm; actor Max von Sydow.

Maximilian Lat. "Greatest." Appropriately enough, used by the emperor of Mexico and the Holy Roman emperor, though a bit of a mouthful for a child. Actor Maximilian Schell.

Mac, Mack, Maks, Maksim, Maksym, Maksymilian, Massimiliano, Massimo, Max, Maxey, Maxemilian, Maxemilion, Maxie, Maxim, Maxime, Maximiliano, Maximilianus, Maximilien, Maximillian, Maximo, Maximos, Maxy, Maxymilian, Maxymillian

Maxwell OE. Place name: Maybe "Maccus's well," though some sources also suggest "large well" or "important

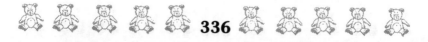

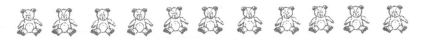

man's well." Mostly Scottish last name, fairly common as a first name. Editor Maxwell Perkins; playwright Maxwell Anderson.

Mayer Lat. "Larger." Var. **Major**. Also Ger. "Farmer."

Mayfield OE. Place name: "Strong one's field."

Mayhew OF. Var. **Matthew**. Heb. "Gift of the Lord."

Maynard OE. "Hard strength." See **Meinhard**. Economist John Maynard Keynes.
   Mayne, Maynhard, Meinhard, Menard

Mayo Ir. Gael. Place name: "Yew tree plain." Mayo is a county in western Ireland. It is also most commonly the short name for a condiment used in sandwiches, a fact parents should bear in mind.

Mead OE. Place name: "Meadow."
   Meade, Meed

Medwin OG. "Strong friend."

Meinhard Ger. "Hard strength." Maynard is the anglicized form.
   Maynard, Meinhardt

Meinrad Ger. "Strong counsel."

Mel Dim. **Melvin** and other "Mel-" names. Actor Mel Gibson; filmmaker Mel Brooks.

Melbourne OE. Place name: "Mill stream." Also the name of a prominent city in Australia. Occasional use.
   Mel, Melborn, Melburn, Milbourn, Milbourne, Milburn, Millburn, Millburne

Melchior Pol. "King." Traditionally the name of one of the Three Kings, along with Caspar and Balthasar.
   Melker, Melkior

Meldon OE. Place name: "Mill hill."
   Melden

Meldrick OE. "Mill ruler."

Melville OE./OF. Place name: "Industrious one's town."

Melvin Could come from a number of sources: possibly Ir. Gael. "polished chief," OE. "sword friend," or an adaptation of Melville.
   Malvin, Malvyn, Malvynn, Mel, Melvyn, Melwin, Melwyn, Melwynn, Vinnie

Menachem Heb. "Comforter." Israeli statesman Menachem Begin.

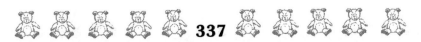

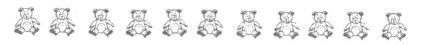

Menahem, Nachum, Nahum

Mendel Semitic. "Wisdom, learning."

Mendell, Mendeley

Mercer Middle English. Occupational name: "Store-keeper." Choreographer Merce Cunningham.

Merce

Meredith Welsh. "Great ruler." More commonly a girl's name, but still clung to for boys in Wales. Composer Meredith Willson.

Meredyth, Merideth, Meridith

Merle Fr. "Blackbird." Very rare for boys.

Merlin Middle English. "Small falcon." Also the name (via a mistranslation: see **Mervin**) of the wizard of the Arthurian legends. Use dates from the 20th century.

Marlin, Marlon, Merle, Merlen, Merlinn, Merlyn, Merlynn

Merrick Anglicization of a Welsh variant of **Maurice**. Used from time to time in this century.

Merrik, Meyrick

Merrill Origin disputed, perhaps OF. "famous" or a phonetic variation of the girl's name Meryl. Its status as a surname probably depends on the medieval use of its antecedent, Muriel.

Meril, Merill, Merrel, Merrell, Merril, Meryl

Merritt OE. "Little renowned one."

Merrett, Merit, Meritt

Merton OE. Place name: "Town by the lake." Theologian Thomas Merton.

Merwyn, Murton

Mervin Old Welsh. "Sea hill." Mervyn is more common in Britain. Merlin the wizard of Arthurian legend was known in Welsh as Myrddin, translated into Latin as Merlin. The name was mildly popular around the turn of the century.

Mervyn, Mervynn, Merwin, Merwinn, Merwyn, Murvin, Murvyn

Meshach Heb. Meaning unknown. Old Testament name: one of three Hebrew men (along with the now obsolete Shadrach and Abednego) thrown into a fiery furnace by King Nebuchadnezzar and rescued by an angel. Used

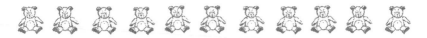

sparingly in the 19th century, even more rare today. Actor Meshach Taylor.

Meyer Ger. "farmer"; Heb. "bringer of light." Architect Richard Meier.

Mayeer, Mayer, Mayor, Meier, Meir, Myer

Micah Heb. Var. **Michael**. Very easily confused with Michael when it is spoken.

Mike, Mikey, Mikal, Mycah

Michael Heb. "Who is like the Lord?" In the New Testament, Michael is the name of the archangel who defeats the dragon. Usage was steady until a period of neglect that lasted from the early 19th to the early 20th century. The subsequent revival was immense, and Michael was, according to many listings, the most popular name for American boys in the 1970s and 1980s. Baseball star Mickey Mantle; actors Mickey Rooney, Michael Caine, Michael J. Fox; singers Michael Jackson, Mick Jagger; cartoon star Mickey Mouse; Soviet president Mikhail Gorbachev.

Micael, Mical, Michal, Micheal, Michel, Michele, Michiel, Mickey, Micky, Miguel, Mihail, Mihaly, Mikael, Mike, Mikel, Mikey, Mikhail, Mikhalis, Mikhos, Mikkel, Mikol, Mischa, Misha, Mitch, Mitchell, Mychal, Mykal, Mykell

Miles Several possible origins, including Lat. "soldier," OG. "merciful," or variant of **Emil** (Lat. "eager to please"). Since the end of the 18th century, it has been quite unusual. Pilgrim leader Miles Standish; musician Miles Davis.

Milo, Myles

Milford OE. Place name: "Mill-ford."

Millard OE. "Guardian of the mill." U.S. President Millard Fillmore.

Millward, Milward

Miller OE. Occupational name. Use as a first name began in the late 19th century, is now sparing. Playwright Arthur Miller.

Millar, Myller

Mills OE. Place name "near the mills," or possibly a contraction of "Miles's son."

Milo Ger. Var. **Miles**. Very unusual. Actor Milo O'Shea.

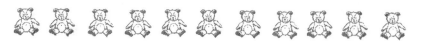

Milton OE. Place name: "Mill town" or perhaps "middle town." One of the more commonplace names transferred to a first name, dating from the early 19th century. Poet John Milton; comedian Milton Berle.
Milt, Mylton

Minor Lat. "Younger." Photographer Minor White.
Mynor

Misha Rus. Var. **Michael**. Given some modern exposure as the nickname of superstar dancer Mikhail Baryshnikov.
Mischa

Mitchell Middle English. Var. **Michael**. The last name evolved in the Middle Ages, when surnames began to be regularly used, and it was transferred back to a first name in the 19th century. It was popular in the middle of the 20th century, but now less common. Band leader Mitch Miller.
Mitch, Mitchel, Mytch

Modred OE. "Brave counselor." In the Arthurian legend, Modred is Arthur's illegitimate son who tries to claim his father's throne, and engineers his ultimate downfall.
Mordred

Mohammed Arab. "Highly praised." The name of the prophet and founder of Islam. Boxer Mohammed Ali.
Mahomet, Mohammad, Muhammad, Muhammed

Monahan Ir. Gael. "Monk."
Monaghan, Monoghan

Monroe Ir. Gael. Place name: May mean "mouth of the Roe River" or possibly "the red marsh." U.S. President James Monroe.
Monro, Munro, Munroe

Montague Fr. Place name: "Sharply pointed mount." More common as first name in the 19th century.
Montagu

Montgomery OE. Place name: "Mount of the rich man." Unusual as a first name, and very likely to be shortened to "Monty." Actor Montgomery Clift.
Montgomerie, Monty

Monty Dim. "Mont-" names like Montague and Montgomery, used rarely as a given name. Given slightly ri-

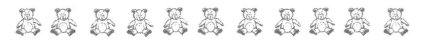

diculous connotations by TV master of ceremonies Monty Hall and British comedy troupe Monty Python.

Moore OE. Place name: "the moors" or OF. "dark-skinned" (as in "Moorish").
More

Mordecai Heb. Meaning not clear, but possibly "follower of Marduk" (who was a god of the Babylonians). An Old Testament name revived by the Puritans and neglected since the 19th century.
Mordechai, Mordy, Mort

Moreland OE. Place name: "Moor-land." Moor is a British term referring to a large, rolling expanse of scrubby, infertile wild land.
Moorland, Morland

Morgan Different sources give several meanings, including Welsh. "great and bright" and OE. "bright or white sea dweller." The name is most common in Wales, however, as both a first and a last name. Actor Morgan Freeman.
Morgen, Morgun, Morrgan

Morley OE. Place name: "Meadow on the moor." TV commentator Morley Safer.
Moorley, Moorly, Morlee, Morleigh, Morly, Morrley

Morris Anglicization of **Maurice**. Now more common as a surname, though it was once interchangeable with **Maurice**.
Morice, Moris, Morrison, Morrisson

Morse OE. "Son of Maurice." Contracted from **Morrison**. Inventor Samuel F. B. Morse.
Morrison

Mortimer OF. Place name: "Still water." Literally, "dead sea" *(mort mer)*. First-name use, as with so many of these place names, dates from the 19th century.
Mort, Morty, Mortymer

Morton OE. Place name: "Moor town." Like Mortimer, used as a first name since the 19th century, though probably more common.
Morten

Morven Scot. Gael. "Huge mountain." First-name use is mostly Scottish, and generally confined to girls.

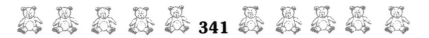

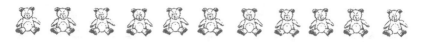

Morfin, Morfinn, Morfyn, Morvyn

Moses History unclear. Some sources suggest Heb. "savior," while others claim it means "taken from the water." The latter definition clearly comes from the biblical story of the infant Moses afloat in the bulrushes, whence he was rescued by Pharaoh's daughter, later to become the great leader of the exiled Israelites. Always current in Jewish families, adopted by the Puritans in the 17th century, now uncommon. Israeli defense minister Moshe Dayan.

Mo, Moe, Moise, Moises, Mose, Moshe, Mosheh, Mosie, Moss, Moyses, Mozes

Muhammad Arab. "Greatly praised." Name of the prophet and founder of Islam.

Hamid, Hammad, Mahmoud, Mahmud, Mahomet, Mohamet, Mohammed, Muhamet, Muhammed

Muir Scot. Gael. Place name: "Moor." Naturalist John Muir.

Murdock Scot. Gael. "Sea fighter" or "sailor." Generally Scottish usage; in the U.S., occurs mainly as a transferred surname.

Murdo, Murdoch, Murtagh, Murtaugh

Muriel Ir. Gael. "Sea bright."

Murphy Ir. Gael. "Sea fighter." A quintessentially Irish last name, in occasional use as a first name.

Murfey

Murray Scot. Gael. Place name, or possibly "mariner." Somewhat common as a first name in the 1930s and 1940s, but now little used.

Moray, Murrey, Murry

Myron Gk. "Fragrant oil." Not, despite its sound, related to myrrh (as carried by the Three Kings). Like Murray, most common in the middle third of the 20th century.

Nabil Arab. "Highborn."
  Nabeel
Nachman Heb. "Comforter."
  Menachem, Menahem, Nahum
Nadim Arab. "Friend."
Nairn Scot. Gael. Place name: "River with alder trees."
Nairne
Naldo Sp. Dim. **Reginald.** OG. "Powerful advice."
Najib Arab. "Of highborn parentage."
  Najeeb
Napoleon OG. Meaning unclear, though tradition says it means "lion of Naples." Napoleon Bonaparte (who obviously inspired its use) came not from Naples, but from Corsica.
  Leon, Nap, Napoleone
Narcisse Fr. "Daffodil." Not, as it would be in English, a flower name, but the name of a beautiful Greek youth who became enamored of his own reflection—hence "narcissism."
  Narcissus, Narkissos
Nasser Arab. "The winner."
Nat Dim. **Nathan, Nathaniel.**
Natal Sp. "Birthday." Referring, of course, to the birthday of Jesus, or Christmas.
  Natale, Natalino, Natalio, Nataly
Nathan Heb. "Given." Old Testament name, revived in the 18th century and quite popular in the last 40 years. Nathan Hale was the American spy who declared, just before he was hanged by the British in 1776, "I regret that I have but one life to lose for my country."
  Nat, Nate, Nathen
Nathaniel Heb. "Given by God." New Testament name of one of the apostles (who was also called Bartholomew). Used by the Puritans, and a steady presence ever since. Author Nathaniel Hawthorne; musician Nat "King" Cole; slave insurrectionist Nat Turner.
  Nat, Natanael, Nataniel, Nate, Nathan, Nathaneal,
  Nathanial, Nathanyal, Nathanyel, Nethaniel, Nethanyel,
  Thaniel

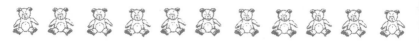

Neal Ir. Var. **Neil.**
Neale, Neall, Nealle, Neel

Ned Dim. **Edward** OE. "wealthy defender"; **Edmund** OE. "wealthy protector."

Nehemiah Heb. "The Lord's comfort." Old Testament prophet, Puritan name, rare in this century.
Nechemya

Neil Ir. Gael. "Champion." Although the name of the most famous Celtic king of Ireland (Niall of the Nine Hostages), it has been used mostly in Scotland until the middle of this century. Astronaut Neil Armstrong; singers Neil Diamond and Neil Young; playwright Neil Simon.
Neal, Neale, Neall, Nealle, Nealon, Neel, Neile, Neill, Neille, Neils, Nels, Nial, Niall, Niel, Niles

Nels Scan. Var. **Nicholas.**

Nelson Eng. "Son of Neil." Established by parents who admired the exploits of English Admiral Nelson at the Battle of Trafalgar. Used consistently, if never widely, since then. Actor Nelson Eddy; New York Governor and U.S. Vice President Nelson Rockefeller; South African activist Nelson Mandela.
Nealson, Neils, Nels, Niles, Nils, Nilson, Nilsson

Nemesio Sp. "Justice."

Neptune Roman god of the sea, and a fanciful name for sea-loving parents.

Nesbit OE. Place name: "Bend shaped like a nose." Refers to a bend in a road, or else to a plot of land.
Naisbit, Naisbitt, Nesbitt, Nisbet, Nisbett

Nestor Gk. "Traveler, voyager." Cinematographer Nestor Almendros.

Neville OF. Place name: "New town." More common in Britain, but very rare in the U.S. Musical conductor Neville Marriner.
Nev, Nevil, Nevile, Nevyle

Nevin Ir. Gael. "Holy, sacred."
Nev, Nevan, Nevins, Niven

Newell OE. Place name: "New hall." The "hall" was often a term for the local manor in early England.
Newall, Newel, Newhall

Newland OE. Place name: "New land."

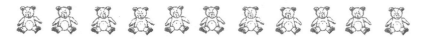

Newlin Old Welsh. Place name: "New pond."

Newman OE. "Newcomer." Began to be used as a first name in England in the 19th century, perhaps influenced by the fame of reforming cleric John Henry (Cardinal) Newman. Now scarce.

Newton OE. Place name: "New town." Like many place names turned last names, made the move to a first name in the 19th century, and has now drifted back to last-name status. Entertainer Wayne Newton.

Niall Ir. Gael. "Champion." A less common variant of **Neil**.
Nial

Nicholas Gk. "People of victory." A New Testament name given even greater fame by the 4th-century Saint Nicholas, patron saint of children and (via his Dutch name, Sinte Klaas) the original Santa Claus. The name was widespread in the Middle Ages through the 17th century, then had a long period of disuse which ended in the middle of the 20th century. Theater director Nikos Psacharapolous; Dickens novel *Nicholas Nickleby*; actors Nicholas Cage, Nickolas Grace, Nicol Williamson; composer Nicolai Rimsky-Korsakov; political philosopher Niccolò Machiavelli.

Claas, Claes, Claus, Colas, Cole, Colet, Colin, Collin, Klaas, Klaes, Klaus, Nic, Nicanor, Niccolo, Nichol, Nichole, Nicholl, Nichols, Nick, Nickey, Nickie, Nicklas, Nickolas, Nickolaus, Nicky, Nicol, Nicola, Nicolaas, Nicolai, Nicolas, Nicolao, Nicolis, Nicoll, Nicolls, Nicolo, Nik, Niki, Nikita, Nikki, Nikky, Niklaas, Niklas, Nikolai, Nikolas, Nikolaus, Nikolay, Nikolos, Nikos, Nilos

Nicodemus Gk. "Victory of the people." New Testament name, very scarce.
Nikodema

Niels Dan. Var. **Neil**.
Niel, Niles, Nils

Nigel Ir. Gael. "Champion." Related not, as many sources claim, to the Latin *niger* ("black"), but to the Latin form of Neil, Nigellus. Almost exclusively a British name, popular in this century. Actor Nigel Havers.

Nissim Heb. "Wondrous things."

Nixon OE. "Son of Nicholas." A contraction of "Nicolas's

son," or "Nick's son." After the disgrace of President Nixon in the early 1970s, unlikely to be used as a first name.

Noah Heb. Meaning unclear, possibly "rest" or "wandering." The latter would be appropriate for the patriarch who drifted in the ark for 40 days. Steadily but not widely used since the 17th century. Lexicographer Noah Webster.
Noach, Noak, Noé

Noble Lat. "Aristocratic." Use as a first name may derive from surnames, or from the use of the adjective as a name. Mostly 19th century.

Noel Fr. "Christmas." Used since the Middle Ages, but not very widespread. More likely to be used for girls. Playwright and actor Noel Coward.
Nata, Natale, Nowel, Nowell

Nolan Ir. Gael. "Renowned." A last name transferred to first name. Baseball star Nolan Ryan.
Noland, Nolen, Nolin, Nollan

Norbert OG. "Renowned northerner." Saint's name that was mildly popular in the middle of the 20th century.
Bert, Bertie, Berty, Norberto

Norman OE. "Northerner." The Normans of France were originally from Scandinavia, or the North, but the name was also used in England even before the Norman Conquest. After medieval use, it was neglected until a substantial 19th-century revival, which has long since faded. Artist Norman Rockwell; authors Norman Vincent Peale, Norman Mailer; TV producer Norman Lear.
Norm, Normand, Normen, Normie

Norris OF. "Northerner." May also derive from the French word for "nurse." Modern use dates from the 19th century.

Northcliff OE. Place name: "Northern cliff."
Northcliffe, Northclyff, Northclyffe

Northrop OE. Place name: "Northern farm." Critic Northrop Frye.
Northrup

Norton OE. Place name: "Northern town." Revived as a first name in the mid–19th century.

Norville Old Anglo/Fr. Place name: "Northern town."

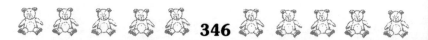

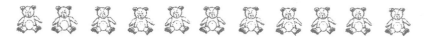

Norval, Norvel, Norvell, Norvil, Norvill, Norvylle
Norvin OE. "Northern friend."
  Norvyn, Norwin, Norwinn, Norwyn, Norwynn
Norward OE. "Warden of the north."
  Norwerd
Norwell OE. "Northern well."
Norwood OE. "Woods in the north."
Nuncio It. "Messenger." Comes from the same root that
  gives us the word "announce."
  Nunzio
Nuri Arab. "Light."
  Noori, Nur, Nuriel, Nuris

Oakes OE. Place name: "Near the oak
  trees." Transferred surname.
  Oak, Oaks, Ochs
Oakley OE. Place name: "Oak-tree
  meadow." The equally unusual Ackerley
  and Acton also refer to landmark oak trees.
  Oak, Oakes, Oakleigh, Oaklee, Oakly
Obadiah Heb. "Servant of God." One of the lesser Old
  Testament prophets. The name has faded gradually from
  sight after its revival by the Puritans in the 17th century.
  Obadias, Obed, Obediah, Obie, Ovadiah, Ovadiach
Oberon OG. "Highborn and bearlike." This is its more
  famous (though little-used) form, as used by Shake-
  speare for the King of the Fairies in *A Midsummer Night's
  Dream*. It also occurs (very rarely) as Auberon.
Obert OG. "Wealthy and bright."
Octavius Lat. "Eighth child." In English-speaking coun-
  tries the name had its heyday in the Victorian era of
  large families. It has survived slightly better in Latin
  countries. Mexican poet Octavio Paz.
  **Octave, Octavian, Octavien, Octavio, Octavo, Octavus,
  Ottavio**
Odell Derivation disputed. Some sources relate it to either

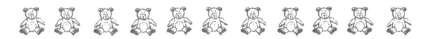

German "rich" or Greek "song," but *The Facts on File Dictionary of First Names* claims that it derives from an Old English place name: "Woad hill." Woad is a blue dye reputedly used by the ancient Druids in their religious rites.

Dell, Odall, Odie

Odolf OG. "Prosperous wolf." In the Middle Ages, to allude to a man as a "wolf" was to compliment his fierceness and courage.

Odolff

Ogden OE. Place name: "Oak valley." Launched as a first name in the 19th century, but never widely used. Poet Ogden Nash.

Ogdan, Ogdon

Olaf Scan. "Ancestor." A royal name in Norway, but when it came to the British Isles with Norse invaders, it did not catch on. Novelist Ole Edvart Rolvaag.

Olaff, Olav, Olave, Ole, Olin, Olle, Olof, Olov

Oleg Rus. "Holy." Fashion designer Oleg Cassini.

Olin Eng. Var. **Olaf**.

Olen, Olyn

Oliver Lat. "Olive tree" is the most common meaning assigned, but some scholars suggest ONorse. "kindly" or "ancestor," among other possibilities. It came to Britain from France, and the controversial Lord Protector Oliver Cromwell made it unpopular for generations. A mild revival occurred in the late 19th century. Charles Dickens's *Oliver Twist*; director Oliver Stone; comic actor Oliver Hardy.

Noll, Oliverio, Olivero, Olivier, Oliviero, Olivor, Olley, Ollie, Olliver, Ollivor

Omar Arab. "Elevated; follower of the Prophet." Heb. "expressive." Currently popular in Arab countries and among Muslims in the U.S. Poet Omar Khayyam; actor Omar Sharif; General Omar Bradley.

Onslow OE. Place name: "Enthusiast's hill."

Ounslow

Oran Ir. Gael. "Green."

Oren, Orin, Orran, Orren, Orrin

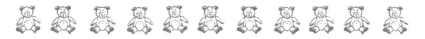

Oren Heb. "pine tree"; Ir. Gael. "fair, pale-skinned." Very unusual. U.S. Senator Orrin Hatch.
Orin, Orren, Orrin

Orestes Gk. "Man of the mountain." An important figure in Greek myth, the son of Agamemnon and the brother of Electra, with whose help he murdered his mother (to avenge his father, whom *she* had murdered). Orestes appears in 8 of the classic Greek tragedies.
Aresty, Oreste

Orford OE. Place name: "Ford of cattle."

Orion Gk. "Son of fire or light." In Greek myth, Orion was a mighty hunter who was turned into the constellation of the same name.

Orlando Sp. Var. **Roland**. OG. "Famous land." Mostly literary and minor late–19th-century use. Composer Orlando Gibbons.
Land, Lanny, Orlan, Orland, Roland, Rolando

Orman OG. "sea-man" or OE. "spear-man."
Ormand

Ormond OE. place name "mountain of bears," or "spear or ship protector"; Ir. Gael. "red." Irish last name, occasionally transferred.
Ormand, Ormonde

Oro Sp. "Golden."

Orrick OE. Place name: "Old oak tree." Poet Orric Johns.
Orric

Orson Lat. "Like a bear." In an old French story, a child named Orson is reared in the forest by a bear. The name is very unusual, though it may be used by ardent fans of director Orson Welles. Actor Orson Bean.
Orsen, Orsin, Orsini, Orsino, Sonny, Urson

Orton OE. Place name: "Shore settlement." Playwright Joe Orton.

Orval OE. "Strength of a spear." Also variant of **Orville**.

Orville OF. Place name: "Town of gold." Though the name translates this way, it may actually have been coined by an 18th-century novelist. Never widespread. Flight pioneer Orville Wright.
Orv, Orval, Orvell, Orvil

Orvin OE. "Spear-friend."
Orwin, Orwynn

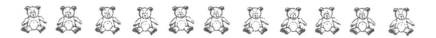

Osbert OE. "Divine and bright." Anglo-Saxon name revived mildly with the antiquarian craze of the 19th century, but now extremely rare. Poet Osbert Sitwell.

Osborn OE. "Divine bear." The 19th-century revival of this Anglo-Saxon name was followed by another small spurt of use in the middle of the 20th century. Rock star Ozzy Osbourne.

Osborne, Osbourn, Osbourne, Osburn, Osburne, Ozzie

Oscar Scan. "Divine spear." Anglo-Saxon name revived by 18th-century literary use, reaching substantial popularity by the late 19th century. Fans of "Sesame Street" would hesitate to name a baby for the curmudgeonly Oscar the Grouch. Lyricist Oscar Hammerstein II; playwright Oscar Wilde; fashion designer Oscar de la Renta.

Oskar, Osker, Ossie, Ozzy

Osgood OE. "Divine Goth."

Osmar OE. "Divine and wonderful."

Osmond OE. "Divine protector." Anglo-Saxon name revived in the 19th century, but scarcely found now.

Osman, Osmonde, Osmont, Osmund, Osmunde

Osred OE. "Divine counsel."

Osric OE. "Divine ruler."

Osrick

Osten Var. **Austin.** Lat. "Worthy of respect."

Austen, Austin, Ostin, Ostyn

Oswald OE. "Divine power." Another Anglo-Saxon name that endured partially because of the fame of two saints of the name. Use has been mostly 19th century, though actor Ozzie Nelson's real name was Oswald.

Ossie, Osvald, Oswaldo, Oswell, Ozzie, Waldo

Oswin OE. "Divine friend."

Osvin, Oswinn, Oswyn, Oswynn

Othman OG. "Wealthy man."

Otis OE. "Son of Otto." Use is mostly American. Actor Otis Skinner; composer Otis Redding.

Oates, Otess

Otto OG. "Prosperous." German name that was fairly common in English-speaking countries until Otto von Bismarck's German armies became threateningly pow-

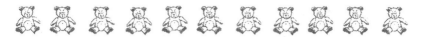

erful at the turn of the 20th century. The Second World War against Germany further limited the name's use.
Odo, Othello, Otho

Oved Heb. "Worshiper, follower."

Owen Welsh. Var. **Eugene**. Gk. "wellborn." Fairly common outside Wales since the 18th century. Author Owen Wister.
Ewen, Owain, Owin

Oxford OE. Place name: "Ford of the oxen." To parents, either a kind of laced shoe or a famous English university.

Pablo Sp. Var. **Paul** Lat. "Little." Artist Pablo Picasso; cellist Pablo Casals.

Paco Sp. Var. **Francis**. Lat. "From France." A diminutive of Francisco. Fashion designer Paco Rabanne.

Paddy Ir. Var. **Patrick**. Unusual as a given name, though so common as a nickname that it used to be used as a term for Irishmen. Author Paddy Chayefsky.
Paddey, Paddie, Padraic, Padraig

Page Fr. A young boy in training as a personal assistant to a knight. Usually a transferred surname, possibly indicating an ancestor who was a page. In the U.S., more often used as a girl's name.
Padget, Padgett, Paget, Pagett, Paige, Payge

Palmer OE. "One who holds a palm." Usually indicates a pilgrim, who would have carried a palm branch on his pilgrimage.
Pallmer, Palmar

Paquito Sp. Dim. **Francis**. Lat. "From France."
Paco

Paris OE. Place name: "From Paris," the city. Also a figure in Greek myth who was Helen of Troy's lover. Use is predominantly American.
Parris

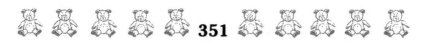

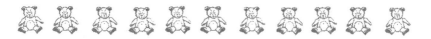

Parker OE. "Park keeper." Occupational name turned surname, popular in the 19th century as a given name but now more scarce. Actor Parker Stevenson.
Parke, Parkes, Parks

Parkin OE. "Little Peter."

Parnell OF. "Little Peter." Made famous by the 19th-century Irish politician Charles Parnell, who campaigned for home rule in Ireland.
Parrnell, Pernell

Parr OE. Place name: "Castle park."

Parrish OF. "Ecclesiastical locality." A parish is the area under the care of one pastor or priest. The name would originally have been a last name based on a place name.
Parish

Parry Old Welsh. "Son of Harry." Composer Hubert Parry.
Parrey, Parrie

Pascal Fr. "Child of Easter." Used as a first name in English-speaking countries only since the 1960s. Philosopher Blaise Pascal.
Pascale, Pascalle, Paschal, Paschalis, Pascuale, Pasquale

Patrick Lat. "Noble, patrician." A Roman name made famous by the 5th-century missionary (and patron of Ireland) Saint Patrick, whose feast day on March 17 is celebrated with parades in the United States, an honor accorded to no other saint. The name spread outside of Ireland in the 18th century and was widely used in the middle of the 20th century, but has now lost some popularity. U.S. statesman Patrick Henry; actor Patrick Swayze.
Paddey, Paddie, Paddy, Padhraig, Padraic, Padraig, Padriac, Pat, Patric, Patrice, Patricio, Patrik, Patrizio, Patrizius, Patryk, Pats, Patten, Patton, Patty

Patton OE. Place name: "Fighter's town." Almost too appropriate a meaning for the name of General George Patton. Author Alan Paton.
Paten, Patin, Paton, Patten, Pattin

Paul Lat. "Small." Popular Roman and medieval name whose tremendously widespread modern use dates from

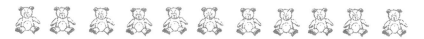

the 18th century. For parents of the nineties, Paul is the name of the cute Beatle, as well as the name of the pope who spearheaded Vatican II. It is somewhat neglected in the current vogue for original names. Artists Paul Cézanne, Paul Gauguin; actor Paul Newman; Revolutionary War hero Paul Revere; musician Paul Simon.

Paavo, Pablo, Paolo, Paulie, Paulin, Paulus, Pauly, Pavel, Pawel, Pol, Poll, Poul

Paxton Lat./OE. Place name: "Peace town." Actor Paxton Whitehead.

Packston, Paxon, Paxten, Paxtun

Payne Lat. "Countryman."

Paine

Pedro Sp. Var. **Peter.**

Pell Middle English. "Skin, parchment." As in parchment that legal documents would be written on; this may be an occupational name, indicating an ancestor who was a clerk.

Pall

Pembroke Celt. Place name: "Bluff, headland."

Pembrook

Penley OE. Place name: "Enclosed meadow."

Penlea, Penleigh, Penly, Pennlea, Pennleigh, Pennley

Penn OE. "Enclosure." In the U.S., tied to the eminent Quaker and founder of Pennsylvania, William Penn.

Pen

Percival OF. "Pierce the vale." Invented by a medieval poet for one of King Arthur's knights, and its meaning is not completely clear. Adopted with some enthusiasm, however, and was particularly well used in the late 19th century, along with more genuinely ancient names. Now scarce.

Parsafal, Parsefal, Parsifal, Perce, Perceval, Percevall, Percey, Percivall, Percy, Purcell

Percy Fr. "From Percy." A Norman place name that became associated with an immensely powerful aristocratic family in the North of England. Its greatest popularity coincided with that of Percival, and like that name, Percy is now widely neglected. Author Walker Percy; poet Percy Bysshe Shelley.

Pearcy, Percey, Percie

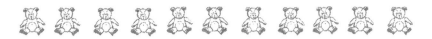

Peregrine Lat. "Traveler, pilgrim." "Peregrinations" is a synonym for "wanderings." Peregrine is also the name of a kind of falcon. The name persists in a small way in Britain. English writer Peregrine Worsthorne.
Peregrin, Peregryn

Perkin OE. "Little Peter."
Perkins, Perkyn, Perrin

Perry Dim. **Peregrine**; or OE. Place name "pear tree." Modern use seems mostly to be inspired by fictional detective Perry Mason. Singer Perry Como.
Parry, Perrie

Pesach Heb. "Spared." The Hebrew name for the great holiday of Passover, which commemorates the fact that Jehovah spared the Israelites in a plague that killed many Egyptians.
Pessach

Peter Gk. "Rock." New Testament name; the saint who, tradition has it, guards the gates to Heaven. The name's greatest popularity came in the first three-quarters of this century, prompted, some sources suggest, by the play *Peter Pan*. Artists Piero della Francesca, Peter Paul Rubens; Russian emperor Peter the Great; actor Peter O'Toole; Peter Rabbit; film director Peter Bogdanovich.
Peadar, Pearce, Peder, Pedro, Peerus, Peirce, Per, Perkin, Pero, Perrin, Perry, Pete, Petey, Petr, Pierce, Piero, Pierre, Pierson, Piet, Pieter, Pietrek, Pietro, Piotr, Pjotr, Pyotr

Peverell OF. "Piper."
Peverall, Peverel, Peveril

Peyton OE. Place name: "Fighting-man's estate." Probably related to **Patton**. Primarily American use, probably as a transferred last name, i.e., a mother's maiden name.
Payton

Phelan Ir. Gael. "Wolf." Mostly Irish use.

Phelps OE. "Son of Philip."

Philip Gk. "Lover of horses." The name of one of the twelve apostles, and a staple since early Christian times, though it receded somewhat in the 19th century. A 20th-century resurgence peaked in the 1960s. Britain's Prince

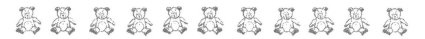

Philip; painter Filippo Lippi; playwright Philip Barry; talk show host Phil Donahue; author Philip Roth.
Felipe, Filip, Filippo, Fillip, Fyllip, Phil, Philipp, Philippe, Phillip, Phillips, Phyllip, Phyllip, Pippo

Philo Gk. "Loving."

Phineas Derivation and meaning unknown, though many sources offer Heb. "oracle." Another possible meaning is "mouth of brass," which would be appropriate for showman Phineas T. Barnum. Violinist Pinchas Zuckerman.
Fineas, Pincas, Pinchas, Pinchos, Pincus

Pickford OE. "From the ford at the peak."

Pierce Var. **Peter.** Actor Pierce Brosnan.
Pearce, Pears, Pearson, Pearsson, Peerce, Peirce, Piers, Pierson, Piersson

Pierre Fr. Var. **Peter.** Canadian Prime Minister Pierre Trudeau.

Piers Gk. "Rock." Peter is actually the Latin form of the name that the Normans took to Britain as Piers. This form, along with Pierce, has been an alternate form more popular in Britain.
Pearce, Pears, Pearson, Pierce, Pierson, Piersson

Pio Lat. "Pious." A name used by several popes, but not found much among English-speaking children.
Pius

Pitney OE. Place name: "Island of the stubborn one."
Pittney

Pitt OE. Place name: "Pit or ditch."

Placido Sp. "Serene." Made famous currently by opera star Placido Domingo.
Placidus, Placyd, Placydo

Plato Gk. "Broad-shouldered." Its occasional use in English-speaking countries may be inspired by admiration for the famous Greek philosopher.
Platon

Platt OF. Place name: "Flat land."
Platte

Pollard Middle English. "Shorn head." "Poll" was originally a term for head, hence our expression "take a poll." A pollard tree's branches have been cut back to

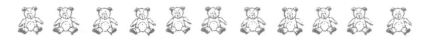

the trunk to promote a bushy growth at the top. Thus the name may either be a place name (for someone who lived near a pollard tree) or a descriptive name (for someone whose head had been closely cropped).

Poll, Pollerd, Pollyrd

Pollock OE. Var. **Pollux**. Artist Jackson Pollock.

Pollack, Polloch

Pollux Gk. "Crown." Along with Castor, one of the Heavenly Twins, the constellation also known as Gemini.

Pomeroy OF. Place name: "Apple orchard." The French word for apple is *pomme*.

Pommeray, Pommeroy

Ponce Sp. "Fifth." Made famous by Spanish explorer Ponce de Leon, but no more common than Quintus, its Latin equivalent.

Porfirio Gk. "Purple stone." The English term is "porphyry." Very rare, but borne by one of the 20th century's great playboys, Porfirio Rubirosa.

Porphirios, Prophyrios

Porter Lat. "Gatekeeper." Occupational name.

Powell OE. Surname related to **Paul**. Author Anthony Powell.

Powel

Prentice Middle English. "Apprentice."

Prentis, Prentiss

Prescott OE. Place name: "Priest's cottage." The middle name of President George Bush, but not widespread.

Prescot, Prestcot, Prestcott

Presley OE. Place name: "Priest's meadow." In the Middle Ages, when these names came into use, the priest was a very important figure in any community. Of course, in the late 20th century the name is associated with another important figure, Elvis Presley.

Presleigh, Presly, Presslee, Pressley, Prestley, Priestley, Priestly

Preston OE. Place name: "Priest's estate."

Prewitt OF. "Brave little one."

Prewet, Prewett, Prewit, Pruitt

Price Welsh. "Son of Rhys." Rhys is a common Welsh name meaning "ardent."

Brice, Bryce, Pryce

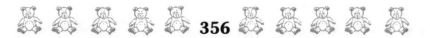

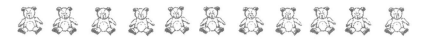

Primo It. "First; firstborn." Number names usually refer to children born with quite a number of older siblings (Quintus, Octavian), and tend to indicate exhaustion of the imagination, but Primo may allude to great pride in the firstborn, especially a son. Author Primo Levi.
Preemo, Premo

Prince Lat. "Prince." As a last name, it may have indicated someone who worked in a prince's household, and occasional first-name use is generally transferred from the last name. There are, of course, exceptions, like the musician formerly known as Prince, who undoubtedly cherished the name for its royal connotations. Comedian Freddie Prinze.
Prinz, Prinze

Proctor Lat. "Official, administrator." Occupational last name.
Prockter, Procter

Prosper Lat. "Fortunate," as in "prosperous." Poet Prosper Mérimée.
Prospero

Pryor Lat. "Monastic leader." A prior is the monk in charge of a monastery, so this might be an occupational name. On the other hand, the tradition of monastic chastity would seem to prevent such a name's being handed down to children.
Prior

Purvis Eng./Fr. "Purveyor." Originally indicated someone who provided food, or provisions.
Purves, Purviss

Quennell OF. Place name: "Small oak."
Quennel

Quentin Lat. "Fifth." The most common of the Q names, but still something of an oddity. Author Quentin Crisp.
Quent, Quenten, Quenton, Quint, Quintin, Quinton, Quintus

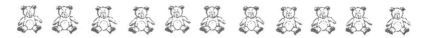

Quigley Ir. Gael. Meaning disputed: possibly "distaff," or "one with messy hair."

Quillan Ir. Gael. "Cub."
  Quillen

Quimby ONorse. Place name: "Estate of the woman." A woman's estate would have been quite a rarity in the Old Norse era.
  Quinby

Quincy OF. Place name: "Estate of the fifth son." Last name of a prominent Massachusetts family whose name is borne by a town and by the 6th U.S. President, John Quincy Adams.
  Quincey

Quinlan Ir. Gael. "Fit, shapely, strong."
  Quindlen

Quinn Ir. Gael. Meaning unknown. Very common Irish last name, occasionally transferred to first-name status, especially in the U.S. Actor Aidan Quinn.

Rabi Arab. "Gentle wind."
  Rabbi, Rabee
Rad OE. "Adviser."
Radbert OE. "Bright adviser."
Radburn OE. Place name: "Red brook."
  Radborn, Radborne, Radbourn, Radbourne, Radburne

Radcliff OE. Place name: "Red cliff." In America, most likely to be associated with the renowned women's college that is now part of Harvard.
  Radcliffe, Radclyffe

Radford OE. Place name: "Red ford" or "ford with reeds."
  Radferd, Radfurd

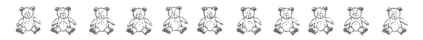

Radley OE. Place name: "Red meadow." As in **Radford**, the first element could also refer to reeds.
Radlea, Radlee, Radleigh, Radly

Radnor OE. Place name: "Red shore" or "reedy shore."

Rafael var. **Raphael**.
Rafe, Rafel, Rafello, Rafer, Raffaelo, Raphael

Rafferty Ir. Gael. "Prosperity wielder." Irish last name occasionally used as a first name.
Raferty, Raffarty

Rafi Arab. "Holding high." The name of the preeminent recording artist for children, which some parents may not consider a drawback.
Rafee, Raffi, Raffy

Ragnar Nor. "Powerful army." Though the Scandinavian form is very rare in the U.S., the anglicized versions are seen from time to time. The most famous Rainier, of course, is the Prince of Monaco, husband of Grace Kelly.
Ragnor, Rainer, Rainier, Rayner, Raynor

Rainart Ger. "Mighty judgment."
Rainhard, Rainhardt, Reinart, Reinhard, Reinhardt, Reinhart, Renke

Raleigh OE. Place name: "Meadow of roe deer." Commemorates Sir Walter Raleigh, explorer and court favorite of Queen Elizabeth I, who is supposed to have spread his cape over a puddle so she could cross with dry feet. The city in North Carolina was named for him.
Ralegh, Rawleigh, Rawley, Rawly

Ralph OE. "Wolf-counsel." A name that has been steadily, if not enormously, popular for the last thousand years (though today's parents might not recognize it immediately in older forms like Rathulf or Radolphus). Its greatest vogue in the U.S. occurred at the turn of the century. Now uncommon. Poet Ralph Waldo Emerson; consumer activist Ralph Nader.
Rafe, Raff, Ralf, Raoul, Raul, Rolf, Rolph

Ralston OE. Place name: "Ralph's settlement."

Ramiro Port. "Great judge."
Ramirez

Ramon Sp. Var. **Raymond**. Given its greatest exposure by the silent-movie star of the 1920s, Ramon Novarro.

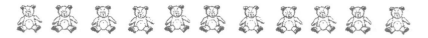

Ramsay OE. Place name: "Raven island" or "ram island." Originally a last name common in Scotland.
Ramsey

Ramsden OE. Place name: "Ram valley." Like most of these place names turned last names, this was transferred to a first name in the 19th century.

Rand OE. "Shield, fighter." Generally a diminutive of **Randolph** and related names.

Randall OE. "Shield-wolf." This is the medieval spoken form of Randolph. Enjoyed some popularity with parents in the baby boom era.
Randal, Randel, Randell, Randle

Randolph OE. "Shield-wolf." From the same root as **Randall**, which has been more popular in the U.S. English politician Lord Randolph Churchill.
Randal, Randall, Randell, Randolf, Randy

Randy Dim. **Randall, Randolph**. Used mostly in the middle of the 20th century, and mostly in America. In British slang, "randy" means "amorous."

Ranger OF. "Forest guardian."
Rainger, Range

Rankin OE. "little shield" or Celt. "son of Francis." A last name found in Scotland and Ireland, rarely transferred as a first name.

Ransford OE. Place name: "Raven ford."

Ransley OE. Place name: "Raven meadow."
Ransleigh, Ransly

Ransom Opinions differ: possibly OE. "shield's son," possibly a diminutive of Randolph. First-name use is mostly a late-Victorian phenomenon.
Ransome

Raoul Fr. Var. **Ralph**. Uncommon among English-speaking parents. Actor Raul Julia.
Raul

Raphael Heb. "God has healed." The name of one of the archangels, possibly (because of his name) the one who stirred the waters at the pool of Bethesda to give it healing powers. Most common in very religious eras (16th and 17th centuries) and the 19th century, which cherished the picturesque. May become more popular (as

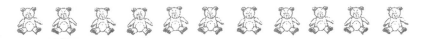

Gabriel has) in the current quest for the unique. Painter Raphael Sanzio; author Rafe Yglesias.

Falito, Rafal, Rafael, Rafaelle, Rafaello, Rafe, Rafel, Rafello, Raffael, Raffaello, Raphaello, Raphello

Rashid Turk. "Righteous, rightly advised." Rashida is used for girls, perhaps a little more frequently.

Rasheed, Rasheid, Rasheyd

Rasmus Dim. Erasmus. Gk. "Loved, desired." Used occasionally in German-speaking countries.

Ravi Hindi. "Sun." Made familiar to today's parents by the eminent sitar player Ravi Shankar.

Ravee

Rawlins OF. Ultimately a diminutive of Roland. A name like this was originally an oral contraction (Rolandson to Rawlinson to Rawlins), then became a last name, and was revived in the late 19th century as a first name.

Rawlinson, Rawson

Ray Dim. Raymond. Quite firmly rooted as an independent name, used mostly in the 20th century. Singer Ray Charles; boxer Sugar Ray Leonard; author Ray Bradbury.

Rae, Raye

Rayburn OE. Place name: "Roe-deer brook."

Raeborn, Raeborne, Raebourn, Raeburn, Rayborn, Raybourne, Rayburne

Raymond OG. "Counselor-protector." Old Teutonic name that was used in the Middle Ages, then forgotten until a very strong 19th-century revival, especially in America. It has been reconsigned to near oblivion. Author Raymond Chandler; actors Raymond Massey, Raymond Burr.

Raemond, Raemondo, Raimond, Raimondo, Raimund, Raimundo, Rajmund, Ramon, Ramond, Ramonde, Ramone, Ray, Rayment, Raymondo, Raymund, Raymunde, Raymundo

Raynor Nor. "Mighty army." An anglicized version of **Ragnar**. Also the name of the huge extinct volcano in Washington State, Mount Rainier. Poet Rainer Maria Rilke.

Ragnar, Rainer, Rainier, Rainor, Ranieri, Raynar, Rayner

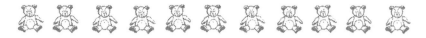

Read OE. "Red-haired." Descriptive name that long ago became a last name, and thence a first name, especially in the U.S.
Reade, Reed, Reid, Reide

Reading OE. "Son of the red-haired." Also a place name.
Redding, Reeding, Reiding

Redford OE. Place name: "Red ford." Hard to use today without invoking the ultrafamous blond actor, Robert Redford.

Redley OE. Place name: "Red meadow."
Radley, Redlea, Redleigh, Redly

Redman OE. Obscure: could mean either "man of counsel" or "man who rides." Never a common choice for parents.

Redmond Ir. Var. **Raymond.**
Radmond, Radmund, Redmund

Reece Welsh. "Fiery, zealous." The native Welsh form is **Rhys**, and it is fairly common in Wales. Actor Roger Rees.
Rees, Reese, Rhys, Rice

Reed OE. "Red-haired." This is the most common spelling of this name, which had a mild flourish of popularity in the baby boom era.
Read, Reade, Reid, Reyd

Reeve Middle English. Occupational name: "Bailiff." A reeve was an administrator for the king or someone of high position, who collected rents and maintained order on the lord's estates. Actor Christopher Reeve.
Reave, Reeves

Regan Ir. Gael. "Little king." Mostly 20th-century use.
Reagan, Reagen, Regen

Reginald OE. "Counsel power." Ronald and Reynolds are just two of the names that come from the same source; Reginald's popularity was mainly British and 19th century. Actor Judge Reinhold; baseball star Reggie Jackson.
Naldo, Rainault, Rainhold, Reg, Reggie, Reginalt, Reginauld, Reginault, Regnauld, Regnault, Reinald, Reinaldo, Reinaldos, Reinhold, Reinold, Reinwald, Renault, Rene, Reynaldo, Reynaldos, Reynold, Reynolds, Rinaldo, Ronald

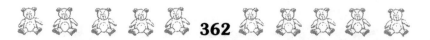

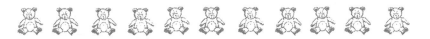

Remington OE. Place name: "Raven-family settlement." Familiar to Americans as a brand of razors, and as the name of a TV action hero of the eighties, Remington Steele. Artist Frederick Remington.

Remy Fr. "From Rheims." Champagne, and the fine brandies made from champagne, are the principal product of Rheims, a town in central France. The name is used for both boys and girls. Author Remy Charlip.
Remee, Remi, Remie, Remmy

Remus Lat. "Swift." The name of one of the legendary twins (the other was Romulus) who founded Rome. At the turn of the century Joel Chandler Harris's "Uncle Remus" stories (including the famous one about the Tar Baby) were very popular.

René Fr. "Reborn." The modern form of Renatus, which did not survive as a male name. Unlike the female version, René has not really spread beyond French-speaking families. Actor René Auberjonois.
Renat, Renato, Renatus

Renfred OE. "Powerful peace."

Renfrew Old Welsh. Place name: "Calm river."

Renny Ir. Gael. "Small and mighty."

Renshaw OE. Place name: "Raven woods."
Renishaw

Renton OE. Place name: "Settlement of the roe deer."

Renzo Dim. **Lorenzo**. Lat. "Laurel." Interior designer Renzo Mongiardino.

Reuben Heb. "Behold, a son." Old Testament name that came into general use in the 18th century. Also a sandwich that features corned beef, sauerkraut, and Swiss cheese. Singer Ruben Blades.
Reuban, Reubin, Reuven, Rouvin, Rube, Ruben, Rubin, Ruby

Rex Lat. "King." Mostly 20th-century use, possibly influenced by actor Rex Harrison. Probably most common as a name for a dog.

Rexford OE. Place name: "King's ford."

Rey Sp. "King." The Hispanic equivalent of Rex or Leroy. Not in general use.
Reyes

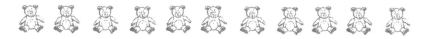

Reynard OF. "Fox" or OG. "Powerful and courageous." Some of the variations (like Renaud) come close to variations of the Reynold/Reginald names, but are not as common.
Raynard, Reinhard, Reinhardt, Renard, Renaud, Renauld, Rennard

Reynold Var. **Reginald**. Probably most familiar in America as a surname, though in the Middle Ages this was the most common form of Reginald.
Reinaldo, Renado, Renaldo, Renato, Renauld, Renault, Reynaldo, Reynolds, Rinaldo

Rhett Var. **Rhys**. Modern parents can hardly use it without thinking of Margaret Mitchell's immortal Rhett Butler, and his great line, "Frankly, my dear, I don't give a damn!"

Rhodes Gk. "Where roses grow." The name of an important Greek island and an important British philanthropist, Cecil Rhodes. He gave his name to both a country (Rhodesia) and a scholarship fund.
Rhodas, Rodas

Rhys Welsh. "Fiery, zealous." This is the native Welsh form of the name that appears more often in English-speaking countries as Reece.

Richard OG. "Dominant ruler." Norman name that went on to be a steady favorite for the last 900 years, with one century (the 19th) of neglect. In the current hunger for the unusual, it is again being overlooked. English Kings Richard I–III; rock star Little Richard; composer Richard Rodgers; actors Richard Burton, Richard Kiley, Richard Gere, Richard Chamberlain; photographer Richard Avedon; U.S. President Richard Nixon.
Dick, Dickie, Dicky, Ric, Richard, Ricardo, Riccardo, Rich, Richardo, Richart, Richerd, Richie, Rick, Rickard, Rickert, Rickey, Ricki, Rickie, Ricky, Rico, Rikard, Riki, Rikki, Riocard, Ritchard, Ritcherd, Ritchie, Ritchy, Ritchyrd, Ritshard, Ritsherd, Ryszard

Richmond OG. "Powerful protector." Most frequently encountered in the U.S. as a place name, like the capital city of Virginia.

Rick Dim. **Richard, Frederick**. Used independently,

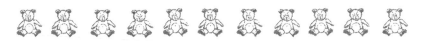

though more common as a nickname. Humphrey Bogart's character in *Casablanca* was named Rick.

Ric, Ricci, Rickey, Rickie, Ricky, Rik, Rikki, Rikky

Rickward OE. "Mighty guardian."

Rickwerd, Rickwood

Rico It. Dim. **Henry.** (OE. "home ruler") via **Enrico.**

Rider OE. "Horseman." Likely to be a transferred last name, for instance a mother's maiden name. Author Rider Haggard.

Ridder, Ryder

Ridge OE. Place name: "Ridge." Referring to a geographical feature in a landscape, as do the following "Ridg-" names.

Rigg

Ridgeway OE. Place name: "Road on the ridge."

Ridgley OE. Place name: "Ridge meadow."

Ridgeleigh, Ridgeley, Ridglea, Ridglee, Ridgleigh

Ridley OE. Place name: "Red meadow." Film director Ridley Scott.

Riddley, Ridlea, Ridleigh, Ridly

Riley Ir. Gael. "Courageous." Irish last name used as a first name for the last 150 years.

Reilly, Ryley

Ring OE. "Ring." Very unusual, though given exposure by author Ring Lardner. Beatles fans will remember that Ringo Starr took his name from the jewelry he favored.

Ringo

Riordan Ir. Gael. "Bard, minstrel."

Rearden, Reardon

Ripley OE. Place name: "Shouting man's meadow."

Ripleigh, Riply

Risley OE. Place name: "Meadow with shrubs."

Rislea, Rislee, Risleigh, Risly, Wrisley

Riston OE. Place name: "Settlement near the shrubs."

Wriston

Ritter Ger. "Knight." Actor John Ritter.

Roald OG. "Famous and powerful." Rare in English-speaking countries. Author Roald Dahl.

Roark Ir. Gael. "Illustrious and mighty." Usually occurs as a last name. Actor Mickey Rourke.

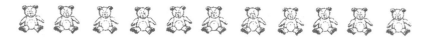

Roarke, Rorke, Rourke, Ruark

Rob Dim. **Robert**. The most common nickname for Robert is probably Bob, but Rob may be given more often as an independent name. Actor Rob Lowe.
Robb, Robbie, Robby

Robert OE. "Bright fame." Another staple male name, common for the last millennium. Its past popularity may be its downfall for this generation of parents. Senator Robert Kennedy; poet Robert Burns; actors Robert DeNiro, Robert Duvall; author Robert Lawson; General Robert E. Lee; author Robert Ludlum.
Bert, Bertie, Bob, Bobbie, Bobby, Rab, Rabbie, Riobard, Rip, Rob, Robb, Robbin, Robbins, Robbinson, Robby, Robers, Roberto, Robertson, Robi, Robin, Robinson, Robyn, Robynson, Rupert, Ruperto, Ruprecht

Robin Dim. **Robert**. Usually a girl's name in America, though A. A. Milne immortalized his son as Christopher Robin in the Winnie the Pooh stories. Comedian/actor Robin Williams; TV personality Robin Leach.
Robbin, Robbyn, Robyn

Robinson OE. "Son of Robert." More commonly a last name. Singer Smokey Robinson; poet Robinson Jeffers; actor Paul Robeson.
Robbinson, Robeson, Robynson, Robson

Rocco Ger./It. "Rest." The most common form (in America, at least) of the name of a popular saint who cured plague victims. He was especially venerated in Italy, which may be why this version of the name is the most common. Rocky is usually a nickname.
Rocco, Roch, Roche, Rochus, Rock, Rocky, Roque

Rochester OE. Place name: "Stone camp or fortress."
Chester, Chet, Rock

Rock Var. **Rocco**. Actor Rock Hudson is the most important precedent for using this name.
Rocky

Rockley OE. Place name: "Rock meadow."
Rocklee, Rockleigh, Rockly

Rockwell OE. Place name: "Rock spring."

Rocky Var. **Rocco**. Impossible to use today without invoking Sylvester Stallone's *Rocky* movies.

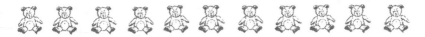

Rod Dim. **Roderick**. Used sparingly as an independent name. Actors Rod Steiger, Roddy McDowall.
Rodd, Roddie, Roddy

Roderick OG. "Renowned rule." Most commonly used in Scotland and other parts of Britain; never a great favorite in America.
Broderick, Brodrick, Brodryck, Rod, Rodd, Rodderick, Roddie, Roddrick, Roddy, Roderic, Roderich, Roderigo, Roderyck, Rodrick, Rodrik, Rodrigo, Rodrigue, Rodrique, Rodryck, Rodryk, Rory, Rurik, Ruy

Rodman OG. "Renowned man."

Rodney OE. Place name: "Island near the clearing." Like many last names, this one began intensive use as a first name in the mid–19th century. This mild popularity endured for some 100 years before fading. Comedian Rodney Dangerfield.
Rodnee, Rodnie

Roe Middle English. "Roe deer." May originally have been an occupational name indicating an ancestor who hunted or trapped such deer.
Row, Rowe

Rogan Ir. Gael. "Red-head." Irish Gaelic has several names to indicate red hair; but then, the Irish people produce many redheads.

Roger OG. "Renowned spearman." At its most popular in the Middle Ages and the 19th and 20th centuries, but on the wane since the 1950s. Actors Rutger Hauer, Roger Moore.
Rodge, Rodger, Rog, Rogelio, Rogerio, Rogers, Rogiero, Ruggiero, Rutger, Ruttger

Roland OG. "Renowned land." Orlando is a common variant in several European languages. Rowland was, for a long time, the preferred version in English. The name dates from the Dark Ages, and the most famous Roland was the valorous nephew of Charlemagne, about whom many romantic tales were written.
Lannie, Lanny, Orlando, Roeland, Rolando, Roldan, Roley, Rolland, Rollie, Rollin, Rollins, Rollo, Rolly, Rowe, Rowland

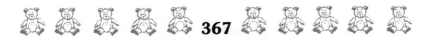

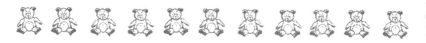

Rolf Var. **Rudolph**. Most common in Scandinavian countries.

Rolfe, Rolle, Rollo, Rolph, Rowland

Roman Lat. "From Rome." The name of several obscure saints and one short-lived pope. The significance of the name no doubt comes from the fact that Rome is the center of the Roman Catholic faith. Football star Roman Gabriel; film director Roman Polanski.

Romain, Romano, Romanos

Romeo It. "Pilgrim to Rome." Cannot be used without reference to the famous romance, and sure to engender a lot of teasing.

Romney Old Welsh. Place name: "Winding river." Painter George Romney.

Romulus Lat. "Man of Rome." Along with Remus, the legendary founder of Rome, though Romulus actually murdered his twin brother in a quarrel over where to situate the city, which he then ruled for 37 years. A rare name. Playwright Romulus Linney.

Ronald OE. "Counsel power." Also from the same source as Reginald and Reynold. Though it was fairly common in the 1940s and 1950s, most parents will associate Ronald with two-term President Ronald Reagan and with clown Ronald McDonald.

Ranald, Ron, Ronnie, Ronny

Ronan Ir. Gael. "Little seal." Mostly Irish use.

Ronson OE. "Son of Ronald."

Rooney Ir. Gael. "Red-haired." Yet another Irish name indicating the traditional Irish coloring. Actor Mickey Rooney.

Rowan, Rowen, Rowney

Roosevelt Old Dutch. Place name: "Rose field." A name that would be simply an ethnic curiosity if it hadn't been borne by two 20th-century presidents, Theodore and Franklin Delano Roosevelt (who were second cousins).

Roper OE. Occupational name: "Rope maker."

Rory Ir. Gael. "Red." Also occurs as a nickname for **Roderick**. Mostly Scottish use, but the name seems highly eligible for 1990s popularity.

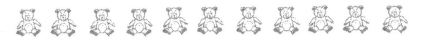

Rosario Port. "The rosary." Most common, for obvious reasons, among Catholic families.

Roscoe Scan. Place name: "Deer woods." Tennis star Roscoe Tanner.
Rosco, Ross

Roslin Scot. Gael. "Little redhead."
Roslyn, Rosselin, Rosslyn

Ross Scot. Gael. "Headland." A place name in Scotland. The name (like so many of the *R* names) may also come from the Gaelic word for "red."
Rosse, Rossell

Roswell OE. Place name: "Rose spring."

Roth OG. "Red." Could apply to hair or complexion, though England's flaxen-haired Teutonic invaders might have used it more for the former, in sheer surprise.

Rothwell ONorse. Place name: "Red spring."

Rover Middle English. "Traveler, wanderer." The term "roving" turns up most often in poetry and songs (as in Byron's poem "So, We'll Go No More A-Roving"), and the name is most commonly given to dogs.

Rowan OE. Place name: "Rowan tree." Also possibly another Gaelic name meaning "red." Presumably, since the term applied to so many people, variations in the name were necessary to tell them apart.
Roan, Rowe

Rowell OE. Place name: "Roe deer well."

Rowley OE. Place name: "Roughly cleared meadow."
Rowlea, Rowlee, Rowleigh, Rowly

Roxbury OE. Place name: "Rook's town or fortress." "Rook" may have referred to a large population of rooks or crows.
Roxburghe

Roy Gael. "Red" or Fr. "king." Most popular earlier in the 20th century, but hard to use because of the Roy Rogers chain of fast-food restaurants. Cowboy Roy Rogers.
Rey, Roi, Ruy

Royal OF. "Royal." Scarce as a name, because of its meaning.
Royall

Royce Meaning and origin unclear: Some sources offer

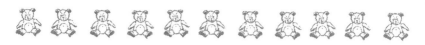

OF./OE. "son of the king"; others suggest OG. "kind fame." The most famous Royce is the man who, along with Mr. Rolls, began turning out England's foremost luxury car.
Roice

Royden OE. Place name: "Rye hill."
Roydan, Roydon

Royston OE. Place name: Not related to Roy at all, but a name whose original meaning varied geographically.

Rudd OE. "Ruddy-skinned." Student leader Mark Rudd.

Rudolph OG. "Famous wolf." Parents would have to have very strong feelings about the name to use it, given the enormous fame of Rudolph the red-nosed reindeer. Actor Rudolph Valentino; ballet star Rudolf Nureyev.
Dolph, Raoul, Rodolfo, Rodolph, Rodolphe, Rolf, Rolfe, Rollo, Rolph, Rolphe, Rudey, Rudi, Rudie, Rudolf, Rudolfo, Rudolphus, Rudy

Rudy Dim. "Rud-" names. Well established by singer Rudy Vallee.

Rudyard OE. Place name: "Red paddock." Preempted by English poet and novelist Rudyard Kipling, though fans of the *Just So Stories* or the *Jungle Book* might want to use it.

Ruford OE. Place name: "Red ford" or "rough ford."
Rufford

Rufus Lat. "Red-haired." Another redhead name, though this one comes from Latin rather than Gaelic. Most common in the 19th century.
Ruffus, Rufous

Rugby OE. "Rook fortress." The name of a famous British school, which in turn gave its name to a famous game.

Rumford OE. Place name: "Wide river-crossing."

Rupert Var. **Robert.** Well established in Britain since the 18th century, but less used here, possibly because to Americans, it has a very English flavor. Actor Rupert Everett; publisher Rupert Murdoch.
Ruprecht

Rushford OE. Place name: "Ford with rushes."

Ruskin OF. "Little red-haired one." Author John Ruskin.

Russell Fr. "Red-head; red-skinned." Originally a last

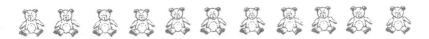

name, but popular as a first name in the middle of the 20th century. Like most fashions of that era, the name is now neglected. Philosopher Bertrand Russell.
Roussell, Russ, Russel

Rusty Fr. "Red-haired." Most commonly a nickname, given when the fact of red hair is well established (which may occur long after a bald baby is given a proper name).

Rutherford OE. "Cattle crossing." Most commonly a family name transferred to first-name use, since passionate admiration for U.S. President Rutherford Hayes seems unlikely to influence parental choice. Use may also be limited by the fact that there is no handy nickname.
Rutherfurd

Rutland ONorse. Place name: "Land of roots" or "red land."

Rutley OE. Place name: "Root meadow" or "red meadow."

Ryan Irish last name. Meaning is unclear, though some sources connect it with "king." Has been mildly popular in recent years. Actor Ryan O'Neal.
Ryon, Ryun

Rycroft OE. Place name: "Rye field."
Ryecroft

Ryland OE. Place name: "Land where rye is grown."
Ryeland

S

Saber Fr. "Sword." The kind of curved sword traditionally used by cavalrymen; also a weapon used in modern-day fencing. Slightly bloodthirsty as a first name.
Sabre

Sabin Lat. "Sabine." The Sabines were a tribe living in central Italy around the time Romulus and Remus established the city of Rome. In an effort to provide wives for the citizens of Rome, Romulus arranged the

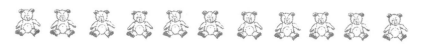

mass kidnapping of the Sabine women, which came to be known (and frequently portrayed in art and literature) as the "Rape of the Sabines." The name is more common in the feminine form.

Sabino

Sacha Rus. Dim. **Alexander**. Gk. "Defender of mankind." Cropped up in English-speaking countries in the last 20 years. The "-a" ending in Russian is not necessarily feminine. French singer Sacha Guitry.

Sascha, Sasha

Sadler OE. Occupational name: "Harness maker." Like most last names turned first names, this one was first transferred in the 19th century.

Saddler

Safford OE. Place name: "Willow river crossing."

Said Arab. "Happy." Currently popular in Arabic countries. Actor Saeed Jaffrey.

Saeed, Sayeed, Sayid

Salim Arab. "Tranquility."

Saleem, Salem

Salton OE. Place name: "Manor settlement" or "willow settlement."

Salvatore It. "Savior." Used mostly by families of Latinate descent. Artist Salvador Dali.

Sal, Salvador, Salvator, Salvidor, Sauveur, Xavier, Xaviero, Zavier, Zaviero

Sam Dim. **Samuel** Heb. "Told by God" or **Samson** Heb. "Sun." Occasionally used on its own, more commonly a nickname. Playwright Sam Shepard; actor Sam Waterston.

Samm, Sammey, Sammie

Samson Heb. "Sun." In the Old Testament, Samson was the warrior whose strength ebbed away when his hair was cut by Delilah. The name was used in the Middle Ages, and the Puritans kept it current with their fondness for Old Testament names, but it has not been fashionable for several hundred years.

Sam, Sampson, Sansom, Sanson, Sansone, Shem

Samuel Heb. "Told by God." A judge and prophet in early Israel; two Old Testament books are named for

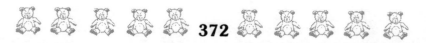

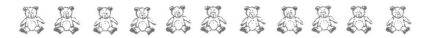

him. The name was used, predictably, by the Puritans and has never really faded since then, though it peaked in the 19th century. Opera singer Samuel Ramey; lexicographer Samuel Johnson; playwright Samuel Beckett; author Samuel Clemens (Mark Twain).

Sam, Sammie, Sammy, Samuele, Samuello, Shem

Sanborn OE. Place name: "Sandy stream."

Sanborne, Sanbourn, Sanburn, Sanburne, Sandborn, Sandbourne

Sancho Lat. "Sacred." Don Quixote's sidekick was called Sancho Panza, which is a little joke, since "Panza" is Spanish slang for "belly."

Sauncho

Sanders Middle English. "Son of **Alexander**." Gk. "Defender of mankind."

Sanderson, Sandor, Saunders, Saunderson

Sandor Hung. Var. **Alexander**. Gk. "Defender of mankind."

Sanditon OE. "Sandy settlement."

Sandy Dim. **Alexander**. Gk. "Defender of mankind." Sometimes also given as a nickname based on a person's coloring, like Rusty. Apparently red or reddish hair is unusual enough to warrant this kind of name, but corresponding names for blonds or brunets don't seem to exist.

Sandey, Sandie

Sanford OE. Place name: "Sandy ford." Acting teacher Sanford Meisner.

Sandford, Sandfurd

Santiago Sp. "Saint James." Catholics are traditionally less reticent about using religious names than Protestants, routinely naming children Salvatore, Socorro, and even Jesus, as well as choosing the names of individual saints.

Santo It./Sp. "Holy." Also a nickname for full saints' names.

Santos

Sargent OF. Occupational name: "Officer." Painter John Singer Sargent; politician Sargent Shriver.

Sarge, Sergeant, Sergent, Serjeant

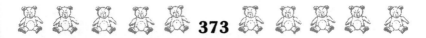

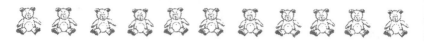

Saturnin Sp. "Saturn." A "saturnine" temperament is moody or sullen, and people born under the sign of Saturn (Capricorns) are generally considered painstaking, reliable, and reserved.

Saul Heb. "Asked for." The name of the first king of Israel, and also the name of the apostle Paul before his conversion to Christianity. Overlooked in the 16th-century revival of Old Testament names, at its peak in the late 19th century. Author Saul Bellow.
Sol, Sollie

Saville Fr. "Willow town." Savile Row, in London, is the worldwide source for fine men's tailoring.
Savil, Savile, Savill, Savylle

Sawyer Middle English. Occupational name: "Woodworker." Most familiar as the name of Mark Twain's boy hero, *Tom Sawyer.*

Saxon OE. "Knife, sword." Used for one of the Germanic tribes that fought with short-bladed weapons.
Saxe, Saxen

Sayer Welsh. "Woodworker." Football star Gale Sayers.
Sayers, Sayre, Sayres

Scanlon Ir. Gael. "Little trapper."
Scanlan, Scanlen

Schuyler Dutch. "Shield, protection" or "scholar." Harks back to the Dutch settlers who brought the name to America in the 17th century.
Schuylar, Skuyler, Skylar, Skyler

Scott OE. "Scotsman." Use is emphatically 20th century, but may be falling away in the 1990s. Actor Scott Glenn; authors Scott Peck, F. Scott Fitzgerald; musician Scott Joplin.
Scot, Scottie, Scotto

Seabert OE. "Shining sea."
Seabright, Sebert, Seibert

Seabrook OE. Place name: "Stream near the sea."
Seabrooke

Seamus Ir. Var. **James.** Heb. "He who supplants." "Shamus" is old-fashioned American slang for a detective, possibly because the urban police force has traditionally been heavily Irish.
Seumas, Shamus

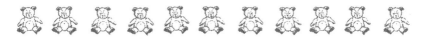

Sean Ir. Var. **John**. Heb. "God is gracious." Spread outside of Ireland only in the 20th century, and popularized by actor Sean Connery.
Shane, Shaughn, Shaun, Shawn

Searle OE. "Armor."

Seaton OE. Place name: "Town near the sea."
Seeton, Seton

Sebastian Lat. "From Sebastia" (an ancient city). Saint Sebastian, an early Christian martyr, was killed in a hail of arrows, and was a favorite subject for Old Master painters. (He is now patron of soldiers.) The name has never been common, though the British have used it somewhat since the 1940s, possibly influenced by a character in Evelyn Waugh's popular *Brideshead Revisited*. To Americans, it may seem a little too rarefied, and it provides no handy nickname.
Bastian, Bastien, Seb, Sebastiano, Sebastien, Sebestyen, Sebo

Sedgley OE. Place name: "Sword meadow." Could indicate a kind of coarse, sharp reedlike grass growing in a meadow, or that the meadow belonged to (or was frequented by) a swordsman. In all cases, refers to a long-ago meadow.
Sedgeley, Sedgely

Sedgwick OE. Place name: "Sword place." As with Sedgley, the sword could refer to grass or an actual weapon.
Sedgewick, Sedgewyck, Sedgwyck

Seeley OE. "Blessed." From the same Germanic root as Selig.
Sealey, Seely

Sefton OE. Place name: "Town in the rushes."

Seger OE. "Sea fighter." Musician Pete Seeger.
Seager, Segar, Seeger

Segundo Sp. "Second." Not common: parents usually have enough imagination to come up with at least two proper names.

Selby OE. Place name: "Manor village."
Shelby

Seldon OE. Place name: "Willow valley."
Selden, Sellden, Shelden

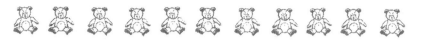

Selig OGer. "blessed."
Seligman, Seligmann, Zelig

Selwyn OE. "Manor-friend." Alternatively, an offshoot of Silvanus. Mostly 19th-century use.
Selwin, Selwinn, Selwynn, Selwynne

Senior OF. "Lord." Hard to use in these days when it has come to mean any individual older than 65.

Sennett Fr. "Elderly."
Sennet

Septimus Lat. "Seventh." Most common in the 19th century, when very large families were the norm.

Seraphim Heb. "Ardent." The seraphim are the highest-ranking angels in Heaven (above angels, archangels, cherubim, etc.). They have six wings and are noted for their zealous love. There have been two Saints Seraphim, one a 17th-century Italian, one an 18th-century Russian mystic.
Serafin, Serafino, Seraphimus

Sereno Lat. "Tranquil." Though the feminine form, Serena, is somewhat popular, the masculine version is very rare.
Cereno

Serge Lat. "Servant, attendant." Strongly associated with Russia, perhaps because of composers Rachmaninoff and Prokofiev, yet it comes from a Latin name and was used by an early pope. Impresario Serge Diaghilev.
Seargeoh, Sergei, Sergey, Sergio, Sergios, Sergiusz, Serguei, Sirgio, Sirgios

Seth Heb. "Set, appointed." In the Old Testament, Adam and Eve's third son (after Cain and Abel). Passed over in the Puritan revival of biblical names, but included in the late–20th-century revival of the same.

Severin Lat. "Severe."
Seweryn

Severn OE. "Boundary." The Severn is an important river running through southern England.

Seward OE. "Sea guardian." Largely 19th century.
Sewerd

Sewell OE. "Sea strong."
Sewald, Sewall

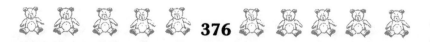

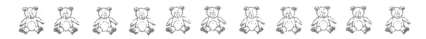

Sexton Middle English. Occupational name: "Church custodian." The sexton (or sacristan) is charged with the upkeep of a church building.

Sextus Lat. "Sixth." Less common than Septimus or Octavius, though five popes have used it. The first one, oddly enough, was actually Christendom's seventh pope.
Sixtus

Seymour OF. "From Saint Maur." Indicates an ancestor who came from a village called Saint Maur, most probably in Normandy. Quite a popular name in the 19th century.
Seamore, Seamor, Seamour

Shadrach Heb. Meaning unknown. Old Testament name: one of three Hebrew men (along with Meshach and Abednego) thrown into a fiery furnace by King Nebuchadnezzar and rescued by an angel. Used steadily in the 16th–19th centuries, but now rare.
Shadrack

Shalom Heb. "Peace." Related to **Solomon**.
Sholom, Solomon

Shamus Var. **Seamus** (Ir. var. **James**: Heb. "the supplanter").

Shanahan Ir. Gael. "Wise, clever."

Shandy OE. "Boisterous, high-spirited."
Shandey

Shane Var. **Sean** (Ir. var. **John**: Heb. "the Lord is gracious"). Popularity in the 1950s and 1960s probably depended on the film *Shane*. Now losing ground.
Shaine, Shayn, Shayne

Shanley Ir. Gael. "Small and ancient."
Shannley

Shannon Ir. Gael. "Old, ancient." The name of an important river, county, and airport in Ireland, used as a first name in this century. Most popular among families with Irish roots, and more common for girls.
Shanan, Shannan, Shannen

Sharif Arab. "Honest." Actor Omar Sharif.
Shareef

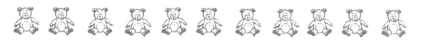

Shaw OE. Place name: "Copse, grove of trees."

Shawn Var. **Sean.** Use of Sean and its variants, feminine and masculine, is on the wane since the late 1970s.

Sheehan Ir. Gael. "Small and tranquil."

Sheffield OE. Place name: "Crooked meadow."

Shelby OE. Place name: "Village on the ledge." Author Shelby Foote.
Shelbey, Shelbie

Sheldon OE. Place name: "Steep valley." Most common in the middle of the 20th century. Author Sidney Sheldon.
Shelden, Sheldin

Shelley OE. Place name: "Ledge meadow." Last name made famous by the poet Percy Bysshe Shelley. Much more commonly used for girls at the moment.
Shelly

Shelton OE. Place name: "Ledge village."

Shem Heb. "Fame." The name of Noah's eldest son in the Old Testament. (Ham and Japheth were the other two.) None of the sons' names are as popular as that of their father.

Shepherd OE. Occupational name: "Shepherd." Mostly 19th-century use, very uncommon now. *Pooh* illustrator Ernest Shepard.
Shep, Shepard, Shephard, Shepp, Sheppard, Shepperd

Shepley OE. Place name: "Sheep meadow."
Sheplea, Shepleigh, Shepply, Shipley

Sherborn OE. Place name: "Bright stream."
Sherborne, Sherbourn, Sherburn, Sherburne

Sheridan Ir. Gael. Unclear meaning, possibly "wild man." Used mostly in Britain. Critic Sheridan Morley; playwright Richard Brinsley Sheridan; Civil War General Philip Sheridan.
Sheredan, Sheridon, Sherridan

Sherlock OE. "Bright hair." Irresistibly reminiscent of Arthur Conan Doyle's fictional detective, Sherlock Holmes.
Sherlocke, Shurlock

Sherman OE. Occupational name: "Shear man." Around the time when last names were coming into being, England's great export was wool. The wool business has

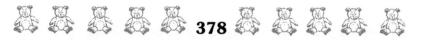

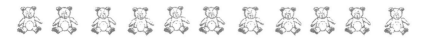

given the modern world a number of occupational names, like Sherman, Shepherd, Fuller, and Weaver.

Scherman, Schermann, Shermann

Sherwin Middle English. "Bright friend."

Sherwind, Sherwinn, Sherwyn, Sherwynne

Sherwood OE. Place name: "Shining forest." Sherwood Forest, a real forest in central England, was the home of the legendary bandit/hero Robin Hood. Playwright Robert Sherwood; Author Sherwood Anderson.

Sherwoode, Shurwood

Shipton OE. Place name: "Sheep village" or "ship village."

Shlomo Var. **Solomon.**

Shelomo

Sidney OE. "From Saint Denis." Famous English last name turned first name in the 18th century, very fashionable in the late 19th century, now little used. To parents of the 1990s, this may seem like a name that belongs to another generation. Author Sidney Sheldon; film director Sydney Pollack; actor Sidney Poitier.

Sid, Sydney

Siegfried OG. "Victory peace." The hero of the last two of Wagner's "Ring" cycle of operas, son of Siegmund, husband of Brunhilde.

Sigfred, Sigfrid, Sigfried, Sigfryd, Sigvard, Sygfried

Sigmund OG. "Victorious protector." Another character from the "Ring" cycle, son of the god Wotan. He fathers Siegfried on his own sister, Sieglinde. The other famous Sigmund is the father of psychoanalysis, Sigmund Freud. A name with many weighty connotations.

Siegmund, Sigismond, Sigismondo, Sigismund, Sigismundo, Sigismundus, Sigmond, Szygmond

Sigwald OG. "Victorious leader."

Siegwald

Silas A contraction of **Silvanus.** New Testament name used in the Puritan era and occurring since then. Has an old-fashioned air that may appeal to parents of the 1990s.

Silvan, Silvano, Silvaon, Silvanus, Silvio, Sylas, Sylvan

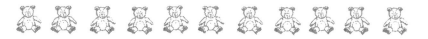

Silvanus Lat. "Wood dweller." Also a New Testament name, but never as widely adopted as its spinoff, **Silas**.
Silvain, Silvano, Silvio, Sylvanus, Sylvio

Silvester Original form of the name we know as Sylvester.
Silvestre, Silvestro, Sylvester

Simon Heb. "Listening intently." Prominent New Testament name, one of the twelve apostles. A common name from the Middle Ages through the 18th century, then revived early in the 20th century. To Americans, it has a rather English air. Simeon, the Old Testament version, has never been as common. Orchestra conductor Simon Rattle.
Shimon, Si, Simen, Simeon, Simmonds, Simmons, Simms, Simone, Simpson, Symon, Symms, Szymon

Sinclair OF. Place name: "From Saint Clair." Still much more familiar as a last name. Author Sinclair Lewis.
Sinclare, Synclair

Siraj Arab. "Light, beam."

Skelly Ir. Gael. "Bard."
Scully

Skerry ONorse. Place name: "Stony isle."

Skip Scand. "Ship boss." The term that has come down to us is "skipper," for the captain of a ship or boat. Skip occurs more commonly as a nickname.
Skipp, Skipper

Slade OE. Place name: "Valley."
Slaide, Slayde

Slavin Ir. Gael. "Mountain man."
Slawin, Slavin, Sleven

Sloan Ir. Gael. "Man of arms." An Irish last name that has become well entrenched in Britain and the U.S. Sometimes makes the leap to first-name status, perhaps as a maternal maiden name.
Sloane

Smedley OE. Place name: "Flat meadow."
Smedleigh, Smedly

Smith OE. Occupational name: "Blacksmith." This extremely common last name occurs as a first name, but

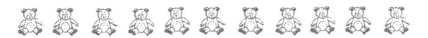

parents would be unlikely to use it unless it was a family name.

Smitty, Smyth, Smythe

Snowden OE. Place name: "Snowy peak." The name of a mountain in Wales, and the title (Earl of Snowdon) of Princess Margaret's ex-husband.

Snowdon

Socrates Gk. Meaning unknown. The name of the great Greek philosopher, used mostly by Greek families.

Sokrates

Solomon Heb. "Peaceable." In the Old Testament, the wise king of Israel. Used in the Middle Ages and the 18th century, but currently a far from common choice.

Salmon, Salomo, Salomon, Salomone, Sol, Solaman, Sollie, Soloman

Somerset OE. Place name: "Summer settlement." A county in England, and a last name given prominence as a first name by author and playwright Somerset Maugham.

Sommerset, Summerset

Somerton OE. Place name: "Summer town."

Somervile, Somerville

Sorrell OF. "Red-brown." A term now used to describe the color of a horse, perhaps applied long ago to the color of an ancestor's hair.

Southwell OE. Place name: "South well."

Spalding OE. Place name: "Divided field." More commonly a last name, rarely transferred to first-name use. Performance artist Spalding Gray.

Spaulding

Spear OE. Occupational name: "Spear-man." Names are sometimes a window into the concerns of a former era, and a number of names from the war-torn Anglo-Saxon age have to do with weapons.

Speare, Spears, Speer, Speers, Spiers

Spencer Middle English. Occupational name: "Provisioner." Used for the person in a large household who dispensed food and drink. Usually a last name, but occurs as a first name, more commonly in Britain. Actor Spencer Tracy.

Spence, Spenser

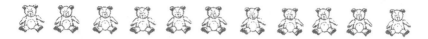

Spiridon Gk. "Basket." The name of a 4th-century Cypriot sheep farmer who became a bishop and a popular Greek saint. The name is little used outside Greek communities. U.S. Vice President Spiro Agnew.
Spiridion, Spiro, Spiros, Spyridon, Spyros

Squire Middle English. Occupational name: "Knight's companion." In more modern terms, perhaps, an aide-de-camp. First-name use mostly 19th century.

Stacy Dim. **Eustace.** Gk. "Fertile." More common as a female name. Actor Stacy Keach.
Stacey

Stafford OE. Place name: "Landing place ford." As with many of these place/last names, used mostly in the 19th century.
Stafforde, Staford

Stanbury OE. Place name: "Stone fortification."
Stanberry, Stanbery, Stanburghe

Stancliff OE. Place name: "Stony cliff."
Stancliffe

Standish OE. Place name: "Stony parkland." The Pilgrims' military leader was Miles Standish, whose courtship Longfellow immortalized in a poem.

Stanfield OE. Place name: "Stony field."
Stansfield

Stanford OE. Place name: "Stony ford." Familiar as the name of the great California railroad magnate Leland Stanford, who founded the university that bears his name. Composer Charles Stanford.
Stamford, Standford

Stanislaus Slavic. Possibly "glorious camp or stand." The patron saint of Poland, Saint Stanislaus, was an 11th-century bishop and martyr.
Stanislas, Stanislav, Stanislaw, Stannes, Stasio

Stanley OE. Place name: "Stony field." It is not clear why some place names, like Sidney and Stanley, became popular enough so that they made the transition to common first names, while others, like Stanford or Sinclair, remain primarily last names. As with Sidney, Stanley's

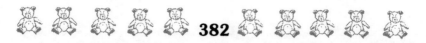

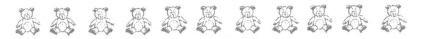

transformation to a first name was the result of great popularity at the turn of the century. Filmmaker Stanley Kubrick.

Stan, Stanlea, Stanlee, Stanly

Stanmore OE. Place name: "Stony lake." On the evidence of this group of "Stan-" names, stones seem to have occupied a great deal of Anglo-Saxon man's attention, perhaps because they had to be cleared from the earth before it could be farmed effectively.

Stanton OE. Place name: "Stony village."
    Stanten, Staunton

Stanway OE. Place name: "Stony roadway."
    Stanaway, Stannaway, Stannway

Stanwick OE. "Dweller at the rocky village."
    Stanwicke, Stanwyck

Stanwood OE. Place name: "Stony woods."

Starr Middle English "Star." Beatle Ringo Starr; football hero Bart Starr.

Stavros Gk. "Crowned." Currently popular in Greece. Greek plutocrat Stavros Niarchos.

Steadman OE. Occupational name: "Farmstead occupant." To many parents of the 1990s, the name will recall Hope and Michael Steadman, characters on the TV series "thirtysomething."
    Steadmann, Stedman

Steel OE. "Like steel." In the rough times when the name was coined, this would have been quite a compliment.
    Steele

Stein Ger. "Stone." Skiing champion Stein Erickson.
    Steen

Stephen Gk. "Crowned." As the name of Christianity's first martyr (Saint Stephen, who was stoned to death), common until the late 18th century. A slow decline was reversed in the middle of the 20th century, and a long period of great popularity is just now waning. Actors Stephen Collins, Steve Martin, Steve McQueen; songwriter Stephen Foster; physicist Stephen Hawking; author Stephen King; filmmaker Steven Spielberg; musician Stevie Wonder.
    Esteban, Estefan, Estevan, Etienne, Staffan, Stefan,

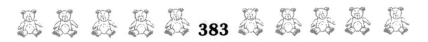

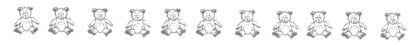

Stefano, Steffen, Stephan, Stephanus, Stephens, Stephenson, Stevan, Steve, Steven, Stevenson, Stevie

Sterling OE. "Genuine, first-rate." As in sterling silver. Not common, but a novel candidate for 1990s popularity.

Stirling

Sterne Middle English. "stern, unbending"; Ger. "star." Authors Laurence Sterne, Thomas Stearns Eliot; violinist Isaac Stern.

Stearn, Stearne, Stearns, Stern

Stewart OE. Occupational name: "Steward." An early variant of Stuart, which finally became the more popular form of the name. It is more common as a first name than many occupational names (Baker, Shepherd, Carpenter), but has never really become a standard first name either. Actor Jimmy Stewart.

Steward, Stuart

Stillman OE. "Silent man."

Stockley OE. Place name: "Tree-stump field." Like the stones in the "Stan-" names, tree stumps would be a hindrance to efficient farming, and thus worthy of note and commemorated in last names.

Stockton OE. Place name: "Tree-stump settlement."

Stockwell OE. Place name: "Tree-stump well."

Stoddard OE. "Horse guard."

Storm OE. "Tempest; storm." The almost too appropriate name of meteorologist Storm Field.

Strahan Ir. Gael. "Minstrel, sage."

Strachan

Stratford OE. Place name: "Street river-crossing."

Strong OE. "Powerful." Originally a name that would characterize its bearer. In the last name, the meaning is lost.

Struthers Ir. Gael. Place name: "Near the brook."

Stuart OE. Occupational name: "Steward." The steward would administer a large feudal household. This was the name of kings of Scotland and England, often considered the most romantic ruling family. (Long curls, a taste for luxury, a reputation for womanizing, and a couple of beheadings all added to the romance.) Most popular in

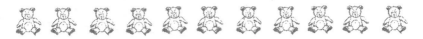

the middle of the 20th century. Portrait painter Gilbert Stuart.

Steward, Stewart

Styles OE. Place name: "Stile." A stile is a set of stairs placed over a wall so it can be crossed easily on foot—an important feature in a rural landscape.

Stiles

Suffield OE. Place name: "Southern field."

Sulaiman Arab. "Peaceable." The Arabic version of **Solomon**. The Turkish sultan Suleiman the Magnificent brought civilization in his country to new heights, but contemporaneous Western rulers would never have characterized him as living up to his name.

Suleiman, Suleyman

Sullivan Ir. Gael. "Black-eyed." Composer Arthur Sullivan; TV host Ed Sullivan.

Sullavan, Sullevan, Sully

Sully OE. Place name: "South meadow."

Sulleigh, Sulley

Sutcliff OE. Place name: "Southern cliff."

Sutcliffe

Sutherland Scan. "Southern land." Sutherland is the name of a county in northern Scotland, which was nevertheless to the south of the Nordic people who called it that.

Southerland

Sutton OE. Place name: "Southern settlement."

Sven Scan. "Youth." Currently popular in Sweden, but not much used in English-speaking countries.

Svein, Svend, Swen, Swenson

Sweeney Ir. Gael. "Small hero."

Sweeny

Swinburne OE. Place name: "Swine stream." Swine, or pigs, were also an important feature of life in the days when last names were being formed. Poet Algernon Swinburne.

Swinborn, Swinbourne, Swinburn, Swinbyrn, Swynborne

Swinford OE. Place name: "Swine ford."

Swynford

Swinton OE. Place name: "Swine settlement."

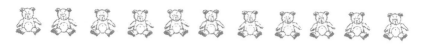

Sylvester Lat. "Wooded." In spite of a distinguished past, the name is now associated with a cartoon cat and an extremely muscular actor, Sylvester Stallone.
Silvester, Sly

Tab Several origins are proposed, including OG. "shining, brilliant" and Middle English "drummer." But the name would be merely a curiosity without the career of fifties teen idol Tab Hunter, whose given name was Arthur.
Tabb, Taber, Tabor

Tabor Hung. "Encampment."
Taber, Taibor, Taybor, Tayber

Tabib Turkish. "Doctor."
Tabeeb

Tad Dim. **Thaddeus** (meaning unknown). Also Old Welsh. "Father." Also used as a nickname in the U.S., where "tad" is slang for "small," probably from "tadpole."
Tadd, Thad

Tadeo Sp. Var. **Thaddeus** (meaning unknown).

Taggart Ir. Gael. "Son of the priest."

Tahir Arab. "Pure, unsullied."
Taheer

Tait ONorse. "Cheerful, gay."
Tate, Tayte

Tal Heb. "Rain."
Talor

Talbot Meaning unknown. An aristocratic last name in England, used as a first name since the 19th century. Tennis star Billy Talbert.
Talbert, Talbott, Tallbot, Tallbott

Tanner OE. Occupational name: "Leather tanner." Hides need to be tanned, or treated with a substance containing tannin, before they become leather. Use as a first name is uncommon; generally a transferred last name.
Tan, Tanney, Tannie

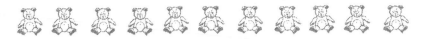

Tanton OE. Place name: "Still river settlement."

Tarleton OE. "Thor's settlement." Margaret Mitchell fans
will remember the Tarleton twins, admirers of Scarlett
O'Hara, in the early pages of *Gone With the Wind.*

Tarrant Old Welsh. "Thunder."
Tarrent

Tate Middle English. "Happy, cheerful."
Tait, Taitt, Tayte

Tavish Ir. Gael. "Twin."
Tavis, Tevis

Taylor Middle English. Occupational name: "Tailor." Like
the rest of the occupational names, used mostly in the
19th century.
Tailer, Tailor, Tayler

Teague Ir. Gael. "Bard, poet."
Teagan

Ted Dim. **Theodore** (Gk. "gift of God") or **Edward** (OE.
"wealthy defender"). Rarely used as an independent
name. Parents tend to give the longer rather than the
shorter version of a name, even if they have decided
ahead of time to use the diminutive form. Newscaster
Ted Koppel; actor Ted Danson.
Tedd, Teddey, Teddie, Teddy

Tedmund OE. "Protector of the land."
Tedmond

Telford OF. "Iron-piercer."
Telfer, Telfor, Telfour

Tempest Fr. "Storm." Occurs as an aristocratic English
last name, and occasionally as a first name, though few
parents could wish for a baby's personality to fit the
name.

Templeton OE. Place name: "Temple settlement." Also
the name of the rat in *Charlotte's Web*, a point that the
young are sure to seize on.
Temp, Temple, Templeten

Tennant OE. "Tenant, renter." Last name used as first
name.
Tenant, Tennent

Tennesee Cherokee place name, used for the state. Made

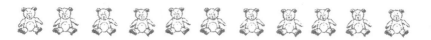

famous by playwright Tennesee Williams (whose given name was Thomas) and likely to be used by nineties parents in homage.

Tennyson Middle English. "Son of Dennis." Used by 19th-century parents in homage to British Poet Laureate Alfred, Lord Tennyson.

Tenny

Terence Lat. Clan name of unknown meaning, though some sources propose "smooth" or "polished." Early Christian name that was never widely adopted until the late 19th century, and even then did not become a standard choice. Actor Terence Stamp.

Tarrance, Terencio, Terrance, Terrence, Terrey, Terri, Terry

Terrill OG. "Following Thor." **Thor**, the god of thunder, was a crucial figure in Norse mythology. The son of Odin, the chief god, Thor was the benevolent intercessor for mankind. His name is an element in many names that have come down to us, the most notable being "Thursday."

Terrall, Terrel, Terrell, Terryl, Terryll, Tirrell, Tyrrell

Terry Dim. **Terence.** Lat. Clan name. Used for both boys and girls, probably more often than Terence itself. Its real heyday was the baby boom era, making it an unlikely choice for the 1990s.

Terrey, Terri, Terrie

Tex Modern name of the Lone Star state, used occasionally as a first name. It has a rakish aura, no doubt from association with cowboys and the Wild West.

Thaddeus Aramaic. Meaning unclear, though "courageous" and "praise" have been suggested. He was one of the more obscure of the twelve apostles, but even this distinction has not popularized the name. Jude is another form of the name.

Tad, Tadd, Taddeo, Taddeusz, Tadeo, Tadio, Tadzio, Thad, Thaddaus

Thane OE. "Landholder." In Old England a thane fit, socially, between the serfs and the nobility. He held his own land, but owed service to his lord. Rare even as a last name.

Thaine, Thayne

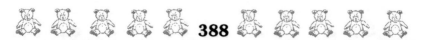

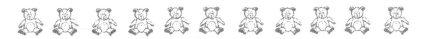

Thatcher OE. Occupational name: "Roof thatcher." In the 1990s bound to be associated with the recent British Prime Minister, Margaret Thatcher.

Thacher, Thatch, Thaxter

Thaw OE. "Melt." Found more often as a last name.

Theobald OG. "Courageous people." Unusual, though some of its foreign variants like Thibault are more common in their countries of origin.

Dietbald, Dietbold, Ted, Teddy, Teobaldo, Thebault, Theo, Thibaud, Thibault, Thibaut, Tibold, Tiebold, Tiebout, Tybald, Tybalt, Tybault

Theodore Gk. "Gift of God." Early Christian name and saint's name, but only mildly popular until President Theodore Roosevelt brought it to prominence. (The teddy bear, of course, is named for him.) The name is now neither popular nor unpopular. Authors Theodore Dreiser, Theodore Sturgeon; painter Théodore Rousseau.

Fedor, Feodor, Fyodor, Teador, Ted, Teddie, Teddy, Tedor, Teodoor, Teodor, Teodoro, Theo, Theodor, Theodorus, Theodosios, Todor, Tudor

Theodoric OGer. "People's ruler." This is the original form of Dietrich and the more common Derek or Dirk. In this version it is extremely rare.

Derek, Derrick, Dieter, Dietrich, Dirck, Dirk, Rick, Ted, Teodorico, Thedric, Thedrick

Theophilus Gk. "Loved by God." A New Testament name that is very rare, though Thornton Wilder entitled one of his most popular novels *Theophilus North*.

Teofil, Théophile

Thierry Fr. Var. **Theodoric**. Not, as one might suppose, the French version of Terry. Fashion designer Thierry Mugler.

Thomas Aramaic. "Twin." One of the apostles, known as Doubting Thomas because he refused to recognize the risen Christ unless he could see and feel the marks of the crucifixion. In spite of this skeptical example, the name has been hugely popular since the 12th century martyrdom of Thomas à Becket. Other Saints Thomas include Thomas Aquinas and Thomas More, but the

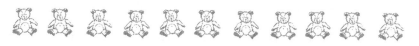

name has been so widely used that it has no religious aura to it. The recent vogue for unusual names, however, has somewhat eclipsed this old standard. President Thomas Jefferson; inventor Thomas Edison; actors Tom Cruise, Tom Hanks; dancer Tommy Tune.

Tam, Tamas, Thom, Thomason, Thomson, Thompson, Tom, Tomas, Tomaso, Tomasso, Tomasz, Tome, Tomek, Tomey, Tomie, Tomislaw, Tomkin, Tomlin, Tommaso, Tommey, Tommie, Tommy

Thor ONorse. "Thunder." The Norse god of thunder, Thor, holds an important place in the Norse pantheon, but in the Anglo-Saxon world the name appears more often in derivative forms, as in Terrill. Explorer Thor Heyerdahl.

Thorin, Thorvald, Tor, Tore, Torre, Tyrus

Thorald ONorse. "Follower of Thor."

Terrell, Terrill, Thorold, Torald, Tyrell

Thorbert ONorse. "Thor's brightness."

Torbert

Thorburn ONorse. "Thor's bear."

Thorbjorn

Thorley OE. Place name: "Thor's meadow" or "thorn meadow."

Thorlea, Thorlee, Thorleigh, Thorly, Torley

Thormond OE. "Defended by Thor."

Thurmond, Thurmund

Thorndike OE. Place name: "Thorny bank."

Thorndyck, Thorndyke

Thorne OE. Place name: "Thorn thicket."

Thorn

Thornley OE. Place name: "Thorny meadow."

Thornlea, Thornleigh, Thornly

Thornton OE. Place name: "Thorny village or town." Used as a first name since the 19th century. Writer Thornton Wilder.

Thorpe OE. Place name: "Hamlet, village."

Thorp

Thurlow OE. Place name: "Thor's hill."

Thurston Scan. "Thor's stone." Parents who watched a lot of TV in the 1960s might shy away from a name that

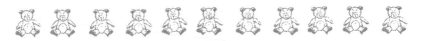

recalled Thurston Howell, the effete millionaire cast-away on "Gilligan's Island." Social critic Thorstein Veblen.

Thorstan, Thorstein, Thorsten, Thurstain, Thurstan, Thursten, Torsten, Torston

Tibor Slavic. "Sacred place."

Tiernan Ir. Gael. "Lord."

Tierney

Tilden OE. Place name: "Fertile valley."

Tilford OE. Place name: "Fertile ford."

Tilton OE. Place name: "fertile estate." All three of these "Til-" names were last names, used occasionally as first names starting in the 19th century.

Till Ger. "People's ruler." Another form of **Theodoric**, vaguely familiar to American ears from the German legends about Till Eulenspiegel, inspiration for an opera by Richard Strauss.

Thilo, Tillman, Tilmann

Timothy Gk. "Honoring God." New Testament name, correspondent with Saint Paul. Scanty use until the 18th century, then increased gradually to the middle of the 20th. After a baby boom peak, it has faded. Radical thinker Timothy Leary; actor Timothy Hutton.

Tim, Timmy, Timmothy, Timo, Timofei, Timofeo, Timofey, Timon, Timoteo, Timothé, Timotheo, Timothey, Timotheus, Tymmothy, Tymon, Tymoteusz, Tymothy

Tino Sp. Dim. **Agostino** and other "-tin" names.

Titus Lat. Unknown meaning. New Testament character. Use is mostly 18th and 19th centuries. Has nothing to do, in spite of its sound, with titans or giants.

Tito, Titos

Tobias Heb. "The Lord is good." Old Testament name that faded after the Puritans used it, and was revived in the 19th century. The diminutive, Toby, is more common now.

Tobe, Tobey, Tobia, Tobiah, Tobie, Tobin, Tobit, Toby

Todd Middle English. "Fox." Used mostly in this century, and fashionable for a spell in the 1970s.

Tod

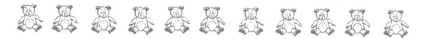

Tom Dim. **Thomas**. Most common in the 19th century as an independent name.
Thom, Tomm, Tommy

Tomlin OE. "Little Tom."
Tomlinson

Tony Dim. **Anthony**. Lat. "Beyond price." Used independently only since the middle of the 20th century. Actors Tony Curtis, Tony Danza.
Toney, Tonie

Tor Nor. "Thunder." Var. **Thor.**
Thor

Torquil ONorse. "Thor's kettle." Use is almost exclusively British.

Torr OE. Place name: "Tower."
Tor

Torrance Ir. Gael. Place name: "Little hills."
Tore, Torin, Torr, Torrence, Torrey, Torrin, Torry

Townley OE. Place name: "Town meadow."
Townlea, Townlee, Townleigh, Townlie, Townly

Townsend OE. Place name: "End of town."

Tracy OF. Place name. Almost always a girl's name now.
Trace, Tracey, Treacy

Trahern Welsh. "Strength of iron."
Traherne

Travis OF. Occupational name: "Toll taker." Most common in the U.S. Fictional Detective Travis Magee.
Traver, Travers, Travys

Tremain Celt. Place name: "Stone house."
Tremaine, Tremayne

Trent Lat. "Gushing waters." Name of an important river in England, thus a place name.
Trenten, Trentin, Trenton

Trevor Welsh. "Large homestead." Use expanded outside of Wales in the mid-Victorian era, but the name was most popular in the middle of the 20th century. Actor Trevor Howard.
Trefor, Trevar, Trever

Trey Middle English. "Three." Related to the French *trois* for "three." Very unusual. Actor Trey Hunt.

Tristan Welsh. The name's Welsh meaning is unclear, but

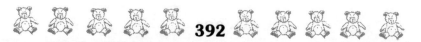

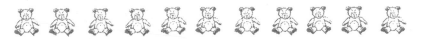

since *triste* is French for "sad," that explanation is often given. Tristan, in the medieval legends, is the knight who is in love with Isolde, wife of his uncle. The tale has been told in many forms, including an epic poem by Tennyson and an opera by Wagner.

Tris, Tristam, Tristram

Trowbridge OE. Place name: "Bridge by the tree."

Troy Ir. Gael. "Foot-soldier." The name of the famous Greek city where the Trojan wars were fought, and a fairly common place name in America (as in Troy, NY). Actor Troy Donahue may have been behind the name's surge of popularity in the 1960s and 1970s. Jane Fonda named one of her children Troy.

Troi, Troye

Truman OE. "Loyal one." Unusual as a last name or a first name, in spite of the greatly admired author Truman Capote or U.S. President Harry S. Truman.

Trueman, Trumaine, Trumann

Trumble OE. "Powerful."

Trumball, Trumbell, Trumbull

Tucker OE. Occupational name: "Fabric pleater." Another occupational name relating to one of medieval Britain's principal industries, the woolen trade.

Tudor Welsh. Var. **Theodore**. Famous as the name of the English dynasty of kings.

Turner Middle English. Occupational name: "Woodworker." "Turning" referred to use of a lathe, which provided the decorative elements on much furniture in the 16th and 17th centuries. Painter J. M. W. Turner.

Twain Middle English. "Divided in two." The most famous bearer of this name, the American writer Mark Twain, took it from the calls of riverboatmen. His original name was Samuel Clemens.

Twaine, Twayn

Twyford OE. Place name: "Double river crossing."

Tyler OE. Occupational name: "Maker of tiles." The name of one of the country's less memorable presidents (John Tyler, 1841–1845). Still, the name is mildly popular in the early 1990s, along with other unusual names like **Hunter** and **Max**.

Tilar, Ty, Tylar

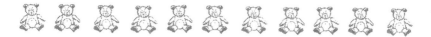

Tynan Ir. Gael. "Dark, dusky."

Tyrone Ir. Gael. "Land of Owen." Given prominence almost entirely by the actors Tyrone Power, Sr., and Jr., around the middle of the 20th century.

Tyson OF. Meaning unclear. Parents in the late 1980s may have used it in admiration of the boxing star Mike Tyson.

Ubadah Arab. "Serves God."

Udell OE. Place name: "Valley of yew trees." Arizona politician Morris Udall.
   Dell, Eudel, Udel, Udall, Yudale, Yudell

Udo Dim. Ulric.

Udolf OE. "Wolf-wealth."
   Udolfo, Udolph

Ugo It. Var. **Hugh**. OG. "Mind, intellect."

Ulf OG. "Wolf." Currently very popular in Sweden.

Ulmer OE. "Fame of the wolf."
   Ullmar, Ulmar

Ulric OG. "Power of the wolf" or "power of the home." Used in Britain before the Norman invasion, but barely known in the last 900-odd years.
   Rick, Udo, Ullric, Ulrich, Ulrick, Ulrik

Ulysses Lat. Var. **Odysseus**, which may mean "wrathful." American use was spurred by the presidency of Civil War hero Ulysses S. Grant. Now rare.
   Ulises, Ulisse

Umberto It. Var. **Humbert**. OG. "Renowned Hun." A royal name in Italy, though very scarce in English-speaking countries. Author Umberto Eco.

Unwin OE. "Nonfriend."
   Unwinn, Unwyn

Upton OE. Place name: "Upper settlement." Mostly last-name use. Author Upton Sinclair.

Upwood OE. Place name: "Upper forest."

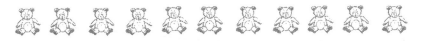

Urban Lat. "From the city." We have a modern word, "urbane," from the same root. Apparently in ancient times city-dwellers had better manners than their rural contemporaries. Though the name was used by eight popes, it is scarce today in English-speaking countries.
Urbain, Urbaine, Urbane, Urbano, Urbanus

Uriah Heb. "The Lord is my light." Prominent Old Testament name at its most popular in the 19th century, though literary parents will be reminded of the smarmy, hand-wringing Uriah Heep in Dickens's *David Copperfield*. Dickens may have killed off the name, in fact; it is very scarce today.
Uri, Uria, Urias, Yuri, Yuria

Uriel Heb. "Flame of God." The Muslim version of the name is Israfil; he is the Muslim angel of music and appears in the Koran along with Gabriel and Michael. In Christian terms he is one of seven named archangels.

Usamah Arab. "Like a lion."

Uziel Heb. "Strength, power."
Uzziah, Uzziel

Vachel OF. "Small cow." Something of a curiosity, brought to public notice by the poet Vachel Lindsay.
Vachell

Vail OE. Place name: "Valley." Famous now as a ski resort in Colorado. Generally a transferred last name.
Bail, Bale, Vaile, Vaill, Vale

Val Dim. **Valentine**. Actor Val Kilmer.

Valdemar OG. "Renowned leader."

Valentine Lat. "Strong." This name and Valerian come from the same root. Valentine is used for both boys and girls, although the early Christian martyr for whom the holiday is named was male.
Val, Valentijn, Valentin, Valentino, Valentyn

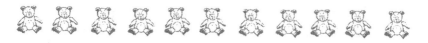

Valerian Lat. "Strong, healthy." Far less common than the feminine version, Valerie. Designer Valerian Rybar.
Valerien, Valerio, Valery, Valeryan

Van Dutch. "Of." A particle of many Dutch names, as in Vandyke. Also possibly a nickname for Evan. Originally may have been used as a nickname for children with transferred Dutch last names, but it became generally popular in the middle of the 20th century. Neglected now. Pianist Van Cliburn; actor Van Johnson.
Vann

Vance OE. Place name: "Marshland." Author Vance Packard.

Vandyke Dutch. Place name: "Of the dyke." The New York area was originally settled by Dutch colonists, and a few Dutch names survive, though not many are used as first names. A "Vandyke" is also the name of a small beard or goatee, from the beards portrayed in portraits by the 17th-century Flemish painter Anthony Van Dyck. Actor Dick Van Dyke.

Vanya Rus. Dim. **John** (Heb. "the Lord is gracious") via **Ivan.** Rare outside of Russia.

Vardon OF. Place name: "Green knoll." The second half of the name comes from the French word that gives us "dune."
Varden, Verdon, Verdun

Varick OG. "Leader who defends."
Varrick, Warick, Warrick

Vasilis Gk. "Royal, kingly." More familiar in its anglicized form, **Basil.**
Vasileios, Vaso, Vasos, Vassilij, Vassily, Vasya, Wassily

Vaughn Welsh. "Small." Appeared as a first name at the turn of the 20th century, at its peak popularity in the baby boom era. Never especially common, though. Actor Robert Vaughn; composer Ralph Vaughan Williams.
Vaughan

Vere Fr. Place name of unknown meaning. It was an upper-class last name in England, and took on near-caricature connotations of nobility, especially after Tennyson published "Lady Clara Vere de Vere," a poem praising the simple values of simple folk. (It contains the

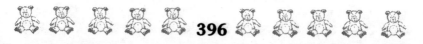

396

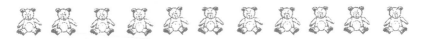

famous line "Kind hearts are more than coronets.") Vere
has not been used much in the U.S.

Vernon OF. Place name: "Alder grove." A Norman name
that took root as an English last name and, by the 19th
century, a first name.
Lavern, Vern, Verne, Vernen, Vernin, Verney

Verrill OF. "Loyal" or OG. "masculine."
Verill, Verrall, Verrell, Verroll, Veryl

Victor Lat. "Conqueror." Extremely common in Christian
Rome, as was its female form, Victoria. Revived during
the reign of Queen Victoria, but not extremely popular
(except among her numerous descendants and godchil-
dren). It was used most during the baby boom era, but
not very widely. Cinematographer Vittorio Storaro; actor
Victor Mature; author Victor Hugo.
**Vic, Vick, Victorien, Victorin, Vidor, Viktor, Vitorio,
Vittorio, Vittorios**

Vilmos Hung. "Determined fighter."

Vincent Lat. "Conquering." From the same root as **Victor,**
but used much more steadily since early Christian days.
It has not suffered neglect, but neither has it ever been
truly popular. Saint Vincent de Paul, a 17th-century
priest, founded an order of missionary brothers, and the
Saint Vincent de Paul Society, an international charitable
organization, was founded in his honor in the 19th cen-
tury. Painter Vincent Van Gogh; film director Vincente
Minnelli; actor Vincent Gardenia.
**Vicente, Vicenzio, Vincenzo, Vin, Vince, Vincens,
Vincentius, Vincents, Vincenty, Vincenz, Vincenzio,
Vincenzo, Vincien, Vinnie, Vinny, Vinzenz**

Vine OE. Occupational name: "Vineyard worker."

Vinson OE. "Son of Vincent."

Virgil Lat. Clan name: possibly meaning "staff bearer."
(The staff would have been part of official insignia in
ancient Rome.) The name is usually homage to the Roman author of *The Aeneid*.
Verge, Vergil, Virgilio

Vito Lat. "Alive." Generally used by Spanish families.
Vital, Vitale, Vitalis, Vitus, Witold

Vivian Lat. "Full of life." Used occasionally for boys in

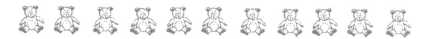

Britain, but an American infant named Vivian would be assumed to be a girl.

Vivyan, Vyvian, Vyvyan

Vladimir Slavic. "Renowned prince." Pianist Vladimir Horowitz.

Vladamir, Vladimeer, Wladimir, Wladimyr

Vladislav Old Slavic. "Splendid rule."

Volker Ger. "People's defender." From the German word that gives us "folk."

Volney OG. "Spirit of the folk."

Wade OE. Place name: "River ford." Transferred last name with a certain popularity in old southern families, after Confederate General Wade Hampton.

Wayde

Wadley OE. Place name: "Ford meadow."

Wadleigh, Wadly

Wadsworth OE. Place name: "Village near the ford." Transferred last name of a family that has long been prominent on the American cultural scene. Poet Henry Wadsworth Longfellow.

Waddsworth

Wagner Ger. Occupational name: "Wagon-builder." New York City Mayor Robert Wagner.

Waggoner

Wainwright OE. Occupational name: "Wagon-builder." Quite a mouthful as a first name, and most likely to be used when it's a family name, such as a mother's maiden name.

Wainright, Wayneright, Waynewright, Waynright

Waite Middle English. Occupational name: "Guard, watchman." In other words, one who waited. Actor/musician Tom Waits.

Waits, Wayte

Wakefield OE. Place name: "Damp field."

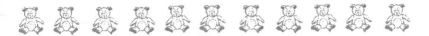

Wakeley OE. Place name: "Damp meadow."
Wakelea, Wakeleigh, Wakely
Wakeman OE. Occupational name: "Watchman." Or one who was awake when others slept. All too appropriate for most babies.
Wake
Walcott OE. Place name: "Cottage by the wall." Could originally have referred to the great Roman wall that still stands in the north of England.
Wallcot, Wallcott, Wolcott
Waldemar OG. "Renowned ruler." Many of these Old German names (William is another) are actually made up of two particles that are both nouns: in this case they are "fame" and "power."
Valdemar
Walden OE. Place name: "Wooded valley." Could also be another variant of one of the Old German names that include the "Wald-" ("power") element, like Walter. Many literature-loving parents may think of Thoreau's book and the pond *Walden*.
Waldi, Waldon
Waldo Dim. **Waldemar**, etc. The "-o" ending is a particularly Germanic diminutive. Though more common than some of the longer forms like Waldemar, it's still unusual. Poet Ralph Waldo Emerson.
Waldron OG. "Powerful raven."
Walford OE. Place name: "Brook ford." Composer Walford Davies.
Walfred OG. "Ruler of peace."
Walker OE. Occupational name: "Cloth-walker." The era that saw the rise of last names was also the great English era of the wool trade, giving us such cloth-manufacturing names as Fuller, Dyer, and Weaver. In that medieval era, workers trod on the wool to clean it. Author Walker Percy; photographer Walker Evans.
Wallace OE. "Welshman." Originally a Scottish name, used to identify foreigners from the south. Like many last names, it was most popular as a first name in the 19th century. Poet Wallace Stevens.

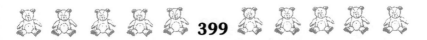

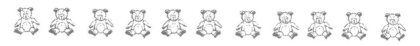

Wallach, Wallas, Wallie, Wallis, Wally, Walsh, Welch, Welsh

Waller OE. Occupational name: "wall maker" or OG. "powerful one."

Wally Dim. **Walter, Wallace,** etc. Actors Wally Shawn, Wally Cox.

Walter OG. "People of power" or "army of power." Norman name that took root strongly in Britain and has been used quite steadily for the last 900 years (with the occasional century of neglect). Not particularly fashionable now. Cartoonist Walt Disney; poet Walt Whitman; journalist Walter Cronkite; actors Walter Brennan, Walter Matthau.

Gaultier, Gauthier, Gautier, Gualterio, Gualtiero, Valter, Valther, Walder, Wally, Walt, Walther, Wat, Watkins

Walton OE. Place name: "Walled town." Composer William Walton.

Walworth OE. Place name: "Walled farm."

Walwyn OE. "Welsh friend."

Walwin, Walwinn, Walwynn, Walwynne, Welwyn

Warburton OE. Place name: "Long-standing fortress town."

Ward OE. Occupational name: "Watchman." Like many of these occupational or place names turned last names, **Ward** was revived as a first name in the 19th century. It is still somewhat more common as a first name than most other occupational names (Smith, Baker, Turner, etc.). Author Ward Just.

Warde, Warden, Worden

Wardell OE. Place name: "Watchman's hill."

Wardley OE. Place name: "Watchman's meadow."

Wardlea, Wardleigh

Ware OE. "Watchful, aware."

Warfield Middle English. Place name: "Field by the weir." A weir was a kind of enclosure built into a stream to trap fish.

Warford Middle English. "Ford near the weir."

Warley Middle English. "Meadow near the weir."

Warner OG. "Fighting defender." Philosopher Wernher Erhardt.

Werner, Wernher

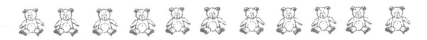

Warren OE. "watchman" or Middle English. "park warden." A warren was originally an area devoted to breeding game, especially rabbits. By extension, the word is now used to describe human dwellings that resemble the haphazard and overcrowded rabbits' tunnels. As a name, Warren was used in the late 19th century and given a boost by the career of President Warren G. Harding. Actor Warren Beatty; U.S. Supreme Court Chief Justice Warren Burger.
Ware, Waring, Warrin, Warriner

Warton OE. Place name: "Town near the weir."

Warwick OE. Place name: "Buildings near the weir."
Warick, Warrick

Washburn OE. Place name: "Flooding stream."

Washington OE. Place name: Possibly "clever man's settlement." Author Washington Irving, born in 1783, was in all likelihood named for the first U.S. president, but the name has not been used as much as one might think, possibly because of its length.

Watson OE. "Son of Walter." Last name used as a first name primarily in the 19th century. Most famous as the name of the sidekick to whom Sherlock Holmes perpetually condescended: "Elementary, my dear Watson."

Waverly OE. Place name: "Meadow of quivering aspens."
Waverlee, Waverley

Wayland OE. Place name: "Land by the path." Singer Waylon Jennings.
Way, Waylan, Waylen, Waylin, Waylon, Weylin

Wayne OE. Occupational name: "Wagon builder or driver," as in Wainwright. Its period of popularity coincided with the popularity of the actor Marion Morrison, better known as John Wayne. Performer Wayne Newton.
Wain, Wayn

Webb OE. Occupational name: "Weaver." Mostly 19th-century use. Actor Clifton Webb.
Web, Weber, Webster

Webley OE. Place name: "Weaver's meadow."
Webbley, Webbly, Webly

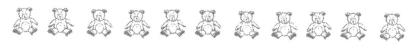

Welborne OE. Place name: "Spring-fed stream." Not, alas, indicative of patrician origins.
Welborn, Welbourne, Welburn, Wellborn, Wellbourn, Wellburn

Welby OG. Place name: "Well-farm." Many parents will think of the long-running TV serial "Marcus Welby, M.D."
Welbey, Welbie, Wellbey, Wellby

Weldon OE. Place name: "Well-hill."
Welden, Welldon

Welford OE. Place name: "Well-ford."
Wellford

Wellington OE. Place name of unclear meaning. Has aristocratic connotations, no doubt from the famous Duke of Wellington, who defeated Napoleon and gave his name to tall, waterproof boots and filet of beef wrapped in pastry.

Wells OE. Place name: "Wells." The name of a famous cathedral town in western England. First-name use was mostly 19th century.

Welton OE. Place name: "Well-town."

Wenceslaus Old Slavic. "Glorious garland." King Wenceslas, the patron saint of Czechoslovakia, was a 10th-century monarch of Bohemia and a martyr for the faith. The famous Christmas carol (written in the 19th century) refers to an entirely imaginary episode, but the name would be unknown to us without it.
Wenceslas, Wenzel, Wiencyslaw

Wendell OG. "Wanderer." Quite rare. Attorney Wendell Willkie.
Wendall, Wendel

Wentworth OE. Place name: "Pale man's settlement."

Werner OG. "Defense army." Closely related to Warner. Use is mostly confined to the U.S.
Wernhar, Wernher

Wesley OE. Place name: "Western meadow." Used in honor of John and Charles Wesley, who founded the Methodist church in the 18th century.
Wesly, Wessley, Westleigh, Westley

Westbrook OE. Place name: "Western stream." This

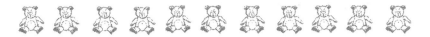

group of place names illustrates one way last names came into use: They described the location of someone's dwelling.

Brook, Brooke, Wesbrook, West, Westbrooke

Westby OE. Place name: "Western farmstead."

Westcott OE. Place name: "Western cottage."

Wescot, Wescott, Westcot

Weston OE. Place name: "Western settlement."

Westen, Westin

Wetherby OE. Place name: "Wether-sheep farm." A wether is a male sheep that has been castrated; a bellwether is a wether who wears a bell and leads a flock. Again, the importance of the wool trade in England when last names were formed gives these "Wether-" names unusual prominence.

Weatherbey, Weatherbie, Weatherby, Wetherbey, Wetherbie

Wetherell OE. Place name: "Wether-sheep corner."

Weatherell, Weatherill, Wetherill, Wethrill

Wetherly OE. Place name: "Wether-sheep meadow."

Weatherley, Weatherly, Wetherleigh, Wetherley

Wharton OE. Place name: "Shore or bank settlement."

Warton

Wheatley OE. Place name: "Wheat field."

Wheatlea, Wheatleigh, Wheatly

Wheaton OE. Place name: "Wheat settlement."

Wheeler OE. Occupational name: "Wheel maker."

Whistler OE. Occupational name: "Whistler or piper." Artist James Whistler.

Whitby OE. Place name: "White farm." All of these "Whit-" names are more commonly last names, though some were used more regularly as first names in the 19th century.

Whitbey, Whitbie

Whitcomb OE. Place name: "White valley." Poet James Whitcomb Riley.

Whitcombe, Whitcumb

Whitelaw OE. Place name: "White hill." Diplomat Whitelaw Reid.

Whitlaw

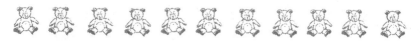

Whitfield OE. Place name: "White field."

Whitford OE. Place name: "White ford."

Whitley OE. Place name: "White meadow."

Whitlock OE. "White lock of hair."

Whitman OE. "White man." The description would refer to hair or complexion. Poet Walt Whitman.

Whitmore OE. Place name: "White moor."
   Whitmoor, Whittemore, Witmore, Wittemore

Whitney OE. Place name: "White island." Last name that was annexed as a girl's name in the 1980s. It is much more popular for girls than it ever was for boys. Railroad millionaire William Collins Whitney.

Whittaker OE. Place name: "White field."
   Whitacker, Whitaker

Wickham OE. Place name: "Village paddock."

Wilbert OG. "Brilliant and resolute." Not the same as Wilbur, despite the similar sound. Used sporadically in the 19th and 20th centuries.
   Wilburt

Wilbur OG. Last name of obscure meaning. Probably confused with Wilbert over the years. E. B. White fans will associate it with the protagonist of *Charlotte's Web*, Wilbur the Pig. Aviator Wilbur Wright.
   Wilber, Willbur

Wiley OE. Place name: "Water meadow." Indicates a meadow that would be flooded from time to time.
   Willey, Wylie

Wilford OE. Place name: "Willow-ford." Actor Wilford Brimley.

Wilfred OE. "Purposeful peace." Like Waldemar, another name whose two elements are both nouns (in this case "will" and "peace"), to the confusion of the translator. Neglected after the Norman invasion, but revived in the 19th century to some popularity, which never spread as far as the U.S. Author Wilfred Sheed.
   Wilfredo, Wilfrid, Wilfried, Wilfryd, Will, Willfred, Willfredo, Willfried

Wilkinson OE. "Son of little Will."
   Wilkins, Willkins, Willkinson

Willard OG. "Bold will." Most common in the U.S.,

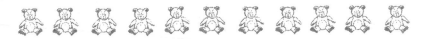

though far from a household word. TV weatherman Willard Scott.

William OG. "Will-helmet." Another two-noun name, more often translated as "resolute protection" or the like. Given a great boost in Norman England by William the Conqueror and succeeding English kings. Between the 17th and 20th centuries, one of the top handful of boy's names, but its popularity has diminished considerably since 1900. The young Prince William of Wales may bring it back into use. Playwright William Shakespeare; actors William Hurt, Willem Dafoe; film director Wim Wenders; poet William Blake; author William Faulkner; U.S. Presidents William H. Harrison, William H. Taft, William McKinley.

Bill, Billie, Billy, Guglielmo, Guillaume, Guillermo, Liam, Vilhelm, Villem, Wilek, Wiley, Wilhelm, Wilhelmus, Wilkes, Wilkie, Wilkinson, Will, Willem, Willhelmus, Willi, Williamson, Willie, Willis, Willkie, Wills, Willson, Willy, Wilmar, Wilmot, Wilmott, Wilson, Wim

Willoughby OE. Place name: "Willow farm."

Willoughbey, Willoughbie

Wilmer OG. "Determined fame."

Willmer, Wylmer

Wilson OE. "Son of Will." Last name turned first name, possibly in compliment to President Woodrow Wilson. Composer Robert Wilson.

Willson

Wilton OE. Place name: "Well settlement."

Windsor OE. Place name: "Riverbank with a winch." Famous from the town and castle of that name in England, and above all from the fact that it is the British royal family's last name. Also the name of a standard way to tie a necktie, invented by the Duke of Windsor, who was a great dandy.

Wyndsor

Winfield OE. "Friend's field." Baseball player Dave Winfield.

Winnfield, Wynfield, Wynnfield

Wingate OE. Place name: "Winding gate." May refer to a gate like a turnstile.

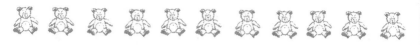

Winslow OE. Place name: "Friend's hill." Painter Winslow Homer.

Winston OE. Place name: "Friend's town" or "wine's town." For modern parents, recalls both English statesman Winston Churchill and a popular brand of cigarettes.
Winsten, Winstonn, Wynstan, Wynston

Winthrop OE. Place name: "Friend's village." In the U.S., it hearkens back to the Puritan governor of Massachusetts, John Winthrop, and his numerous Bostonian descendants.

Winton OE. Place name: "Friend's settlement." Closely related to Winston.

Wolcott OE. Place name: "Wolf's cottage." Wolf, in this case, would be a first name.

Wolfe OE. "wolf."
Woolf

Wolfgang OG. "Wolf quarrel." A very Germanic name that would not be considered by English-speaking parents without the fame of composer Wolfgang Amadeus Mozart.

Woodrow OE. "Row by the woods." "Row" could refer to a row of houses or trees or bushes (as in a hedgerow). The name has been given prominence beyond the usual place name by admirers of U.S. President Woodrow Wilson.
Woody

Woodward OE. Place name: "Woods warden." Actor Edward Woodward.
Woodard

Woody Dim. **Woodrow,** etc. A particularly American name adopted by actor Allen Konigsberg, now better known as Woody Allen. Folk singer Woody Guthrie.

Worth OE. Place name: "Fenced farm." Used since the 19th century.
Worthey, Worthington, Worthy

Wright OE. Occupational name: "Carpenter." Again, mostly 19th-century use. The astounding feats of aviators Orville and Wilbur Wright apparently did not in-

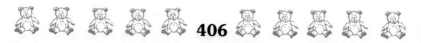

spire parents to use their name in homage. Painter Joseph Wright of Derby.

Wyatt OF. "Small fighter." Last name occasionally used as a first name, notably by Wild West Sheriff Wyatt Earp.
Wiatt, Wye

Wycliff OE. Place name: "White cliff."
Wycliffe

Wylie OE. "Clever, charming, full of wiles."
Wiley, Wye

Wyndham OE. Place name: Either "Wyman's hamlet" or "hamlet near the winding way." Used as a first name in the 19th century and into the 20th, but very unusual today. Author Wyndham Lewis.
Windham, Wynndham

Wynn Welsh. "fair, white" or OE. "friend." Used more frequently for girls in the past few years, but still uncommon.
Win, Winn, Wynne

X

Xan Dim. **Alexander**. Gk. "Defender of mankind."

Xanthus Gk. "Golden-haired."
Xanthos

Xavier Basque. "New house." Most often found as a middle name following Francis, in honor of Saint Francis Xavier, a 16th-century Jesuit missionary who took Christianity to the East Indies and Japan. Band leader Xavier Cugat.
Javier, Xever, Zavier

Xenophon Gk. "Foreign voice." Xenophon was a Greek historian of the 4th century B.C.
Xeno

Xenos Gk. "Hospitality."
Zeno, Zenos

Xerxes Per. "Monarch." Xerxes was the title of several Persian rulers. One (in the 5th century B.C.) made war

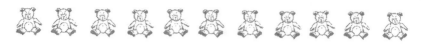

on the Greeks and also appears in the biblical Apocrypha as Ahasuerus, husband of Esther.

Ximenes Sp. Var. **Simon.** Heb. "Listening intently."
Jimenes, Jimenez, Ximenez

Yaakov Heb. Form of **Jacob** ("he who supplants"). Comedian Yakov Smirnov.
Iago, Yaacob, Yachov, Yacov, Yago, Yakob, Yakov

Yale OE. Place name: "Fertile moor." Familiar as the name of one of the Ivy League universities, founded by Elihu Yale.

Yancy Origin unclear. Several sources suggest this was an Indian word for "Englishman," and propose that this was the origin of the word "Yankee." But the *Facts on File Dictionary of First Names* claims the name is used to honor a Southern proslavery politician of the 19th century. Rare, in any case.
Yance, Yancey, Yantsey

Yannis Gk. Var. **John.** Heb. "The Lord is gracious."
Ioannis, Yanni, Yannakis

Yaphet Heb. "Comely." Actor Yaphet Koto.
Japhet, Japheth, Yapheth

Yardley OE. Place name: "Fenced meadow."
Yardlee, Yardlea, Yardleigh, Yardly

Yasahiro Jap. "Serene."

Yasir Arab. "Well to do." Palestinian leader Yasser Arafat.
Yaseer, Yasser

Yates Middle English. Place name: "The gates." Poet W. B. Yeats.
Yeats

Yehudi Heb. "Praise." Related to the feminine Judith, and to the nearly obsolete Jude. Violinist Yehudi Menuhin.
Judah, Yechudi, Yechudit, Yehuda, Yehudah, Yehudit

Yeoman Middle English. "Attendant, servant."
Youman

Yitzhak Heb. Var. **Isaac** ("laughter"). Violinist Itzhak Perlman.
Itzak, Izaak, Yitzchak

Yochanan Heb. "The Lord is gracious." A form of **John**.
Johanan, Yohannan

York OE. Place name: "Boar settlement" or "yew settlement." Also familiar as an American place name, which makes it a bit difficult to use as a first name.
Yorick, Yorrick, Yorke

Yule OE. "Winter solstice." The time of year around Dec. 21, the pagan winter feast. Now, of course, it means Christmas. Rarely used, even for Christmas babies.
Euell, Ewell

Yuri Rus. Var. **George**. Lat. "Farmer."
Yurii, Yury

Yusuf Var. **Joseph**. Heb. "The Lord increases." Currently very popular in Arabic-speaking countries. The "-uf" ending is more typically Arab, the "-ef" ending more often Hebrew.
Yosef, Yoseff, Yusef, Yusuff

Yves Fr. Var. **Ivo**. OG. "Yew wood." Since yew wood was used for bows, the name may have been an occupational one meaning "archer." This form is almost exclusively found in France. Singer Yves Montand; fashion designer Yves Saint Laurent.
Ives, Ivo, Yvo

Zachariah Heb. "The Lord's has remembered." Biblical name occurring in both Old and New Testaments. As might be expected, it was revived by the Puritans and found fairly constantly through the 19th century. Less common in the 20th, but boys named Zack are turning up in more and more nursery schools in the 1990s. President Zachary Taylor.
Zacaria, Zacarias, Zacary, Zaccaria, Zaccariah, Zaccheus,

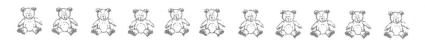

Zach, Zachaios, Zacharia, Zacharias, Zacharie, Zachary, Zacheriah, Zachery, Zacheus, Zack, Zackariah, Zackerias, Zackery, Zak, Zakarias, Zakarie, Zakariyyah, Zakery, Zecheriah, Zekariah, Zekeriah, Zeke

Zadok Heb. "Fair, righteous."
Zadoc, Zaydok

Zale Gk. "Sea-strength."
Zayle

Zalman Heb. "Peaceable." The more common form in English is Solomon. Author Salman Rushdie.
Salman, Zalomon

Zahir Arab. "Brilliant." Currently popular in Arabic-speaking countries.
Zayyir

Zane Eng. Var. **John**. Heb. "The Lord is gracious." Made famous by author Zane Grey, who wrote many westerns, among them *Riders of the Purple Sage*.
Zain, Zayne

Zared Heb. "Trap."

Zebadiah Heb. "Gift of Jehovah." In the New Testament, the father of apostles John and James. The name is all but obsolete today.
Zeb, Zebedee, Zebediah

Zebulon Heb. "To give honor to." Old Testament name of one of Jacob's sons. Extremely rare.
Zebulen, Zebulun, Zevulon, Zevulun

Zedekiah Heb. "The Lord is just." Name of an Old Testament king of Judah. Mostly 19th-century use.
Zed, Zedechiah, Zedekias

Zeke Heb. "Strength of God." Dim. **Ezekiel**. Ezekiel was an important Old Testament prophet.

Zelig Yiddish: "Blessed, holy." In German, "selig" means holy.
Selig, Zeligman, Zelik

Zenas Gk: "Hospitable"
Zeno, Zenon

Zephaniah Heb: "Precious to the Lord." A minor Old Testament prophet. Sparing 19th-century use.
Zeph, Zephan

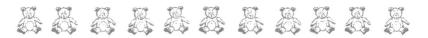

Zero Arab. "Void." A rather daunting name for a baby, though actor Zero Mostel seems to have survived it.

Zeus Gk. "Living." The name of the chief of the Olympian gods, who was also father of many gods and goddesses including Athena, Ares, Apollo and Artemis.

Zindel Yiddish. Var. **Alexander**. Gk. "Defender of mankind."
Zindil

Ziv Heb. "Full of life."
Ziven, Zivon

Zoltan Hung. "Life." Composer Zoltan Kodaly.

Zuhayr Arab. "Brilliant, shining." Currently popular among Arabic-speaking parents.

Zuriel Heb. "The Lord my rock."